Ounces

6	7	8	9	10	11	12	13	14	15	
170	198	227	255	283	312	340	369	397	425	**0** Pounds
624	652	680	709	737	765	794	822	850	879	**1**
077	1106	1134	1162	1191	1219	1247	1276	1304	1332	**2**
531	1559	1588	1616	1644	1673	1701	1729	1758	1786	**3**
984	2013	2041	2070	2098	2126	2155	2183	2211	2240	**4**
438	2466	2495	2523	2551	2580	2608	2637	2665	2693	**5**
892	2920	2948	2977	3005	3033	3062	3090	3118	3147	**6**
345	3374	3402	3430	3459	3487	3515	3544	3572	3600	**7**
799	3827	3856	3884	3912	3941	3969	3997	4026	4054	**8**
252	4281	4309	4337	4366	4394	4423	4451	4479	4508	**9**
706	4734	4763	4791	4819	4848	4876	4904	4933	4961	**10**
160	5188	5216	5245	5273	5301	5330	5358	5386	5415	**11**
613	5642	5670	5698	5727	5755	5783	5812	5840	5868	**12**
067	6095	6123	6152	6180	6209	6237	6265	6294	6322	**13**
520	6549	6577	6605	6634	6662	6690	6719	6747	6776	**14**
973	7002	7030	7059	7087	7115	7144	7172	7201	7228	**15**
427	7456	7484	7512	7541	7569	7597	7626	7654	7682	**16**
881	7909	7938	7966	7994	8023	8051	8079	8108	8136	**17**
335	8363	8391	8420	8448	8476	8504	8533	8561	8590	**18**
788	8816	8845	8873	8902	8930	8958	8987	9015	9043	**19**
242	9270	9298	9327	9355	9383	9412	9440	9469	9497	**20**
695	9724	9752	9780	9809	9837	9865	9894	9922	9950	**21**
149	10177	10206	10234	10262	10291	10319	10347	10376	10404	**22**
6	7	8	9	10	11	12	13	14	15	

Ounces

MANAGEMENT OF HIGH-RISK PREGNANCY AND INTENSIVE CARE OF THE NEONATE

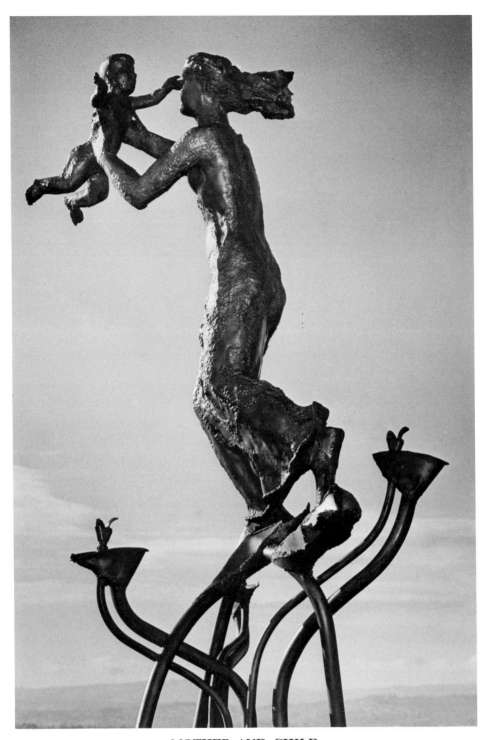

MOTHER AND CHILD
by Frederick Littman in Council Crest Park, Portland, Oregon.

MANAGEMENT OF HIGH-RISK PREGNANCY AND INTENSIVE CARE OF THE NEONATE

S. GORHAM BABSON, M.D.

Professor of Pediatrics and Director of Neonatal
Intensive Care Center, Doernbecher Memorial Hospital
for Children, University of Oregon Health
Science Center, Portland, Oregon

RALPH C. BENSON, M.D.

Professor and Chairman, Department of Obstetrics
and Gynecology, University of Oregon Health
Science Center, Portland, Oregon

MARTIN L. PERNOLL, M.D.

Associate Professor of Obstetrics and Gynecology
and Head of Division of Perinatology, University of
Oregon Health Science Center, Portland, Oregon

GERDA I. BENDA, M.D.

Assistant Professor of Pediatrics and Associate
Director of Neonatal Intensive Care Center, Doernbecher
Memorial Hospital for Children, University of Oregon
Health Science Center, Portland, Oregon

THIRD EDITION

with 82 *illustrations*

THE C. V. MOSBY COMPANY

Saint Louis 1975

THIRD EDITION

Copyright © 1975 by The C. V. Mosby Company

All rights reserved. No part of this book may be reproduced in any manner without written permission of the publisher.

Previous editions copyrighted 1966, 1971

Printed in the United States of America

Distributed in Great Britain by Henry Kimpton, London

Library of Congress Cataloging in Publication Data

Main entry under title:

Management of high-risk pregnancy and intensive care of the neonate.

First-2d editions by S. G. Babson and R. C. Benson published under titles: Primer on prematurity and high-risk pregnancy, and Management of high-risk pregnancy and intensive care of the neonate, respectively.
  Bibliography: p.
  Includes index.
  1. Infants (Premature) 2. Pregnancy, Complications of. I. Babson, Sydney Gorham. Management of high-risk pregnancy and intensive care of the neonate.
[DNLM: 1. Infant, Newborn, Diseases—Therapy.
2. Infant, Premature, Diseases—Therapy. 3. Intensive care units. 4. Pregnancy complications—Therapy.
WS410 M266]
RJ250.B3 1975   618.3′97   75-2429
ISBN 0-8016-0414-1

CB/CB/B 9 8 7 6 5 4 3 2 1

PREFACE

High perinatal morbidity and mortality levels are no longer acceptable natural hazards of childbirth. Limitation in family size and expectation of normal progeny have become the goals of every society regardless of position or race. Fortunately, this concept can now be supported in view of the spectacular advances in perinatal medicine. Systems have been developed to recognize those at risk and to deliver the proper sophistication of care. High-risk pregnancy is benefited not only by the expanded attention to general factors such as maternal hygiene, nutrition, and social aspects of family relationship, but also by specific newer methodology, including antenatal genetic and biochemical diagnosis, physiologic maturity testing of the fetus, and ultrasonic scanning for fetal growth and development. These tests focus on the optimum time for interrupting pregnancy for some or delaying parturition in others so that the fetus will have the best chance of survival. Proper utilization of these diagnostic tools should eliminate iatrogenic prematurity from elective induction and cesarean section. In addition, it is becoming increasingly clear that labor, delivery, and transitional nurseries must be intensive care areas with critical care monitoring. This is provided during labor by continuous fetal heart rate monitoring and, when indicated, by fetal scalp blood sampling. Obstetric anesthesia is much improved,

and traumatic modes of delivery are being abandoned.

Early efficient resuscitation of the neonate and appropriate respiratory support on the basis of blood gas levels have diminished the sequelae of hypoxia and acidosis. Efficient temperature control and early nutritional support have minimized abnormal catabolism and dehydration. These advances have without question improved the quality of surviving infants.

The obstetrician trained in maternal-fetal medicine and the pediatrician trained in neonatology are using their combined knowledge in bridging the gap in fetal and neonatal care. What has been fragmented care in the past has become a sophisticated team approach including the nurse specialist, social worker, public health nurse, and laboratory and paramedical personnel as participating team members.

This edition has been largely rewritten in view of the rapid developments in the field of perinatal medicine. New chapters have been added and include regionalization of perinatal care on the basis of levels of skills and equipment required commensurate with degree of fetal and neonatal jeopardy; fetal and neonatal transport including methods and equipment; how to identify in a practical manner the fetus at risk and what standards should apply to justify transfer to centers for continuous sophisticated care; and feeding the infant at high risk, including alimentation by peripheral vein.

This third edition continues to use a concise approach to diagnosis and management in outline form with both physician and nurse in mind. As a team they must be prepared to give skilled care, especially for unexpected perinatal hazards that develop at the community hospital level, as well as for the multitude of problems not requiring transfer to the specialized center.

S. Gorham Babson
Ralph C. Benson
Martin L. Pernoll
Gerda I. Benda

CONTENTS

MANAGEMENT OF HIGH-RISK PREGNANCY AND INTENSIVE CARE OF THE NEONATE

1

What is a high-risk perinate?

Between 5 and 10 million conceptions occur yearly in the United States. Of these, 2 to 3 million are early, spontaneous abortions. This loss may be fortuitous because as many as half of these conceptuses demonstrate on study aberrations of chromosome structure or number. Others may suffer from fetal viremia such as rubella or from damage by unidentified pathogens. Nearly 1 million pregnancies are legally or illegally terminated. Of the more than 3.2 million pregnancies each year that reach 20 weeks of gestational age, approximately 40,000 fetuses die before delivery. Almost the same number of neonates succumb in the first month of life after birth. Another 40,000 have severe (but often correctable) congenital malformations. Complications of pregnancy and delivery will contribute heavily to at least 90,000 who will be mentally retarded (IQ of 70 or below) and to another 150,000 who will have great difficulty in school because they are "poor learners." These handicapped individuals will be unable to compete fully in our increasingly complex society. Once viability is reached, perinatal death and permanent damage measured in terms of man-years of loss of life and productive living exceeds that from other major catastrophes, for example, cardiovascular disease, cancer, or accidents. Indeed, yearly perinatal deaths exceed all other causes of death combined until 65 years of age. Certainly the morbidity occurring during the perinatal interval of life is among the most urgent problems of modern medicine.

Other factors also contribute to making perinatal safety more pressing at the present time. For example, sweeping social changes have altered the size of families. Until recently, large families were in vogue, and death or perinatal wastage was unfortunate but not considered a major tragedy. Today, the situation is different, and current concepts stress quality of life. The majority of families consist of one to three children. Deliberate family planning is increasing, and abortion is being used to eliminate unwanted pregnancies. Every child is increasingly becoming a wanted child. Consequently, the health care worker is asked, with intensified urgency, to protect the individual from damage before, during, and after birth. To provide perinatal safety, it is mandatory to define those who are at risk and then provide the specific care necessary to prevent death or damage.

DEFINITION OF PERINATAL JEOPARDY

Perinatal jeopardy is the hazard of death or disability that occurs in human growth and development from viability until 28 days after birth. The risk may be subdivided into the portion of life that is intrauterine and that which is extrauterine. This division allows better delineation of those factors with which there is perinatal risk.

1

FACTORS RELATING TO INTRAUTERINE JEOPARDY

The mother may have a serious health problem, obstetric disorder, poor social environment, or biologic handicap—all potentially inimical to perinatal health. Some fetuses may be damaged early, others late; many infants will be born before their due date, or they may be unusually small for their gestational age. A few will have grown too large or will have remained in utero too long; each situation has its special hazards.

Women who are likely to have a higher incidence of perinatal mortality or morbidity during pregnancy must be identified. Completely unexpected complications are infrequent in women who have had a thorough evaluation and careful longitudinal observation, in which significant variations are recognized and problems treated during pregnancy and anticipated at delivery. The obstetric nurse, public health nurse, and social worker should complement physician and clinic care in promoting maternal and fetal health, especially in the case of illness, when the family is under stress, or when social conditions are poor.

A list* of high-risk factors in women contributing to perinatal mortality and morbidity in infants and children is presented here. About 10% to 20% of women fall into these groupings and account for over half the fetal and neonatal deaths.

1. A family history of serious hereditary and familial abnormalities, for example, osteogenesis imperfecta, mongolism
2. A history of prematurity or small-for-dates birth in self or most recent child
3. Significant congenital anomalies involving the central nervous system, heart, or skeletal system; pulmonary abnormalities; also blood dyscrasias, including anemia (hematocrit under 32%)
4. A severe social problem, for example, teen-age pregnancy, drug addiction, or absence of father
5. Long delayed or absent prenatal care
6. Age under 18 or over 35 years
7. A height under 60 inches and a prepregnant weight of less than 20% under or over the standards for weight and height
8. A fifth or subsequent pregnancy, especially when gravida is over 35 years of age
9. A subsequent gestation within 3 months of a previous pregnancy
10. A history of prolonged infertility and/or essential drug or hormone treatment
11. Teratogenic viral illness in the first trimester
12. Stressful events, for example, severe emotional tensions, hyperemesis gravidarum, general anesthesia, shock, critical accidents, or extensive exposure to radiation
13. A habit of heavy smoking
14. Obstetric complications past or present, for example, toxemia, placental separation, isoimmunization, hydramnios, or amniotic fluid leak
15. A multiple pregnancy
16. A fetus that fails to grow normally or is disparate in size from that expected
17. Minimal or no weight gain
18. Abnormal presentation, for example, breech, transverse; unengaged presenting part at term
19. A fetus over 42 weeks' gestational age

Demographic studies have identified special maternal and fetal complications that are related significantly to fetal and neonatal death. Tables 1-1 and 1-2 present

---

*Modified from Wigglesworth, R.: "At risk" registers, Dev. Med. Child Neurol. **10**:679, 1968.

Table 1·1. High-risk pregnancy and related hospital perinatal mortality*

Cause of death	Incidence/ 1,000 total births†	Stillbirths/ 1,000 total births	Live-born infants, deaths/ 1,000 total births	Perinatal mortality/ 1,000 total births
Breech (single)	36.5	3.4	3.1	6.5
Premature separation	12.6	2.7	1.6	4.3
Twin birth	22.7	0.8	1.4	2.2
Preeclampsia (grade 1)	34.8	1.5	0.5	2.0
Hydramnios	4.7	0.8	1.0	1.8
Urinary tract infection	32.7	0.7	0.7	1.4
Preeclampsia (grade 2)	6.2	0.9	0.4	1.3
Placenta previa	5.7	0.4	0.8	1.2
Prolapsed cord	4.8	0.9	0.3	1.2
Diabetes mellitus	6.0	0.4	0.6	1.0
Hypertension and proteinuria	13.9	0.7	0.1	0.8
Pyelonephritis	6.3	0.2	0.2	0.4
Phlebitis	5.7	0.3	0.1	0.4
Eclampsia	0.8	0.2	0.1	0.3
Total hospital perinatal mortality		16.1	14.9	31.0

*From Butler, N. R., and Bonham, D. G.: British perinatal mortality survey, 1958, perinatal mortality report of the survey under auspices of the National Birthday Trust Fund, vol. 1, Edinburgh, 1963, E. & S. Livingstone, Ltd.
†30,765 total births.

Table 1-2. High-risk pregnancy and mortality rate according to diagnosis*

Diagnosis	Incidence/1,000 total births	Mortality (%)		
		Stillbirths	Live births	Totals
Eclampsia	0.8	28.0	12.0	40.0
Hydramnios	4.7	17.2	22.1	39.3
Premature separation	12.6	21.2	12.7	33.9
Prolapsed cord	4.8	19.7	6.1	25.8
Preeclampsia (grade 2)	6.2	14.7	6.8	21.5
Placenta previa	5.7	7.5	13.8	21.3
Breech (single)	36.5	9.2	8.5	17.7
Diabetes mellitus	6.0	6.0	9.2	15.2
Twin birth	22.7	4.3	6.3	10.6
Hypertension and proteinuria	13.9	5.4	0.7	6.1
Preeclampsia (grade 1)	34.8	4.2	1.5	5.7
Urinary tract infection	32.7	2.1	2.1	4.2
All hospitalized patients	30,765	1.6	1.5	3.1

*From Butler, N. R., and Bonham, D. G.: British perinatal mortality survey, 1958, perinatal mortality report of the survey under auspices of the National Birthday Trust Fund, vol. 1, Edinburgh, 1963, E. & S. Livingstone, Ltd.

data from the British Perinatal Mortality Survey that indicate the incidence of specific complications and the perinatal mortality rate according to each diagnosis. In Table 1-2 breech presentation, premature separation of the placenta, toxemia, twinning, and urinary tract infection are associated with over 60% of fetal and 50% of neonatal mortality. Much of this perinatal mortality and morbidity in survivors can be avoided by skillful diagnosis and available therapy.

Some of these disorders, for example, eclampsia or nephritis, are uncommon, but they may account for a perinatal mortality of as much as 40%, an extremely high attrition. Twins make up about 23 of each 1,000 births. Although their perinatal mortality is about 11%, this is nearly four times that of pregnancy in general. Death that occurs before or after early delivery can often be ascribed to the same etiology. It is obvious that potential fetal and neonatal jeopardy demands delivery in a fully equipped maternity center where expert team support will be available.

FACTORS PLACING THE NEWBORN AT INCREASED JEOPARDY

After delivery, additional environmental factors may augment or reduce the ultimate capabilities of the offspring. The incidence of congenital anomalies, premature birth, cerebral palsy, and mental retardation is related to and often caused by undesirable antecedents preceding delivery and even conception. Identification of these harmful influences and their avoidance or neutralization must be the goals of everyone interested in obstetrics, pediatrics, and public health. Some deleterious factors will remain unknown; others may

be known to exist but thus far defy elimination; but many can be identified, excluded, or controlled.

The following associations before and after birth place the infant at increased risk and therefore require special care and observation:

1. History in the mother of previously listed pregnancy risk factors, particularly
   a. Prolonged rupture of membranes
   b. Abnormal presentation and delivery
   c. Prolonged, difficult labor or precipitous delivery
   d. Prolapsed cord
2. Birth asphyxia as suggested by
   a. Fetal heart rate fluctuations
   b. Meconium staining, particularly aspiration
   c. Fetal acidosis (pH below 7.2)
   d. Apgar scores below 7—particularly if present at 5 minutes
3. Preterm birth (before 38 weeks)
4. Postterm birth (after 42 weeks) with evidence of fetal wasting
5. Small-for-dates infants (below 5th percentile)
6. Large-for-dates infants (below 95th percentile), especially the large preterm infant
7. Any respiration distress or apnea
8. Obvious congenital anomalies
9. Convulsions, limpness, or difficulty in sucking or swallowing
10. Distention and/or vomiting
11. Anemia (less than 45% hemoglobin) or bleeding diathesis
12. Jaundice in first 24 hours or bilirubin levels above 15 mg/100 ml

The identification of unexpected neonatal problems and classification by weight/gestation parameters are discussed in

Table 1-3. Death rates by age: Oregon and United States, 1970*

Age	Oregon	United States
All ages	933.8	940.4
Under 1 yr	1,638.7	2,045.0
1- 4 yr	92.2	79.0
5-14 yr	42.9	41.4
15-24 yr	134.4	126.7
25-34 yr	120.2	159.8
35-44 yr	256.9	314.1
45-54 yr	627.4	724.9
55-64 yr	1,475.0	1,662.4
65-74 yr	3,234.2	3,665.8
75-84 yr	7,528.8	7,769.3
85+ yr	15,555.2	17,875.5

*All rates per 100,000 population in specified group.

Chapter 6. Regionalization of neonatal care and the levels of care necessary for infants at varying degrees of risk are discussed in Chapter 12.

The importance of the enormous morbidity and mortality during the perinatal interval of life cannot be overemphasized. Table 1-3 illustrates death rates by age in Oregon and the United States (1970 census). Considering that two thirds of all deaths that occur under 1 year of age occur in the first 27 days and that an equal number of fetuses succumb after viability is reached (stillborn), it can be appreciated that deaths related to the perinatal interval exceed the combined number of deaths from all other causes to 65 years of age. Dramatic as the mortality rate is, it represents just the tip of the iceberg; the larger portion is the morbidity incurred in this interval of life, when as many as 1 out of every 10 Americans is to a greater or lesser degree impaired for the remainder of his life.

2

Standard prenatal care and identification of risk factors

Ideally if a gravida participates in prenatal care, identification and treatment of problems that may threaten the patient or her fetus will be accomplished. Thus antenatal care is actually a screening procedure to differentiate those at jeopardy (high risk) from those in little danger (low risk). For that system to be effective, it must be based on an uncompromising search for those factors which may endanger the pregnancy.

This chapter outlines a routine antenatal care program designed to search for risk factors. Once identified, the endangered individuals require highly specialized care, which will be discussed in later chapters.

STANDARD PRENATAL CARE

Pregnancy is a multifactorial dynamic state. We believe the following steps are essential for discrimination of patients at high risk, moderate risk, or low risk:
1. A careful screening history
2. A general and specific physical examination designed to exclude risk factors
3. Routine laboratory screening
4. Individually indicated maternal laboratory evaluation
5. Careful fetal assessment during the course of pregnancy
6. Specialized studies to ascertain fetal well-being and/or fetal maturity

Standard records

Concise, problem-oriented obstetric records are necessary to document the progress of each pregnancy. The format and amount of information contained in various standard chart forms vary considerably. Appendix B contains the record system (medical, nursing, dietary) that has proved useful at University of Oregon Health Science Center. These forms are designed for screening of specific risk factors and indicate the data base for the first visit as well as subsequent visits.

Standard antenatal visits

Following is a standard schedule of prenatal office visits:

Weeks of gestation	Frequency of visits
0-32	Once every 4 weeks
32-36	Once every 2 weeks
36-delivery	Once a week

An additional essential practice at each visit is to query the patient about her general health and answer any complaints or questions she may have.

Routine laboratory screening

Laboratory tests assist in detection or confirmation of the presence of certain risk factors. All the following studies should be obtained as early in pregnancy as possible and some (indicated in italics) should be repeated at the twenty-eighth and thirty-fourth weeks of pregnancy:

1. *Hematocrit and/or hemoglobin*
2. White blood count
3. Differential white blood count
4. Urinalysis
5. Culture of urine (with bacterial sensitivities if there are at least 10^5 bacteria/ml)
6. Serologic test for syphilis
7. Rubella antibody titer
8. Toxoplasmosis antibody titer
9. Blood grouping and Rh determination
10. *Screening test for antibodies* (Hemantigen or comparable screening test)
11. Papanicolaou cervical, vaginal smear
12. Cervical culture for *Neisseria gonorrhoeae*

The other essentials of standard prenatal care, including the individually indicated laboratory evaluation, close and comprehensive fetal assessment, and special studies to ascertain fetal well-being, are discussed in later chapters.

NUTRITION DURING PREGNANCY

Increased nutritional requirements during pregnancy are multiple, and diet is only a part of nutrition. The stress of pregnancy, as well as other intrinsic and extrinsic factors, can be only roughly appraised. Unfortunately, extrapolation from animal studies are in most instances merely suggestive.

Pregnancy on the average will account for about 24 lb of weight gain during the entire gestation. It is recommended this be accomplished by a steady weight gain of 0.5 to 1 lb/wk. It is unlikely that an obese, sedentary patient should gain 24 lb in addition to her excessive weight, however. Obviously, one should not attempt this correction on a crash basis, especially during the first or last trimester, to avoid harm to the fetus. Similarly, a gravida con-

siderably underweight may do well to gain more than 24 lb. An attempt should be made, then, to help the patient reach her ideal weight for height and age 4 to 6 weeks post partum.

More than one third of the total weight gain of 24 lb (11 kg) during a term pregnancy represents fetal weight: approximately 7.7 lb (3,500 gm). The placenta, amniotic fluid, and uterine weight each account for between 1.4 and 2 lb (650 and 900 gm). Increased interstitial fluid and blood volume contribute 2.7 to 4 lb (1,200 to 1,800 gm), respectively. Breast enlargement adds at least 0.9 lb (400 gm). The remaining 3.5 lb (1,640 gm), otherwise unspecified, represents fat and other maternal stores.

Standard weight for height is given in Table 2-1. It should be noted also that Table 2-1 applies to patients of medium body build who are 25 years of age or

Table 2-1. Standard weight for height of women*

Height	Weight
4' 10"	104
4' 11"	107
5' 0"	110
5' 1"	113
5' 2"	116
5' 3"	118
5' 4"	123
5' 5"	128
5' 6"	132
5' 7"	136
5' 8"	140
5' 9"	144
5' 10"	148
5' 11"	152
6' 0"	156

*The above weights were taken from the Metropolitan Life Insurance Company, Actuarial Tables, 1959, and adjusted to comply with instructions appearing on the Gain in Weight Grid—height in inches without shoes plus 1 inch to establish a standard for heels. Patients should be weighed with shoes as normally worn. Table 2-1 is for medium body build and, except for extreme body build deviations, these figures should be used.

older. For patients less than 25 years old, deduct 1 lb for each year. For the young adolescent, however, individualization will be necessary, especially if maximal growth has not yet been achieved.

Proper weight gain does not guarantee optimal nutrition. In general, about 4 lb of weight gain in the first trimester, 10 to 12 lb in the second, and 8 to 10 lb in the last are reasonable. Nevertheless, a gain of more than 2 to 3 lb/mo in the last 3 to 4 months suggests fluid retention and may presage a developing toxemia of pregnancy.

Few individuals are capable of counting calories consistently, nor are they generally willing to be specific. Nonetheless, the caloric intake and weight gain or loss are rough correlates. Hence the adequacy of the caloric intake can be estimated by the trend in body weight. Importantly, a number of other variables pertain, including the basal metabolic rate, the lean body mass, and the physical activity of the individual, as well as the stage of the pregnancy.

Poor maternal nutrition (low hemoglobin level or protein deficiency) is a contributory cause of abnormal bleeding and spontaneous premature labor and delivery. It is the underweight gravida who is more likely to delivery early. Moreover, preeclampsia and eclampsia probably are the result, at least in part, of nutritional, most likely protein, deficiency.

The popular belief that intrauterine growth can be satisfactorily maintained despite maternal deprivation is no longer tenable as a generality. The mother's health and that of her offspring depend in large measure on the quality and, to a lesser degree, on the quantity of her food.

Table 2-2. Recommended daily dietary allowances for nonpregnant and pregnant women

	Recommended daily allowances for nonpregnant women					Pregnant	Lactating
Age in years	11-14	15-18	19-22	23-50	51 +		
Energy (kcal)	2,400	2,100	2,100	2,000	1,800	+300	+500
Protein (gm)	44	48	46	46	46	+30	+20
Fat-soluble vitamins							
Vitamin A activity (RE)	800	800	800	800	800	1,000	1,200
(IU)	4,000	4,000	4,000	4,000	4,000	5,000	6,000
Vitamin D (IU)	400	400	400			400	400
Vitamin E activity (IU)	12	12	12	12	12	15	15
Water-soluble vitamins							
Ascorbic acid (mg)	45	45	45	45	45	60	80
Folacin (μg)	400	400	400	400	400	800	600
Niacin (mg)	16	14	14	13	12	+2	+4
Riboflavin (mg)	1.3	1.4	1.4	1.2	1.1	+0.3	+0.5
Thiamin (mg)	1.2	1.1	1.1	1.0	1.0	+0.3	+0.3
Vitamin B_6 (mg)	1.6	2.0	2.0	2.0	2.0	2.5	2.5
Vitamin B_{12} (μg)	3.0	3.0	3.0	3.0	3.0	4.0	4.0
Minerals							
Calcium (mg)	1,200	1,200	800	800	800	1,200	1,200
Phosphorus (mg)	1,200	1,200	800	800	800	1,200	1,200
Iodine (μg)	115	115	100	100	80	125	150
Iron (mg)	18	18	18	18	10	+18	18
Magnesium (mg)	300	300	300	300	300	450	450
Zinc (mg)	15	15	15	15	15	20	25

It is known that the fetus normally doubles its weight during the last 2 months of pregnancy; this may be reduced significantly by a starvation regimen.

Diet and pregnancy

At least fifty nutrients are thought to be essential nutritional needs of the gravid woman. They vary with a patient's requirements during the numerous phases of pregnancy and puerperium. Fetal growth and maintenance are a greater nutritional challenge than the normal recovery period postnatally. Lactation naturally adds another dimension. If pregnancy is complicated by colitis, for example, the amount and type of food would have to be modified accordingly.

The National Academy of Sciences–National Research Council (Table 2-2) has suggested the optimal caloric (more than 36 kcal/kg body weight) and nutritional requirements of proteins, carbohydrates, and fats, together with sixteen other food requirements of the pregnant woman. Regrettably, this is not as easy as it sounds because of gross differences in patient needs, both recognized and unrecognized. Many synergistic processes imply an interplay involving numerous elements. Bone formation, hemoglobin synthesis, and protein conjugation are good examples.

The importance of protein in the anabolism of pregnancy always is emphasized, but the implication that carbohydrates and fats are of little importance, especially in the matter of excess weight reduction, is unfortunate. Protein insufficiency can develop, even with adequate protein ingestion, if insufficient calories are available because a large portion of the amino acids in the protein is deaminated for energy needs. Brief semistarvation (less than 1,500 calories) may reduce body proteins, enzymes, and even hormones. If starvation is extended for weeks or months, fluid retention and weight gain will be noted. Misinterpretations by the obstetrician may

lead to an even stricter diet. By and large, reduction of the caloric intake below 1,500 calories for any length of time is unwise during pregnancy because of probable fetal deprivation.

High-risk obstetric patients having need of special dietary (and medical) counseling include women with the following:

1. Anemia (hemoglobin level of less than 9.5 gm, hematocrit reading = 30) and other chronic metabolic disorders, that is, diabetes mellitus, thyroid dysfunction, colitis, and cardiovascular and renal disease
2. A weight 10% under or more than 20% over the standard for height and age at the onset of pregnancy and considerable gain or any loss during gestation
3. A history of serious obstetric complications in a previous pregnancy or sequentially in several prior pregnancies: repeated abortion, toxemia of pregnancy, premature separation of the placenta, low birth weight babies, and a short interval between pregnancies
4. Socioeconomic problems: adolescents, the poor, and those not knowledgeable about the selection, storage, and preparation of food
5. Obstetric complications: preeclampsia, multiple pregnancy, ulcerative colitis, hyperemesis gravidarum, etc.

A good pregnancy diet is a deceptively simple thing. Lack of knowledge, money, mores, or motivation are a few of the reasons the pregnant woman does not receive a well-balanced, high-protein, high-vitamin, high-mineral diet. Excessive carbohydrates, especially sweets, should be limited. Following are the *daily* basic food requirements in pregnancy and lactation (Brewer):

1. One quart (4 glasses) or more of milk (any kind will do: whole milk, buttermilk, low fat, skim, or powdered skim milk)
2. Two eggs

3. One or two servings of fish, liver, chicken, lean beef, lamb, or pork or any kind of cheese
4. One or two good servings of fresh, green, leafy vegetables: mustard, collard, or turnip greens or spinach, lettuce, or cabbage
5. Two or three slices of whole wheat bread
6. A piece of citrus fruit or a glass of lemon, lime, orange, or grapefruit juice
7. One pat of margarine, vitamin A enriched

The pregnant woman should also include the following in her diet:

1. A serving of whole-grain cereal: Wheatena, Cream of Wheat, farina, or oatmeal, four times a week
2. A yellow or red vegetable five times a week
3. Liver once a week
4. Whole baked potato three times a week

The obstetrician has been obsessed for years with the notion that too much table salt or sodium-containing preparations are at least a contributory cause of eclamptogenic toxemia. Granted that the pre-eclamptic patient cannot "handle" (excrete) sodium once the disorder has developed, there is no convincing evidence that the sodium ion is the culprit. "Everything in moderation" still is an excellent maxim. If one concentrates on a good diet, especially an ample protein intake, the sodium "problem" usually will take care of itself.

Edema is also a bogy during pregnancy. Dependent or physiologic edema occurs in well-nourished, healthy women because of mild circulatory stasis. It is especially common in warm weather, and rest periods and elevation of the legs suffice for relief. This type of edema is a sign of neither cardiac nor renal disease nor toxemia of pregnancy. It is not an indication for diuretic therapy. In contrast, generalized or pathologic edema reflects a disease process. This abnormality, often due to heart or kidney failure or toxemia of pregnancy, cannot be prevented by diuretics, which may be indicated, however, in the treatment of selected patients. Be this as it may, thiazide diuretics are extremely potent and may cause serious maternal or fetal complications, even when used discriminatingly.

Patients will fare better if the physician stresses good diet rather than total weight gain. Many women become so self-conscious and self-critical of poundage that they go on harmful crash diets, take drastic purges, or exhaust themselves in exercise fads. The physician who takes the positive approach of stressing the essential foods in reasonable portions rarely has to be critical or accusatory, and his patients are more relaxed and cooperative.

The fetus and nutrition

Attempts to assess the effect of maternal nutrition on the outcome of pregnancy have been only partially successful. Fetal growth and development and the function of the placenta obviously are dependent on the type and amount of food metabolized.

Many complications of pregnancy are directly or indirectly due to inadequate diet and may reflect the lifelong nutritional experience of the gravida as well as shorter-term dietary deficiency. They include iron- and vitamin-deficiency anemias, infection, probably toxemia of pregnancy, and certain instances of obstetric hemorrhage. Prepregnant nutrition as measured by weight and pregnancy gain markedly affects fetal growth. Poor nutrition may be the primary cause of low birth weight infants throughout the world, particularly those in the weight range of 2,000 to 2,500 gm, most of whom are mature at birth. The possibility that normal central nervous system development may be impaired in poor nutritional states emphasizes the urgent need for adequate and proper food intake during gestation. A favorable nutritional state before conception and in the first trimester before most prenatal care has started is often disregarded as a vital need for the fetus. It is proposed by Drillien that poor environment during the

Table 2-3. Association between prepregnancy weight, birth weight, and percentage of low birth weight infants*

Prepregnancy weight (lb)	Mean birth weight	Birth weight below 2,501 gm (%)
<100	3,144	4.9
100-119	3,285	2.7
120-139	3,427	1.9
140-159	3,531	0.4
160-179	3,625	0.8
≥180	3,776	0.7

*From Eastman, N. J., and Jackson, E.: Weight relationships in pregnancy, Obstet. Gynecol. Survey **23**:1003, 1968.

Table 2-4. Association between maternal weight gain, birth weight, and percentage of low birth weight infants*

Weight gain	Mean birth weight	Birth weight below 2,501 gm (%)
Loss	3,360	3.3
0-10	3,278	4.4
11-20	3,301	3.1
21-30	3,426	1.2
31-40	3,562	0.7
≥41	3,636	0.5

*From Eastman, N. J., and Jackson, E.: Weight relationships in pregnancy, Obstet. Gynecol. Survey **23**:1003, 1968.

mother's childhood is still restrictive on fetal growth of her progency even after improvement in her social and economic status.

Prepregnant weight is directly related to weight gain and inversely related to the percentage of low birth weight infants in women delivered at term. (See Table 2-3.)

Gain in weight during pregnancy also is related to an increase in fetal size at birth, with a fall in the percentage of low birth weight infants concomitant with increasing weight gain (Table 2-4). An exception may occur when loss in weight has occurred during pregnancy. A suggested explanation is the inclusion of a proportionately larger number of obese women whose tendency toward increased fetal weight is only partially blunted by severe dietary control. Women with a low prepregnant weight (under 120 lb) and a limited gain in weight (under 11 lb) produce a high incidence of low-weight newborns. These infants have a much higher neonatal mortality. Such women should be identified early in pregnancy and given helpful specific nutritional advice and longitudinal observation.

More liberal diets for average women during pregnancies, with emphasis on quality of food rather than quantity of calories, particularly in those requiring weight limitation, should improve fetal health and size. Although larger babies may be stronger babies, excessive size is related to an increased likelihood of dystocia, fetal distress, and birth trauma.

In summary:

1. Faulty maternal nutrition, including vitamin and mineral lack, has an adverse effect on fertility, embryogenesis, and fetal growth.

2. Undernutrition and overrestricted weight gain in the mother increases the incidence of low birth weight infants and perinatal mortality.

3. Close spacing of pregnancies may deplete nutritional stores to the disadvantage of subsequent progeny.

4. The mother's health and that of her offspring depend in large measure on the quality rather than the quantity of her food intake.

Nutritional supplementation

Many investigators are challenging the routine administration of minerals and vitamins (except possibly iron and folic acid) during pregnancy. Certainly nutritional supplementation has never been a replacement for sound nutritional counseling. It must be concluded at the present time that routine supplementation of dietary vitamins and minerals is a questionable necessity.

EMOTIONAL ASPECTS OF PREGNANCY

Childbirth still causes much needless fear and anxiety among women. Many obstetric disorders are emotionally induced or are aggravated by psychologic factors.

The antenatal period offers a unique opportunity to study and treat the fears, anxieties, and conflicts related to gestation, parturition, and motherhood. Better understanding and the formation and acceptance of healthy attitudes can make an invaluable contribution to the mental health and happiness of the mother-to-be and her family. Toward that end we believe that more emphasis should be placed on the woman's role in rearing children in our complex society than on the actual delivery of the baby. Counseling will do much to prevent and treat many troublesome psychic or somatic complications. Severe problems will require consultation and definitive therapy.

We have been impressed with many obvious concerns of our patients that really amount to "family distress." Whether tension is a "cause" of early delivery or of fetal deprivation must be considered. Naturally, emotional pressures come long before the birth of the baby. Prenatal care generally reduces stress and its problems, but anxieties and other pressures seem to be reflected in the product of the pregnancy.

Generally a mother gains a special attachment for her baby while she is on the maternity floor with her infant. What happens when her newborn is removed to a nursery for high-risk infants? Babies who remain in an incubator for a long time may become rejected, even if they were wanted. One patient said, "I feel like I never had him; he's almost no one to me."

In our series of small-for-dates and pre-

mature babies, diet was found to be poor in about half the cases. On the other hand, there was a very low incidence of toxemia of pregnancy.

Because emotional stress is a serious problem for many obstetric patients and their husbands, it is important that the physician meet their needs. Certain patients are dependent but not necessarily inadequate. These individuals may require frequent counseling and direction.

There seems to be no substitute for a good physician-patient relationship. Yet certain details may detract from antenatal care—good though it may be fundamentally. For example, does the obstetrician keep the patient in awe? Does he have the ability to counsel the mother *and* the father? The physician may represent a father figure, and fear of judgment and punishment may enter the picture. The physician should not ask, "Have you been taking the iron pills?" He should inquire, "Are you having any trouble taking iron pills?"

Severe, prolonged tension from any cause may alter the fetal environment or the hormonal balance in the delicate maternal-placental-fetal relationship and thus impair fetal development. Pregnancy may come as a surprise, and when the fetus is unwanted, sufficient stress in the mother may interfere with fetal development. The mother's emotions may affect fetal health in other ways: rejection may be the basis for chain-smoking, excessive intake of tranquilizers or other drugs, variations in food intake, and reduced interest in prenatal care or personal health. In extreme cases the mother may try to take her life or that of the fetus.

SOCIAL, CULTURAL, AND ECONOMIC FACTORS THAT INFLUENCE PERINATAL MORBIDITY AND MORTALITY

The many social factors that place the birth of neonates at greater risk are interrelated. Ignorance, poverty, and disinterest in the pregnancy are far too prevalent. We shall attempt to identify specific factors that appear to be related to low birth weight infants.

1. Accidental pregnancy and irresponsible parenthood

   Of all the problems that beset the world, unplanned, unexpected pregnancy is one of the most critical. The majority of such pregnancies, particularly in the lower socioeconomic sector of the population, are unwanted and often rejected by one or both parents. These pregnant women, especially if unwed or teen-agers, neglect antenatal care and leave advice unheeded. Whereas many mothers are unconcerned about the outcome, others hope to abort or pray for the birth of a stillborn. The high incidence of ill-timed and undesired pregnancies is one reason the United States has an unfavorable position relative to infant mortality rates among the so-called advanced countries. In any event, the world's birth rate has far outstripped the death rate now that death control has become more efficient than birth control. At the present rate of growth there will be 7 billion persons in the world by the year 2000. The potential crowding may not be as serious as the loss that will occur with the further encroachment of a technologic society on our living space. We had better think in terms of child limitation as well as in terms of the improvement of the environment for the fetus and the child if the quality of the human race is to be advanced.

2. Race

   Racial difference may be a factor in the proportion of smaller infants born in a comparative population. Blacks have a greater percentage of low birth weight infants as compared to whites, as shown in Table 2-5. Differences in socioeconomic opportunities explain much of the disparity. This factor may not be the only one, however, because "prematurity" rates of American Indians, persons of very low socioeconomic status, also are similar to those of United States white citizens. The mortality rates, however, are strikingly increased in both of the more underprivileged groups.* In contrast, it is of interest that Chinese- and Japanese-American infants have an infant mortality rate one third that of blacks and two thirds that of whites in the United States.

3. Occupational and educational states: social class

   Occupation of the father is related to profound differences in the incidence of "prematurity" and infant mortality. In Table 2-6 the advantages that farmers and professional people have over farm laborers and unmarried mothers are clearly evident. The farmer's limited access to medical care is more than compensated for by an apparently healthier life.

---

*The regionalization of perinatal care for the Navaho Indians in Arizona has brought their neonatal mortality in line with that of white citizens.

Table 2-5. The racial factor in low birth weight fetal and infant mortality*

Birth weight under 2,500 gm		Percentage of live births
Indian (American) (1962)	19,700 births	7.8
Nonwhite (1961)	667,462 births	13.0
White (1961)	3,606,864 births	6.8

*Data from Rosa, F., and Resnick, L.: Birth weight and perinatal mortality of the American Indian, Am. J. Obstet. Gynecol. **91**:972, 1965.

Table 2-6. Births and infant deaths as recorded on birth and death certificates classified by occupation of father and ranked by premature birth rate, Oregon, 1966*

	Number	Percent of total	Premature infants†		Infant death rate for state
			Birth rate‡	Death rate	
Farmer	946	2.7	33.8	4.2	8.5
Professional	4,423	12.6	49.1	9.5	15.6
Clerical	1,414	4.0	55.3	9.2	17.7
Sales	2,208	6.3	60.2	8.6	14.0
Managers	2,730	7.8	60.4	11.4	17.6
Craftsmen	4,740	13.5	61.2	12.9	22.2
Operatives	4,972	14.2	66.6	12.7	22.1
Other	1,509	4.3	67.6	13.3	21.2
Laborers	8,647	24.7	71.8	12.0	23.1
Service workers	1,154	3.3	78.3	15.6	27.7
Farm laborers	590	1.7	88.1	25.4	37.3
Illegitimate births§	1,720	4.9	93.6	19.2	33.7
State total and rates	35,053	100.0	64.8	12.1	21.1

*From Kernek, C., Osterud, H., and Anderson, B.: Patterns of prematurity in Oregon, Northwest Med. 65:639, 1966.
†In this table premature infants include all births under 5 lb 8 oz.
‡All birth and death rates are based on 1,000 live births.
§Illegitimate births are included for completeness.

a. The incidence of "prematurity" and perinatal death is increased with menial occupational states (Table 2-6).
b. Ward patients in many hospitals have more than a 50% higher incidence of low birth weight infants than private patients of the same race in the same institution.
c. College women have half as many low birth weight infants as those with a grade school education.

Whether these differences are due to better pregnancy planning, living conditions, and personal habits or faulty nutrition remains unanswered, but all seem to be important.

4. The teen-ager and the unwed
The pregnant teen-age girl, whether married or not, presents a serious problem. She and her partner usually are emotionally and intellectually immature and often are unable to successfully cope with the difficult social, economic, and educational problems created. Re-

striction of the child's developmental potential is likely. Moreover, increase in tax dollars for aid to dependent children has created serious budget deficits in government. The following observations generally apply:
a. Age at first pregnancy is decreasing.
b. A greater proportion of births out of wedlock occur in young parents.
c. Teen-age marriage, particularly after conception, is notably unstable and, in the majority, ends in dissolution.
d. Infants weighing under 1,501 gm born to teen-agers are double the percentage born to women 25 to 30 years of age.
e. The low birth weight in illegitimate pregnancy is more than doubled.
f. Perinatal mortality in the unwed is almost twice that of married women.

Hence teen-age pregnancy is a serious handicap to family fulfillment and solidity and to the achievement of independence from parental and government aid. Children born to more mature

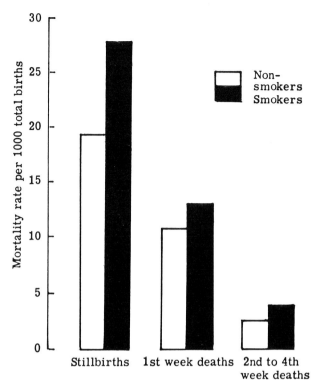

Fig. 2-1. Stillbirth, early and late neonatal mortality rates by maternal smoking habit. (From Butler, N. R., and Alberman, E. D., editors: Perinatal problems. The second report of the 1958 British Perinatal Mortality Survey, Edinburgh and London, 1969, E. & S. Livingstone, Ltd.)

parents perform better in school, demonstrate superior emotional balance, and enjoy greater family contentment.

5. Economic factors

   Lack of money can be an important reason why the pregnant woman and her fetus do not receive adequate care, diet, or rest.

MATERNAL SMOKING DURING PREGNANCY

The detrimental effect of cigarette smoking on the fetus is now clear. Although nicotine, carbon monoxide, and tars have been held responsible, smoking could be considered a reflection of stress, like excessive eating or drinking. Although the mechanism of the effect of smoking on the outcome of pregnancy remains obscure, the following associations have been shown in prospective controlled studies:

1. Fetal weight is reduced at least 200 gm on the average, with a significant increase in the incidence of low birth weight infants.

2. Mortality rates are higher, particularly during fetal life (Fig. 2-1).

A distressing factor is the additional detrimental effect of smoking on conditions affecting placental perfusion, such as has been shown to apply to the hypertensive gravida.

The conclusions of the British Perinatal Mortality Survey (Fig. 2-1) indicate that smoking is prejudicial to fetal health. Consequently, the probable survival of fetuses of mothers in the high-risk category who smoke is further reduced.

Every effort should be made to discourage the smoking habit during pregnancy, even though the smoking may be the result of tensions.

PATERNAL INFLUENCES

The paternal role in prematurity and high-risk pregnancy is largely theoretical and is yet to be clarified.

1. Older age of the father has been related to an increased incidence of stillborn infants and infants having a congenital abnormality. However, maternal age is also higher than the mean in most of these cases, which suggests that paternal age is still an uncertain factor in reproductive wastage.

2. The inheritance of Rh-positive genes from the father by the fetus may result in erythroblastosis when the mother is Rh negative.

3. Chronic alcoholism and diabetes mellitus in the father may affect fetal development adversely.

MISCELLANEOUS FACTORS

1. High-altitude exposure may result in small-for-dates babies and perhaps developmental anomaly.

2. Hormonal insufficiency indicated by low or falling chorionic gonadotropin and pregnanediol levels is a poor prognostic sign for the fetus.

3. Narcotic addiction is a serious threat to reproduction.

4. Genetic influences often impair fetal development.

• • •

In summary, the normal development of the fetus is threatened by a myriad of factors, both singly and in combination. Many are "obstetric" in nature in that maternal complications play a threatening role. More are "environmental" in that unfavorable social conditions, educational handicaps, or nutritional deficits are inimical to optimal fetal health. An interaction between many of these factors occurs and adversely affects the perinatal mortality rate and the quality of survivors.

Improvement in fetal health care (both medical and environmental) is an obligation of the community and a right of the patient. Solutions for social, economic, and educational deficiencies are current challenges. Pregnancy by choice rather than chance promises to be most relevant in improving the quality of the fetus as well as the later adequacy of the child. Perinatal death and neurologic sequelae will be reduced, and the chain of succeeding generations of physically and emotionally deprived children may be broken. (See Chapter 27.)

IDENTIFICATION OF SPECIFIC RISK FACTORS

Certain checkpoints must be utilized in the continuum of antenatal care to guarantee that all risks are identified and treated appropriately. We employ the following checkpoints:

1. Initial screening
2. Prenatal visit screening
3. Intrapartum screening
   a. On admission to hospital
   b. On admission to obstetric intensive care area
4. Delivery evaluation
   a. Neonatal
   b. Maternal
5. Postpartum evaluation
   a. Neonatal
   b. Maternal

The patients at risk are then defined by the following criteria at each checkpoint:

1. Initial screening
   Biologic and marital factors
   a. High risk
      1. Maternal age of 15 years or less
      2. Maternal age of 35 years or more
      3. Massive obesity
   b. Moderate risk
      1. Maternal age 15 to 19 years
      2. Maternal age 30 to 34 years

3. Nonwhite
4. Single
5. Obesity (more than 20% of standard weight for height) (Table 2-1)
6. Malnutrition (less than 100 lb)
7. Short stature (60 inches or less)

Obstetric history

a. High risk
   1. Previously diagnosed genital tract anomalies
      a. Incompetent cervix
      b. Cervical malformation
      c. Uterine malformation
   2. Two or more previous abortions
   3. Previous stillborn or neonatal loss
   4. Two previous premature labors or low birth weight infants (less than 2,500 gm)
   5. Two excessively large previous infants (more than 4,000 gm)
   6. Maternal malignancy
   7. Uterine leiomyomas (5 cm or more or submucus in location)
   8. Ovarian mass
   9. Parity of eight or more
   10. Previous infant with isoimmunization
   11. History of eclampsia
   12. Previous infant with
      a. Known or suspected genetic or familial disorders
      b. Congenital anomaly
   13. Previous history of need for special neonatal-infant care or a birth-damaged infant
   14. Medical indications for termination of a previous pregnancy

b. Moderate risk
   1. Previous premature labor, low birth weight infant (less than 2,500 gm), or abortion
   2. One excessively large infant (more than 4,000 gm)
   3. Previous operative deliveries
      a. Cesarean section
      b. Midforceps delivery
      c. Breech extraction
   4. Previous prolonged labor or significant dystocia
   5. Borderline pelvis
   6. Previous severe emotional problems associated with pregnancy or delivery
   7. Previous uterine or cervical operations
   8. Primigravida
   9. Parity of five to eight
   10. Involuntary sterility
   11. Prior ABO incompatibility
   12. Prior fetal malpresentation
   13. Previous history of endometriosis
   14. Pregnancy occurring 3 months or less after the last delivery

Medical and surgical history

a. High risk
   1. Moderate to severe chronic hypertension
   2. Moderate to severe renal disease
   3. Severe heart disease (Class II to IV, or a history of congestive heart failure)
   4. Diabetes (Class B to F)
   5. Previous endocrine ablation
   6. Abnormal cervical cytology
   7. Sickle cell disease
   8. Drug addiction or alcoholism
   9. History of tuberculosis or PPD test revealing a diameter of more than 1 cm
   10. Pulmonary disease
   11. Malignancy
   12. Gastrointestinal or liver disease
   13. Previous cardiac or vascular surgery

b. Moderate risk
   1. Mild chronic hypertension
   2. Mild renal disease
   3. Mild heart disease (Class I)
   4. History of mild hypertensive states of pregnancy
   5. History of pyelonephritis
   6. Diabetes (Class A)
   7. Family history of diabetes
   8. Thyroid disease
   9. Positive serology

10. Excessive use of drugs
11. Emotional problems
12. Sickle-cell trait
13. Epilepsy
2. Prenatal visit screening
Early pregnancy
a. High risk
    1. Failure of uterine growth or disproportionate uterine growth
    2. Exposure to teratogens
        a. Radiation
        b. Infection
        c. Chemicals
    3. Pregnancy complicated by isoimmunization
    4. Need for antenatal genetic diagnosis
    5. Severe anemia (9 gm or less hemoglobin)
b. Moderate risk
    1. Unresponsive urinary tract infection
    2. Suspected ectopic pregnancy
    3. Suspected missed abortion
    4. Severe hyperemesis gravidarum
    5. Positive VDRL test
    6. Positive gonorrhea screening
    7. Anemia not responsive to iron treatment
    8. Viral illness
    9. Vaginal bleeding
    10. Mild anemia (9 to 10.9 gm hemoglobin)
Late pregnancy
a. High risk
    1. Failure of uterine growth or disproportionate uterine growth
    2. Severe anemia (less than 9 gm hemoglobin)
    3. More than 42½ weeks' gestation
    4. Severe preeclampsia
    5. Eclampsia
    6. Breech if vaginal delivery is planned
    7. Moderate to severe isoimmunization (necessitating intrauterine transfusion or neonatal exchange transfusion)

8. Placenta previa
9. Hydramnios or oligohydramnios
10. Antepartum fetal death
11. Thromboembolic disease
12. Premature labor (less than 37 weeks' gestation)
13. Premature rupture of the bag of waters (less than 38 weeks' gestation)
14. Tumor or other obstruction of the birth canal
15. Abruptio placentae
16. Chronic or acute pyelonephritis
17. Multiple gestation
18. Abnormal oxytocin challenge test
19. Falling urinary estriols
b. Moderate risk
    1. Hypertensive states of pregnancy (mild)
    2. Breech if cesarean section is planned
    3. Uncertain presentations
    4. Need for fetal maturity studies
    5. Postdate pregnancy (41 to 42½ weeks)
    6. Premature rupture of the membranes (more than 12 hours without labor if gestation is more than 38 weeks long)
    7. Induction of labor
    8. Suspected fetopelvic disproportion at term
    9. Floating presentations 2 weeks or less from the estimated date of confinement
3. Intrapartum screening (secondary on admission to hospital or tertiary on admission to obstetric intensive care area)
a. High risk
    1. Previous factors indicative of high-risk category
    2. Severe preeclampsia or eclampsia
    3. Hydramnios or oligohydramnios
    4. Amnionitis
    5. Premature rupture of the membranes for over 24 hours
    6. Uterine rupture
    7. Placenta previa

8. Abruptio placentae
9. Meconium staining of amniotic fluid
10. Abnormal presentation
11. Multiple gestation
12. Fetal weight less than 2,000 gm
13. Fetal weight more than 4,000 gm
14. Abnormal presentation
15. Multiple pregnancy
16. Fetal bradycardia (longer than 30 minutes)
17. Breech delivery
18. Prolapsed cord
19. Fetal acidosis (pH 7.25 or less in first stage of labor)
20. Fetal tachycardia (longer than 30 minutes)
21. Shoulder dystocia
22. Fetal presenting part not descending with labor
23. Evidence of maternal distress
24. Abnormal oxytocin challenge test
25. Falling urinary estriols
26. Immature or intermediate lecithin/sphingomyelin or rapid surfactant test

b. Moderate risk
1. Mild hypertensive states of pregnancy
2. Premature rupture of membranes more than 12 hours before labor
3. Primary dysfunctional labor
4. Secondary arrest of dilatation
5. Meperidine (Demerol), more than 200 mg
6. Magnesium sulfate, more than 25 gm
7. Labor longer than 20 hours
8. Second stage of labor longer than 1 hour
9. Clinically small pelvis
10. Medical induction of labor
11. Precipitous labor (less than 3 hours)
12. Elective induction
13. Prolonged latent phase
14. Uterine tetany
15. Oxytocin (Pitocin) augmentation

16. Marginal separation of placenta
17. Operative forceps
18. Vacuum extraction
19. General anesthesia
20. Any abnormality of maternal vital signs
21. Abnormal uterine contractions

4. Postnatal criteria for risk
Postnatally mothers are closely watched in the delivery room for a brief interval before transfer to the postpartum recovery room, where the patient's vital signs, lochia, etc. are observed carefully for the first 6 to 8 hours post partum.

a. Specific factors placing the mother at high risk include
1. Hemorrhage
2. Infection
3. Abnormal vital signs
4. Traumatic delivery

b. The infant is observed briefly in the delivery room, and an initial screening physical examination is completed. The infant is then transferred to the transitional nursery, where postnatally all infants are admitted temporarily for transitional care in incubators and under radiant warmers. Approximately 5% of infants born are at sufficient risk to be transferred to a neonatal intensive care unit. Another 20% are at medium risk and should receive special care. They include infants who are disproportionate in weight, height, and gestational indexes; are light for length (ponderal index of less than 2.25); or have bilirubin over 10 mg/100 ml. The following criteria are used to select high-risk infants for admission to neonatal intensive care units (tertiary centers):
1. Continuing or developing signs of respiratory distress syndrome
2. Asphyxiation (Apgar score of less than 6 at 5 minutes)
3. Less than 33 weeks' gestational age
4. Weight of less than 1,600 gm

5. Cyanosis or suspected cardiovascular disease
6. Major congenital malformations requiring surgery or catheterization
7. Convulsions, sepsis, hemorrhagic diathesis, or shock
8. Meconium aspiration syndrome

In addition, the following infants are at high risk and require intensive care:
1. Prematurity (less than 2,000 gm)
2. Apgar score at 5 minutes of 6 or less
3. Resuscitation at birth
4. Fetal anomalies
5. Respiratory distress syndrome
6. Dysmaturity with meconium stain
7. Congenital pneumonia
8. Anomalies of respiratory system
9. Neonatal apnea
10. Other respiratory distress
11. Hypoglycemia
12. Hypocalcemia
13. Major congenital anomalies that do not require immediate procedures
14. Congestive heart failure
15. Hyperbilirubinemia
16. Hemorrhagic diathesis, mild
17. Chromosomal anomalies
18. Sepsis
19. CNS depression longer than 24 hours
20. Seizures
21. Persistent cyanosis

c. Moderate risk
1. Dysmaturity
2. Prematurity (2,000 to 2,500 gm)
3. Apgar score at 1 minute of 4 to 6
4. Feeding problems
5. Multiple birth
6. Transient tachypnea
7. Hypomagnesemia or hypermagnesemia
8. Hypoparathyroidism
9. Failure to gain weight

10. Jitteriness or hyperactivity with specific causes
11. Cardiac anomalies not requiring immediate catheterization
12. Heart murmur
13. Anemia
14. CNS depression less than 24 hours

SELECTED REFERENCES

Anderson, J. M.: High-risk groups—definitions and identifications, N. Engl. J. Med. **273**:308, 1965.
Anstil, A. O., Joshi, G. B., Lucas, W. E., Little, W. A., and Calligan, D. A.: Prematurity: a more precise approach to identification, Obstet. Gynecol. **24**:716, 1964.
Baird, D.: The epidemiology of prematurity, J. Pediatr. **65**:909, 1964.
Bonner, J., and Goldberg, C.: The assessment of iron deficiency in pregnancy, Scot. Med. J. **14**:209, 1969.
Brewer, T. H.: Human pregnancy nutrition: an examination of traditional assumptions, Aust. N. Z. J. Obstet. Gynaecol. **10**:87, 1970.
Brewer, T. H.: Human maternal-fetal nutrition, Obstet. Gynecol. **40**:868, 1972.
Butler, N. R., and Bonham, D. G.: British perinatal mortality survey, 1958, perinatal mortality report of the survey under auspices of the National Birthday Trust Fund, vol. 1, Edinburgh, 1963, E. & S. Livingstone, Ltd.
Clifford, S. H.: High-risk pregnancy. I. Prevention of prematurity—the sine qua non for reduction in mental retardation and other neurological disorders, N. Engl. J. Med. **271**:243, 1966.
Drillien, C. M., and Wilkinson, E. M.: Emotional stress and mongoloid births, Dev. Med. Child Neurol. **6**:140, 1964.
Emerson, J. K., and others, Caloric cost of normal pregnancy, Obstet. Gynecol. **40**:786, 1972.
Gold, E. M.: Identification of the high risk fetus, Clin. Obstet. Gynecol. **11**:1069, 1968.
Gold, E. M.: Interconceptional nutrition, J. Am. Diet. Assoc. **55**:27, 1969.
Gruenwald, P., Funakawa, H., Mitani, S., Nishimura, T., and Takeuchi, S.: Influence of environmental factors on foetal growth in man, Lancet **1**:1026, 1967.
Hendricks, C. H.: Delivery patterns and reproductive efficiency among groups of differing socio-economic status and ethnic origins, Am. J. Obstet. Gynecol. **97**:608, 1967.
Jacobson, H. N., and Reid, D. E.: II. A pattern

of comprehensive maternal and child care, N. Engl. J. Med. **271**:302, 1964.

Kaminetsky, H. A., and others, Effect of nutrition in teenage gravidas on pregnancy and status of the neonate, I. Nutritional profile, Am. J. Obstet. Gynecol. **115**:639, 1973.

Kitay, J. Z.: Folic acid deficiency in pregnancy, Mod. Med. **38**:77, 1970.

Lewis, B. V., and Nash, P. J.: Pregnancy in patients under 16 years, Br. Med. J. **2**:733, 1967.

Mulcahy, R., and Knaggs, J. F.: Effect of age, parity, and cigarette smoking on outcome of pregnancy, Am. J. Obstet. Gynecol. **101**:844, 1968.

Pitkin, R. M., and others, Maternal nutrition: a selective review of clinical topics, Obstet. Gynecol. **40**:773, 1972.

Rantakallio, P.: Groups at risk in low birth weight infants and perinatal mortality, Acta Paediatr. (Supp. 193), 1969.

Russell, C. S., Taylor, R., and Maddison, R. N.: Some effects of smoking in pregnancy, J. Obstet. Gynaecol. Br. Commonw. **73**:742, 1966.

Russell, J. K.: Pregnancy in the young teenager, Lancet **1**:365, 1969.

Stein, Z., and others, Nutrition and mental performance, Science **178**:708, 1972.

Taylor, R. D., and Swartout, J. W.: Biochemical survey of protein efficiency during pregnancy in urban women, Obstet. Gynecol. **29**:244, 1967.

Terris, M., and Gold, E. M.: An epidemiologic study of prematurity, I and II, Am. J. Obstet. Gynecol. **103**:358, 1969.

Tracy, T., and Miller, G. D.: Obstetric problems of the massively obese, Obstet. Gynecol. **33**:204, 1969.

Utian, W. H.: Obstetrical implications of pregnancy in primigravidae aged 16 years or less, Br. Med. J. **2**:734, 1967.

Von der Ahe, C. V.: The unwed teenage mother, Am. J. Obstet. Gynecol. **104**:279, 1969.

Walter, A. R. P.: Controversy on iron needs, uptake levels, deficiency stigmata and benefits from iron supplementation, Postgrad. Med. J. **45**:747, 1969.

Wilson, M. G., Parmelee, A. H., Jr., and Huggins, M. H.: Prenatal history of infants with birth weights of 1500 grams or less, J. Pediatr. **63**:1140, 1963.

Yerushalmy, J.: Mother's cigarette smoking and survival of the infant, Am. J. Obstet. Gynecol. **88**:505, 1964.

Zackler, J., Andelman, S. L., and Bauer, F.: Young adolescent as an obstetric risk, Am. J. Obstet. Gynecol. **103**:305, 1969.

3

Assessment of fetal health in high-risk pregnancy

FETAL DEVELOPMENT AND GROWTH

Interest in human fetal development and growth is mounting because of the obvious clinical implications. To understand the significance of deviations from established norms, it is necessary to understand the different "phases" of fetal development and growth.

The *ovular phase* comprises the first 4 weeks after fertilization. In that period a series of rapid mitotic divisions (cleavage) ensue that result in the formation of a blastula. Next a blastocyst is formed, and organ anlagen are relatively positioned by the process of gastrulation.

The *embryonic phase* extends from approximately the end of the fourth week until between the eighth and eleventh week. During this interval the organ systems develop from their primordia. This phase is characterized by marked growth and differentiation. The sequence of organogenesis is shown in Fig. 3-1.

The *fetal phase* is the interval from completion of organogenesis until delivery. Obviously, growth proceeds at a rapid rate during this interval.

Since growth in the healthy fetus apparently proceeds in a demonstrable fashion, deviations from this pattern of growth for any fetus may be of clinical significance. Fig. 3-2 shows this growth and the associa-

tions and morbidity factors when fetal growth deviates above the 90th percentile or below the 10th percentile. The type of problem shown depends on the timing of the insult. Interference with development, for example, chromosomal defects or rubella, may inhibit growth throughout gestation, whereas interference with growth has a variable onset that depends on the complication. For example, nutritional impairment usually is imposed after midpregnancy, whereas multiple pregnancy, toxemia, placental insufficiency, and postmaturity have variable onsets.

Fetal growth charts have become valuable as a reference even though at the present time the data used can show only the distribution of measurements of many who were prematurely born, rather than longitudinal data on the presumable healthier population that waits for delivery until term.

Fig. 3-3 shows the fetal growth curves of a Denver population. The Denver curves are primarily representative of a population of low socioeconomic background and are reduced in comparison to the Portland curves (Fig. 3-2), which apply to white, middle-class, private patients. The former were born above a 5,000 feet altitude, and the latter were born at virtual sea level. The Denver grid may be more applicable to general populations, but as such, does

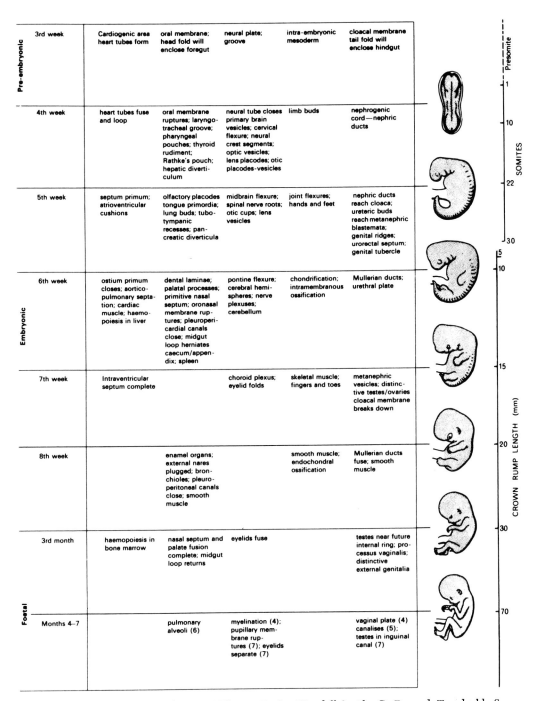

3rd week	Cardiogenic area heart tubes form	oral membrane; head fold will enclose foregut	neural plate; groove	intra-embryonic mesoderm	cloacal membrane tail fold will enclose hindgut
4th week	heart tubes fuse and loop	oral membrane ruptures; laryngo-tracheal groove; pharyngeal pouches; thyroid rudiment; Rathke's pouch; hepatic diverticulum	neural tube closes primary brain vesicles; cervical flexure; neural crest segments; optic vesicles; lens placodes; otic placodes-vesicles	limb buds	nephrogenic cord—nephric ducts
5th week	septum primum; atrioventricular cushions	olfactory placodes tongue primordia; lung buds; tubo-tympanic recesses; pancreatic diverticula	midbrain flexure; spinal nerve roots; otic cups; lens vesicles	joint flexures; hands and feet	nephric ducts reach cloaca; ureteric buds reach metanephric blastemata; genital ridges; urorectal septum; genital tubercle
6th week	ostium primum closes; aortico-pulmonary septation; cardiac muscle; haemo-poiesis in liver	dental laminae; palatal processes; primitive nasal septum; oronasal membrane ruptures; pleuroperi-cardial canals close; midgut loop herniates caecum/appendix; spleen	pontine flexure; cerebral hemi-spheres; nerve plexuses; cerebellum	chondrification; intramembranous ossification	Mullerian ducts; urethral plate
7th week	Intraventricular septum complete		choroid plexus; eyelid folds	skeletal muscle; fingers and toes	metanephric vesicles; distinc-tive testes/ovaries cloacal membrane breaks down
8th week		enamel organs; external nares plugged; bron-chioles; pleuro-peritoneal canals close; smooth muscle		smooth muscle; endochondral ossification	Mullerian ducts fuse; smooth muscle
3rd month	haemopoiesis in bone marrow	nasal septum and palate fusion complete; midgut loop returns	eyelids fuse		testes near future internal ring; pro-cessus vaginalis; distinctive external genitalia
Months 4–7		pulmonary alveoli (6)	myelination (4); pupillary mem-brane rup-tures (7); eyelids separate (7)		vaginal plate (4) canalises (5); testes in inguinal canal (7)

Fig. 3-1. Organogenesis. (From Williams, P. L., Wendell-Smith, C. P., and Treadgold, S.: Basic human embryology, London, 1966, Pitman Medical Publishing Co., Ltd.)

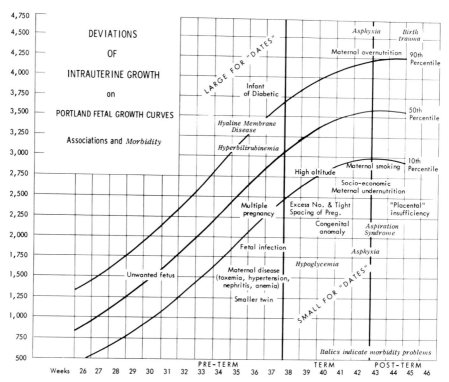

Fig. 3-2. Important associations and morbidity factors of accelerated or reduced fetal growth above the 90th percentile and below the 10th percentile for gestational age using the Portland curves. Fetal growth data obtained from 40,000 single, white, middle-class infants born near sea level.

not reflect optimal fetal growth. The slowing of fetal growth toward the end of the last trimester of pregnancy is a result of the restriction imposed by the fetal environment rather than a declining growth potential. Thus the average fetus is subject to some interference with nutrition. The adequacy of the placenta, the health of the mother, and the nutrition available to the fetus determine the timing of this slowing of fetal growth. In a sequential study of Japanese babies Gruenwald and colleagues show that improvement in the socioeconomic state of the population increases the weight of infants at term. Linear growth of the fetus during World War II continued only until 35 or 36 weeks of gestation,

whereas by 1963-1964, fetal growth continued unchecked to 38 weeks. Similar differences may explain the Denver/Portland comparisons of growth in weight.

When precise measurements of the size of any fetus can be plotted longitudinally against normal growth curves, the physician has a powerful tool to assess the state of health to the perinate. There are clinically applicable techniques for these determinations.

CLINICAL PARAMETERS OF FETAL WELL-BEING
Estimation of fetal age

The duration of pregnancy, more specifically fetal age, has become increasingly

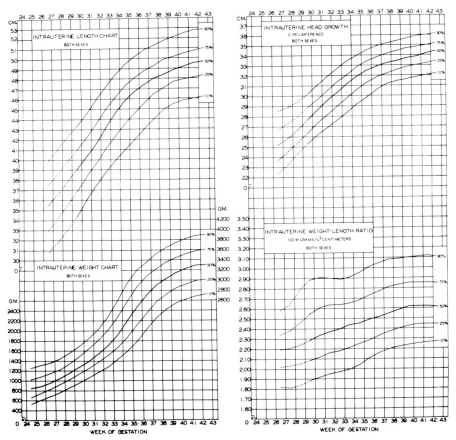

Fig. 3-3. Weight, height, and head circumference of living infants born after 24 weeks' gestation graphed as percentiles. (From Lubchenco, L. O., Hansman, M., and Boyd, E.: Pediatrics **37**:403, 1966.)

important in the determination of fetal prognosis and specific requirements of nursery care after birth. The principal reason is the considerable number of neonates delivered preterm electively. Toxemia of pregnancy and a previous cesarean section each account for about a fourth of all early terminations of pregnancy whereas isoimmunization and diabetes mellitus individually make up approximately one fifth of inductions for early delivery. Obviously, when termination of a pregnancy is not urgently indicated, the physician should delay until fetal maturity has been reached. If compelling reasons exist for premature birth, however, all parties must be apprised of the problems to be faced.

No single method of determining fetal age is precise enough to substantiate a clinical decision. Several procedures, together with an accurate obstetric history and physical examination, increase the accuracy of the estimation of gestational age, however. One should first utilize the simplest and safest methods and progress to more intricate and variable procedures if equivocal results are obtained initially. Regrettably, even when these methods are used, data are still insufficient regarding complicated pregnancy such as toxemia, erythroblastosis, and diabetes, for which early delivery may be required.

Most prenatal gestational age studies were neither prospective, nor was a series of these procedures done on the same patients concurrently. In addition, immediate postnatal studies on the newborns to validate previous determinations are rare. Therefore, for these reasons, few reliable "correlated gestational age determinations" are available to date.

Calculation of pregnancy duration from last menstrual period

An important estimate of gestational age is calculated from the first day of the last menstrual period. This span of time is actually the menstrual age, but it is used synonymously with gestational age, even though conception probably did not occur until approximately 2 weeks later. The time interval is best expressed in whole weeks

rather than as a mixed number of days. The World Health Organization has recommended the use of "completed weeks" rather than rounding to the nearest week.

Numerous problems must be considered when one calculates the duration of gestation from the first day of the last menstrual period (LMP):

1. Many women fail to record their menstrual dates.

2. Menstrual cycles are often irregular and variable.

3. Pregnancies may follow in close sequence without menstruation occurring between gestations.

4. Postconceptual bleeding may be confused with menstruation.

5. Ovulation that occurs during the cycle

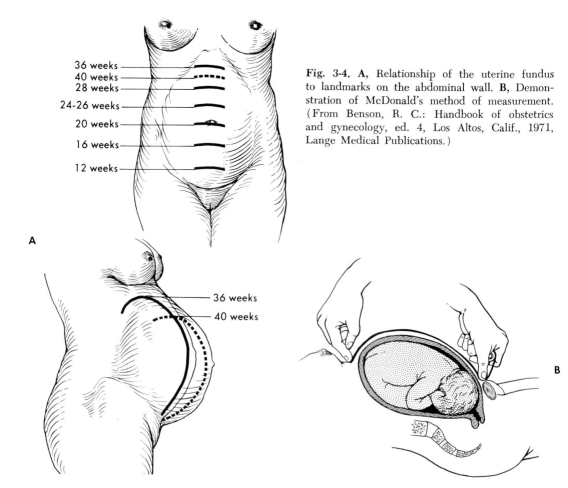

Fig. 3-4. **A,** Relationship of the uterine fundus to landmarks on the abdominal wall. **B,** Demonstration of McDonald's method of measurement. (From Benson, R. C.: Handbook of obstetrics and gynecology, ed. 4, Los Altos, Calif., 1971, Lange Medical Publications.)

immediately after the cessation of ovulation inhibition methods of contraception may be delayed.

These factors may affect the accuracy of reporting in 10% to 40% of women, depending on the population observed. The physician who considers a fetus of questionable menstrual age must estimate the gestational age. This can be done prenatally with increasing accuracy.

Basal body temperature record or single coitus

If a reliable basal body temperature record is available, or if an isolated intercourse can be dated, the precise onset of pregnancy can be documented. Such a rare record may be invaluable.

Measurement of uterine size

The most frequently utilized clinical parameter for estimation of fetal well-being is the serial abdominal measurement of the height of the uterine fundus.

1. Height of fundus in relation to anatomic landmarks
   The anteverted fundus is palpable just above the symphysis pubis at 10 to 12 weeks' gestation. It is halfway between the symphysis and the umbilicus at approximately 20 weeks. These and other relationships of the height of the fundus on the abdominal wall are demonstrated in Fig. 3-4.
2. Mensuration of fundal height
   Because landmarks are less useful in estimation of the duration of pregnancy during the second half of pregnancy, various calculations involving the direct measurement of fundal height have been advocated. One popular approach is *McDonald's maneuver* (Fig. 3-4). It is performed by measuring from the anterosuperior margin of the symphysis pubis with a flexible tape over the circumference of the uterus to its uppermost extent. This distance then allows the calculation of the duration of gesta-

tion: height of fundus in centimeters $\times$ 8/7 = weeks of pregnancy. Although not exact, serial measurements assist in documenting fetal growth.

3. Correlations of uterine fundal measurement with fetal weight
   R. W. Johnson devised a formula for estimating the weight of the fetus.

   $n = 12$, when the station of the fetal head is below the level of the ischial spines
   $n = 11$, if the presenting part is above the level of the ischial spines (and one is added to n for patients over 200 lb)
   $k = $ constant (155)

   Then

   $$(\text{cm of fundal measurement}) - n \times k = \text{approximate fetal weight in gm}$$

   Again, this is only an approximation, since only 50% will be within 240 gm of the calculated weight; moreover, the calculation applies only to vertex presentations.

4. Girth measurements
   Measurements of the abdominal circumference taken at the umbilicus with the patient in the supine position also provide a reproducible method for detecting increase, constancy, or decrease of uterine size. Girth is particularly useful in abnormal conditions when used in conjunction with the fundal height.

5. Correlations of abnormal serial measurements
   a. Unexpectedly large measurements
      1. Incorrect date of last menstrual period or of conception
      2. Multiple gestation
      3. Hydramnios
      4. Tumor
      5. Ascites
   b. Unusually small measurements
      1. Incorrect date of conception or last menses
      2. Intrauterine death
      3. Oligohydramnios
      4. Fetal anomaly
      5. Fetal undergrowth
      6. Missed abortion

Determination of fetal lie, presenting part, and position

In the second half of the pregnancy, systematic examination of the abdomen generally should reveal the intrauterine relationship of the fetus. It should be recorded at each visit and is generally accomplished by the four maneuvers of Leopold. These maneuvers are illustrated in Fig. 3-5 and are designed to determine the following:

1. The fetal poles and uterine fundus
2. The side to which the fetal back is directed
3. The part of the fetus that overlies the pelvic inlet
4. The side of the cephalic prominence

5. The depth of the presenting part in the pelvis

Rigorous application of these maneuvers at each patient visit may allow early determination and favorable management of breech, multiple gestation, hydramnios, malpresentation, and compound presentation.

Fetal heart tones

Identification of the fetal heart, which constitutes positive proof of fetal life, may be accomplished by electronic detection or fetoscope.

1. Electronic detection

   Ultrasonic devices utilizing the Doppler

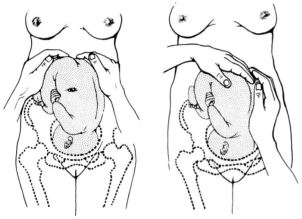

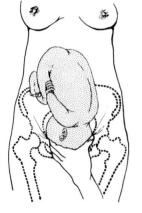

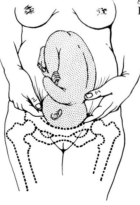

Fig. 3-5. Four maneuvers of Leopold. (From Benson, R. C.: Handbook of obstetrics and gynecology, ed. 4, Los Altos, Calif., 1971, Lange Medical Publications.)

principle may detect the fetal heartbeat as early as the ninth week of gestation. Later in pregnancy these devices may not only pick up fetal heart tones but may document the circulation of blood within large vessels. Equipment of this type is particularly useful early in pregnancy in the proof of fetal life, to rule out molar gestations, and to confirm or reject the clinical diagnosis of multiple gestations. In later pregnancy, such devices are very useful in cases of hydramnios, multiple gestation, massive obesity, and other states in which ausculation is unsatisfactory.

2. Fetoscope

Because the range of sound in which fetal heart tones are best heard involves bone conduction, the head fetoscope generally is a reliable stethoscopic instrument. With the use of the fetoscope, the fetal heart tones generally can first be heard between 18 and 22 weeks of gestation. Because the fetal heart is heard best over the back of the fetus on its left side, the point of maximum intensity of the fetal heartbeat may be used to corroborate impressions gained by Leopold's maneuvers concerning fetal lie and presenting part. For example, if the fetal heart tones are heard best in the area above the umbilicus on the right side, it is a reasonable presumption that the fetus is presenting by the breech, with the back to the mother's right side. The fetal heart rate will gradually slow during the course of pregnancy, but the rate is not a reliable index of the length of gestation.

Fetal motion

Maternal perception of fetal movement, which is termed "quickening," may provide an additional estimate for the duration of pregnancy. Quickening usually is noted at 20 weeks in the primigravida and 14 to 18 weeks in the multigravida.

On combined abdominopelvic examina-

tion about the sixteenth week, fetal parts may be palpable. At about the same time, active fetal movement can be seen or palpated by the examiner. Passive fetal movement may be noted even earlier in pregnancy by internal ballottement, or palpable bobbing during vaginal examination. This evidence of pregnancy is only presumptive, however.

LABORATORY PARAMETERS OF FETAL WELL-BEING
Antenatal genetic diagnosis

Intrauterine diagnosis of many disease processes that may result in a seriously deformed or mentally deficient child is now feasible by amniocentesis and subsequent studies. Nonetheless, there are definite risks to prenatal diagnosis (the two most common being hemorrhage and infection). Therefore a number of prerequisites for patient selection must be established.

Prerequisites for patient selection

1. The pregnancy must be at high risk for a specific disease process.

2. There must be a specific demonstrable chromosome or biochemical marker that will reliably indicate a fetus affected with that disease.

3. The chromosome or biochemical marker must be demonstrable early enough in gestation to permit reasonable options.

4. The available treatment and prognosis of the disorder must be known.

5. The risk of complications from amniocentesis must be less than the hazards of the disease.

In practice, these prerequisites usually are applicable with one of the following:

1. A previous child or close relative with Down's syndrome or other chromosomal disorders

2. Advanced maternal age (40 years of age or more) or a great anxiety regarding anomalies in a somewhat younger mother (35 to 40 years of age)

3. The significant likelihood of a child's having one of the following inherited metabolic disorders, which are now amenable to antenatal diagnosis*:

Acatalasemia	Ketotic hypergly-
Argininosuccinic	cemia
aciduria	Krabbe's disease
Chédiak-Steinbrinck-	Lesch-Nyhan syn-
Higashi syndrome	drome
Citrullinemia	Lysosomal acid phos-
Congenital erythro-	phatase deficiency
poietic porphyria	Mannosidosis
Cystinosis	Maple syrup urine
Fabray's disease	disease
Fucosidosis	Metachromatic leuko-
Galactosemia	dystrophy
Gaucher's disease	Methylmalonic
Glucose-6-PO₄ dehy-	aciduria
drogenase defi-	Mucopolysacchari-
ciency	doses (Types 1
Glycogen storage	to 6)
diseases (Types 2	Niemann-Pick disease
to 4)	Ornithine-α-keto acid
GM₁ gangliosidoses	transaminase defi-
(Types 1 and 2)	ciency
GM₂ gangliosidoses	Orotic aciduria
(Types 1 to 3)	Pyruvate decarbox-
Homocystinuria	ylase deficiency
Hyperlysinemia	Refsum's disease
Hypervalinemia	Xeroderma pigmen-
I-cell disease	tosum

4. A previous child or sibling with a severe sex-linked recessive disease, e.g., the Duchenne type of muscular dystrophy
5. A previous child with a neural tube defect

Certain requirements for providing intrauterine diagnosis must be met, however. Therefore only those with experience should undertake this service, which must be accomplished by a team composed of at least an obstetrician experienced in amniocentesis, a medical genetics group with biochemical and cytogenetic expertise who have proper counseling capability, and a full range of professional referrals.

*From Littlefield, J. W.: Genetics and the perinatal patient, Mead Johnson Symposium on Perinatal and Developmental Medicine 1:29, 1972.

Timing

Amniocentesis is most frequently accomplished between 14 and 16 weeks of gestation. This timing is based on the relative amount of amniotic fluid available and the number of cells in the fluid. Most experts recommend transabdominal amniocentesis, which is generally performed as an outpatient procedure after thorough explanation of the risks as well as advantages and options. Ultrasound is increasingly being used to "map" the area and thus decrease the possibility of transplacental bleeding because of injury. Following is the procedure:

1. Utilize B-scan ultrasound to localize the placenta and identify needle placement.
2. Perform pelvic examination to determine uterine size and position.
3. Shave selected abdominal wall site.
4. Prepare abdomen with tincture of iodine.
5. Drape the sterile area.
6. Infiltrate the skin and subcutaneous tissues with 1 ml of 1% procaine.
7. Insert 3½-inch 22-gauge disposable spinal needle into the uterine cavity.
8. Remove stylet and aspirate amniotic fluid, filling two 10 ml plastic syringes.

Risks

The exact risks for either the patient or her fetus are presently unknown. Happily, short-term and intermediate complications are uncommon (less than 1% in most reported series). The risks we have encountered in a recent series are listed in Table 3-1.

Limitations

Prenatal diagnosis still has numerous limitations. Consequently, counseling regarding interruption or continuation of the pregnancy should consider the following:

1. Diagnosis of metabolic diseases from amniotic fluid, or from uncultured or cultured amniotic fluid cells, has been made in

Table 3-1. Complications of prenatal genetic diagnosis (123 cases)

Complication	Number	Percentage	Comments
Spontaneous abortion	5	4	3 normal (18, 25, and 26 days after tap); 1 affected (I-cell disease) aborted day before therapeutic abortion
Amniocentesis necessary more than once	14	11	2 refused repeat amniocentesis
Bloody tap	17	14	By visual inspection; no complication in any of these
Transient amniotic fluid leakage	2	2	No sequelae
Culture failure	6	5	2 repeat amniocentesis refused 4 repeat amniocentesis with normal results (culture failures were at beginning of study)
Error in diagnosis	1	1	Cultured maternal blood (therefore, wrong sex predicted)
Twins	2	2	Information on one only, but second was also balanced translocation (case 2 identical)
Postabortion depression	1	1	Patient returned for amniocentesis for subsequent pregnancy
Other genetic abnormality not suspected	1	1	43-year-old gave birth to infant with de novo osteogenesis imperfecta congenita, who died
Failure to make diagnosis	4	3	2 culture failures and 1 dry tap in which repeat amniocenteses could not be obtained; 1 lab failure in biochemical determination

relatively few cases for each disease, so that the procedure must be considered quasiexperimental.

2. Culturing amniotic fluid cells is a tedious and complex process. Our mean time from amniocentesis to results was 19 days. This waiting interval is emotionally difficult for families, and when more complex biochemical analyses are required, the diagnosis may take 4 to 8 weeks.

3. Usually only one specific disease process can be investigated in each case.

4. Many autosomal dominant diseases, such as Huntington's chorea and Marfan's syndrome, are not currently amenable to prenatal diagnosis or medical treatment.

One should check with a genetics center regarding newer specific analyses before counseling patients because the capability for diagnosis is increasing rapidly.

Serial measurement of fetal growth

1. Radiography

The experienced radiologist, using combinations of radiographic signs and measurements, can establish fetal age with considerable accuracy. The technical quality of the films and the interpretation given constitute reliability and consistency.

When a radiologic assessment of fetal development is necessary for appropriate treatment of the patient, films must be specifically exposed to demonstrate the ossification centers and bony landmarks for the needed measurements. A

Table 3-2. Estimation of the duration of pregnancy from body and skeletal measurements[*]

Length (cm)	Weight (gm)	Head circumference (cm)	Duration of pregnancy (weeks)	Os calcis†	Talus†	Lower femoral epiphysis†	Upper tibial epiphysis†	Cuboid†
26.2	400	17.6	21					
27.9	480	18.9	22					
29.5	560	20.3	23					
21.2	650	21.5	24	0				
32.8	750	22.8	25	1.4				
34.3	850	24.0	26	2.7				
35.9	990	25.3	27	3.8	0			
37.4	1,140	26.5	28	4.8	1.3			
38.8	1,300	27.6	29	5.6	2.3			
40.2	1,470	28.6	30	6.3	3.1			
41.6	1,670	29.5	31	6.9	3.9	0		
42.9	1,910	30.4	32	7.5	4.6	0.5		
44.1	2,150	31.2	33	8.1	5.2	1.5		
45.2	2,390	32.0	34	8.6	5.7	2.3		
46.3	2,610	32.7	35	9.1	6.2	3.0		
47.4	2,810	33.3	36	9.6	6.7	3.6	0	
48.3	2,990	33.8	37	10.1	7.2	4.1	0.7	
49.2	3,160	34.3	38	10.5	7.6	4.6	1.6	
49.9	3,240	34.7	39	10.9	7.9	5.1	2.4	0
50.5	3,300	35.0	40	11.2	8.2	5.5	3.0	1-2

[*]Data from v. Harnack; from Huntingford, P., Hüter, K., and Saling, E., editors: Perinatal medicine, 1st European Congress, Berlin, Stuttgart, 1969, Georg Thieme Verlag.
†Mean diameter in millimeters in transverse section.

high degree of error must be expected when films obtained for decisions other than fetal age (pelvimetry, presentation, etc.) are used.

Measurement of the length of the fetal lumbar spine can be read directly from an x-ray film of the fetus in procubitus. The figure obtained is multiplied by a correction factor (8.7 for a distance center film of 1 M) for the length of the fetal skeleton.

No measurement can be exact, but, together with other radiologic criteria for dimension and age such as ossification centers, a reasonable assessment of fetal age is possible as is shown in Table 3-2.

Ossification centers in the fetus must be approximately 3 mm in diameter before they are easily visualized on x-ray film.

Radiologic examinations during pregnancy may expose the fetus and mother to undesirable amounts of radiation. Nonetheless, the consequences of such exposure must be contrasted with the need for precision to ensure proper obstetric management.

2. Ultrasound

Assessment of fetal growth on the basis of serial measurements of head and thorax made by using ultrasound is the simplest and most reliable method of determining fetal growth. Fetal weight and week of gestation are predictable from the biparietal diameter obtained near term (Table 3-3). Although some have reported the ultrasonic thoracic measurement to be inaccurate, others have found that one third of the small-for-dates fetuses have a proportionally reduced growth rate that may be noted

Table 3-3. Ultrasonic estimation of fetal weight and maturity*

Biparietal diameter (cm)	Weight gm	Weight lb/oz	Weeks of gestation	Biparietal diameter (cm)	Weight gm	Weight lb/oz	Weeks of gestation
1.0	NA	NA	9	6.0	660.4	1 8	25.5
1.1	NA	NA	9	6.1	737.6	1 10	26.0
1.2	NA	NA	9.5	6.2	814.8	1 13	26.0
1.3	NA	NA	10.0	6.3	892.1	2	26.5
1.4	NA	NA	10.0	6.4	969.3	2 2	27.0
1.5	NA	NA	10.5	6.5	1,046.5	2 5	27.0
1.6	NA	NA	11.0	6.6	1,123.7	2 8	27.5
1.7	NA	NA	11.0	6.7	1,200.9	2 10	28.0
1.8	NA	NA	11.5	6.8	1,278.2	2 13	28.0
1.9	NA	NA	12.0	6.9	1,355.4	3	28.5
2.0	NA	NA	12.0	7.0	1,432.6	3 3	29.0
2.1	NA	NA	12.5	7.1	1,509.8	3 5	29.0
2.2	NA	NA	13.0	7.2	1,587.0	3 8	29.5
2.3	NA	NA	13.0	7.3	1,664.3	3 11	29.5
2.4	NA	NA	13.5	7.4	1,741.5	3 14	30.0
2.5	NA	NA	14.0	7.5	1,818.7	4	30.5
2.6	NA	NA	14.0	7.6	1,895.9	4 3	30.8
2.7	NA	NA	14.5	7.7	1,973.1	4 5	31.0
2.8	NA	NA	15.0	7.8	2,050.4	4 8	31.7
2.9	NA	NA	15.0	7.9	2,127.6	4 11	32.0
3.0	NA	NA	15.5	8.0	2,204.8	4 14	32.7
3.1	NA	NA	16.0	8.1	2,282.0	5	33.0
3.2	NA	NA	16.0	8.2	2,359.2	5 3	33.6
3.3	NA	NA	16.5	8.3	2,436.5	5 6	34.0
3.4	NA	NA	17.0	8.4	2,513.7	5 8	34.6
3.5	NA	NA	17.0	8.5	2,590.9	5 11	35.0
3.6	NA	NA	17.5	8.6	2,668.1	5 14	35.5
3.7	NA	NA	18.0	8.7	2,745.3	6	36.0
3.8	NA	NA	18.0	8.8	2,822.6	6 3	36.5
3.9	NA	NA	18.5	8.9	2,899.8	6 6	37.0
4.0	NA	NA	19.0	9.0	2,977.0	6 8	37.4
4.1	NA	NA	19.0	9.1	3,054.2	6 11	38.0
4.2	NA	NA	19.5	9.2	3,131.4	6 14	38.4
4.3	NA	NA	20.0	9.3	3,208.7	7 2	39.0
4.4	NA	NA	20.0	9.4	3,285.9	7 3	39.0
4.5	NA	NA	20.5	9.5	3,363.1	7 6	39.8
4.6	NA	NA	21.0	9.6	3,440.3	7 10	40.0
4.7	NA	NA	21.0	9.7	3,517.5	7 11	40.8
4.8	NA	NA	21.5	9.8	3,594.8	7 14	41.0
4.9	NA	NA	22.0	9.9	3,672.0	8 2	41.7
5.0	NA	NA	22.0	10.0	3,749.2	8 3	NA
5.1	NA	NA	22.5	10.1	3,826.4	8 6	NA
5.2	42.6	2	23.0	10.2	3,903.6	8 10	NA
5.3	119.9	5	23.0	10.3	3,980.9	8 13	NA
5.4	197.1	6	23.5	10.4	4,058.1	8 14	NA
5.5	274.3	10	24.0	10.5	4,135.3	9 2	NA
5.6	351.5	13	24.0	10.6	4,212.5	9 5	NA
5.7	428.7	14	24.5				
5.8	514.9	1 2	25.0				
5.9	583.2	1 5	25.0				

*Courtesy Timothy G. Lee, M.D., Chief, Section of Ultrasound, Department of Diagnostic Radiology, University of Oregon Health Science Center.

earlier in the thoracic measurement compared to the biparietal diameter of the head. Thus ultrasonic fetal cephalometry combined with thoracic measurement taken serially may offer a better index of fetal well-being and weight than cephalometry alone.

Ultrasonographic examination is safe and reliable and can be used repeatedly throughout pregnancy. It may be useful also for

a. Appraisal of fetal growth
b. Placental localization
c. Volumetric growth of the placenta
d. Diagnosis of molar gestation
e. Identification of multiple gestation
f. Detection of certain fetal abnormalities, that is, anencephaly and hydrocephaly
g. Diagnosis of fetal death
h. Confirmation of fetal lie, presenting part, position
i. Identification of compound presentations

Ultrasonography generally is markedly superior to radiography for visualization of both bony and soft tissues and their mensuration.

Biochemical testing
Human chorionic gonadotropin (HCG)

Human chorionic gonadotropin, a protein hormone, is produced by the cytotrophoblast. The detection and measurement of HCG is of practical importance for the diagnosis of pregnancy and the evaluation of possible trophoblastic disease. The most sensitive method for measuring HCG is by radioimmunoassay. Although a test with this degree of sensitivity may be important in the prognosis of choriocarcinoma, immunologic tests employing hemagglutination, inhibition, or latex agglutination are satisfactory for the diagnosis of pregnancy. Radioimmunoassay techniques may demonstrate HCG as early as 24 hours after implantation, but the more commonly employed urinary tests of pregnancy are

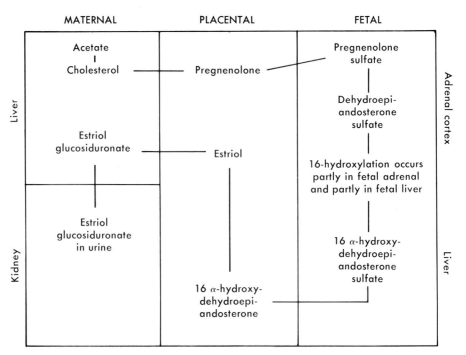

Fig. 3-6. Estriol biosynthesis in late pregnancy.

usually not reliable until about 42 days after the first day of the last menstrual period. The hormone peaks at 60 to 70 days of gestation, followed by a slow fall to a relatively steady titer at 100 to 130 days of pregnancy. Pregnancy tests have not been use-

Table 3-4. Average estriol excretion in normal pregnancy*

Gestation (weeks)	Mean estriol excretion (mg/24 hr)	Standard deviation (mg)	Number of subjects
6	0.05		3
7	0.06		3
8	0.09		4
9	0.15	0.079	7
10	0.16	0.085	7
11	0.23	0.255	7
12	0.28	0.153	8
13	0.58	0.249	9
14	0.70	0.354	10
15	1.15	0.425	7
16	1.95	0.760	8
17	2.40	0.775	10
18	3.65	0.899	15
19	4.36	1.339	29
20	5.59	1.932	31
21	6.70	2.256	11
22	7.59	1.904	9
23	9.36	2.221	12
24	10.04	2.144	11
25	10.57	3.228	11
26	12.98	1.612	11
27	13.75	2.100	10
28	12.96	3.465	19
29	14.67	3.266	42
30	15.21	3.490	41
31	15.24	3.604	18
32	17.51	4.265	11
33	18.12	4.197	15
34	18.82	3.571	16
35	22.55	3.040	15
36	23.39	3.928	19
37	28.61	7.652	24
38	31.33	6.565	42
39	33.34	9.373	46
40	34.49	9.352	25
41	33.22	7.935	16

*From Klopper, A., and Billewicz, W.: Urinary excretion of estriol and pregnanediol during normal pregnancy, J. Obstet. Gynaecol. Br. Commonw. **70:**1024, 1963.

ful in prognosis or for routine fetal evaluation. There is a significant incidence of both false-negative and false-positive results with immunologic pregnancy tests.

Estriol

The biosynthesis of the steroid hormone estriol depends on an intact maternal-fetal placental unit (Fig. 3-6). Urinary estriol determinations are meaningful only if they are determined serially in the latter half of the same pregnancy. A normal range may indicate that the fetus is not in immediate danger; nonetheless, low or significantly decreased estriol excretion has been associated with fetal disease or even impending death. Estriol values are especially useful in the assessment of fetal well-being in pregnancies complicated by diabetes mellitus, hypertension, eclamptogenic toxemia, placental insufficiency (including postmaturity), and suspected intrauterine fetal demise. Estriol excretion is decreased in cases of fetal anencephaly and in gravidas who are taking large doses of corticosteroids, who have severe anemia, who live at high altitudes, who have severe renal disease, or who are taking medications such as ampicillin and chlorothiazide diuretics. In contrast, urinary estriol is elevated in normal multiple gestation.

Neonatal apnea, marked cyanosis, or gross neurologic abnormality may be associated with reduced urinary estriol excretion. Table 3-4 details the average estriol excretion in normal pregnancy. Note that a drop of 40% from a previously obtained value is indicative of fetal distress and warrants assessment and possible intervention.

Human chorionic somatomammotropin (HCS)

Human chorionic somatomammotropin is also called human placental lactogen (HPL). HCS is a protein hormone produced by the syntrophoblast. Generally, this hormone is measured by radioimmunoassay. Abnormally low HCS values are equal to or less than 4 μg/ml maternal serum after 30 weeks' gestation. After the first postpartum day, HCS is no longer detectable in the serum. HCS levels may identify a pregnancy compromised by placental insufficiency because of vascular disease, hypertension, preeclampsia pyelonephritis, essential hypertension, lupus erythematosus, or glomerulonephritis.

Other means of biochemical testing

Heat-stable alkaline phosphatase, diamine oxidase cystine aminopeptidase (oxytocinase), and pregnanediol may become valid methods for assessing fetal viability. These determinations are not, however, recommended at the present time for routine clinical use.

Physiologic maturity testing

Physiologic maturity testing by means of amniotic fluid has proved to be exceedingly useful when pregnancy threatens to terminate prematurely, when gestation is prolonged (over 42 weeks), and in complicating disease states when pregnancy should be terminated. Amniocentesis may be performed as early in pregnancy as one believes there is a reasonable chance of fetal survival. Care should be taken to perform the amniocentesis either behind the fetal neck or below the presenting part (toward the cervix). If blood is encountered, one should determine whether it is of fetal or maternal origin. The Kleihauer stain is useful for this purpose.

1. Rapid surfactant test

A rapid test for surfactant in amniotic fluid to assess the risk of respiratory distress syndrome was described by Clements and colleagues in 1972. This test is of extreme importance because it may be performed by a competent laboratory or physician with minimal effort and equipment, and it has a high degree of reproducibility.

  a. Reagents

    1. 0.9% sodium chloride (9 gm/L distilled water)

    2. 95% ethanol

  b. Equipment

    1. Centrifuge

    2. Vortex mixer

    3. Two 10 × 100 mm tubes

    4. Two No. 0 rubber stoppers

    5. Two 1 ml and one 2 ml pipettes

    6. Test tube rack

    7. Pipette bulb

  c. Procedure

    1. Centrifuge at 2,000 rpm for 10 minutes to settle particulate matter immediately after drawing the amniotic fluid.

    2. Pipette 1 ml from the "clear" supernate into one 14 × 100 ml tube and 0.5 ml into the other.

    3. Draw 0.5 ml saline into the second tube.

    4. Add 1 ml 95% ethanol to each tube, stopper, and shake (Vortex), setting at 5-6 for 15 seconds.

    5. Immediately place the tubes upright in the test tube rack and let them sit for 15 minutes. A ring of bubbles completely around the meniscus after 15 minutes is a positive test result.

    6. Determine fetal maturity from Table 3-5.

Table 3-5. Method of interpretation of fetal lung maturity tests

Predicted fetal status	Lecithin/ sphingomyelin ratio	Rapid surfactant test
Mature	≥2.00	Complete ring of bubbles persisting 15 min at 1:1 and 1:2 dilutions
Intermediate	1.50 to 1.99	Complete ring of bubbles persisting 15 min at 1:1 dilution only
Immature	<1.50	Incomplete ring of bubbles at both dilutions

We have found that fetal lung maturity can be correlated with the results of amniotic fluid analysis (578 samples). The rapid surfactant test was found to be nearly totally reliable in predicting fetal lung maturity, and it was more reliable in predicting fetal lung immaturity (69%) than the lecithin/sphingomyelin (L/S) ratio (38%) discussed below. The rapid surfactant test can be used as a primary method for determining fetal pulmonary maturity, and the L/S ratio can be used as an additional indicator of fetal maturity when the rapid surfactant test is intermediate or the sample contaminated by blood or meconium.

2. Lecithin/sphingomyelin ratio (L/S ratio)
   A method of determining the relative L/S ratio in amniotic fluid was published by Gluck and co-workers in 1971. Most authorities now agree that the L/S ratio is a useful test for fetal maturity. Nevertheless, there are reports of discrepancies between the results of the test and the clinical status of the infant—particularly when the L/S ratio is in the intermediate range. Moreover, it has been argued that the test is not a reliable index of fetal lung immaturity, as was previously noted (38%). This technique, like the rapid surfactant test, is most commonly used prior to repeat cesarean section and in preeclampsia, isoimmunization, diabetes mellitus, fetal postmaturity, premature rupture of the membranes, and potential fetal jeopardy from other causes. This test requires a well-equipped laboratory with capability for thin-layer chromatography. In our hands, the test has been most reproducible if a densitometer is employed. Each laboratory should develop its own standards. The L/S ratio is interpreted as is noted in Table 3-5.

3. Creatinine
   Measurement of the amniotic fluid creatinine correlates well with fetal gestational age. Unfortunately this determination has the inherent limitations of all the methods listed below because none will measure a vital substance necessary for fetal survival. They are correlated only with fetal age. Before the thirty-fourth week it is infrequent to note more than 2 mg/100 ml, and after 37 weeks it is unusual to encounter less than 2 mg/100 ml, (many are 3 to 4 mg/100 ml) of amniotic fluid creatinine.

4. Spectrophotometric analysis
   The $\triangle$ OD 450 mμ in nonisoimmunized patients may also be used to indicate the length of gestation. At less than 35 weeks many are more than 0.01, and if 36 weeks or more, the $\triangle$ OD usually is 0.0.

5. Fetal fat cells
   The number of fetal fat cells identified by a number of staining techniques, such as Nile blue, is of less value than the studies mentioned above.

6. Visual inspection
   Visual inspection of the amniotic fluid may allow certain generalizations. It is yellow or straw colored and slightly turbid early in gestation; as term approaches, it becomes clear and opalescent, and has varying amounts of white particulate matter floating in it (vernix). With isoimmunization, it is yellow and slightly turbid. When it contains blood, amniotic fluid is opaque and varying degrees of dark red. Meconium staining is marked by green-brown coloration and opacity. The yellow-brown "tobacco juice" opaque fluid that accompanies intrauterine death is characteristic.

Stress testing

Antepartum stress testing is now being evaluated clinically as a guide to the tolerance of the high-risk fetus to labor. This technique utilizes the patient's spontaneous uterine contractions or oxytocin-induced uterine contractions. Stress testing presumably determines relative placental "respiratory" reserve. The fetal heart tones must be continuously monitored by means of an external device. A positive test is recorded when a "late deceleration" fetal heart rate pattern occurs (Chapter 4). This pattern probably indicates fetal inability to tolerate labor. A negative test is interpreted as probable capability for tolerating labor. The stress test has been criticized because it is unquantifiable and time-consuming.

Hypoxic stress tests and exercise stress tests are subject to the same criticisms and at the present time are the subject of research.

Other means of fetal assessment
Amnioscopy

Amnioscopy often identifies the passage of meconium, presumably a sequel to hypoxia. Amnioscopy is easy to do in most multiparas near term, but it is satisfactory only occasionally in the primigravida. Unfortunately, amnioscopy is not a screening procedure. Moreover, not all fetuses pass

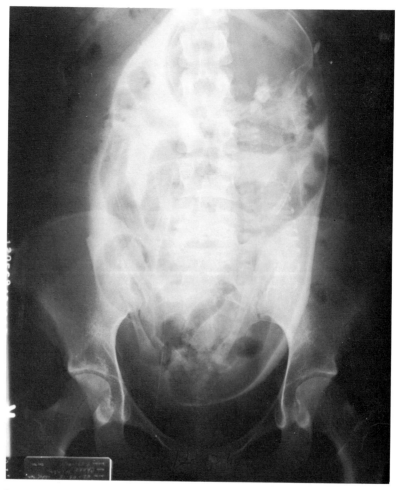

Fig. 3-7. Anteroposterior amniogram showing breech presentation, with placenta on right lateral uterine wall.

meconium, especially prematures, even in the presence of definite hypoxia. The test must be done daily or every few days in questionable cases, and the cervix must be dilated slightly—the assumption being that the patient is at or near term.

Amniotic fluid osmolarity

In early pregnancy the amniotic fluid is virtually isotonic, but near term a decrease in protein concentration and increased chloride ion content, as compared with serum or plasma, results in ever-increasing ismolarity (or freezing-point depression due to solute concentration, assuming no blood contamination). At term an amniotic fluid osmotic pressure of about 250 mOsm/L can be expected. This is 20 to 25 mOsm/L lower than the fetal or maternal plasma. A slow but definite fall in osmolarity after 40 weeks then occurs. This pattern of osmolarity is not altered appreciably, except by severe maternal fluid-electrolyte derangement such as might occur in un-

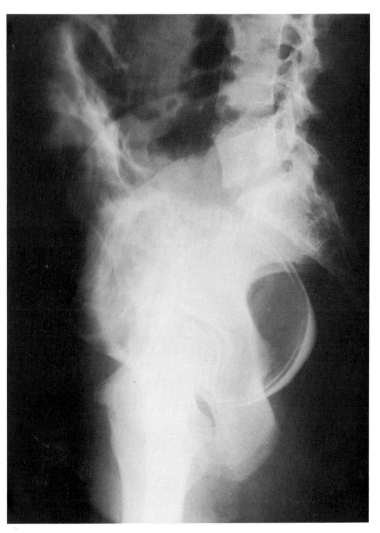

Fig. 3-8. Lateral amniogram showing intact bag of waters, engaged vertex, and absence of placenta previa.

controlled diabetes mellitus or advanced nephritis. Hence decreasing amniotic fluid osmolarity can be equated with advancing gestational age, even in toxemic patients or those with severe isoimmunization. Obviously, several amniocenteses should be done to establish the trend.

Amniography

Amniography contrasts the soft tissues and skeleton of the fetus, the uterine cavity, and the fetoplacental surface (Figs. 3-7 and 3-8). It is particularly useful in the identification of fetal abnormalities, for example, scalp edema, hydrops, and anomalous development such as gastrointestinal atresia. Amniography facilitates fetal transfusion and may confirm fetal jeopardy or demise.

Iothalamate acid (Angio-Conray) or diatrizoate sodium (Hypaque-M), 75%, is the aqueous contrast medium often used. Generally, 10 to 15 ml of amniotic fluid is removed at 22 to 28 weeks and 20 ml from the twenty-ninth week onward, followed by instillation of a similar quantity of the iodine solution.

Opacification of amniotic fluid is seen in the fetal gastrointestinal tract within 15 minutes of injection as early as the twelfth week of pregnancy. Lack of swallowing indicates gastrointestinal obstruction, serious fetal compromise, or death.

Liposoluble contrast media such as iophendylate (Ethiodan), 30 ml, may also be used in amniography. These slightly viscid fluids are absorbed progressively on the vernix and, after 6 to 8 hours, will outline the fetal skin clearly, remaining visible on x-ray films for several weeks after injection.

Prior to the thirty-eighth week, the skin of the fetus is almost completely outlined by iophendylate, 8 ml, injected into the amniotic cavity, even the fingers, toes, and external genitalia. Between the thirty-eighth to fortieth week, the outlines of the extremities and abdomen become patchy,

so that a clear, complete outline does not occur. At term and later, only the outline of the head and back is clearly seen. The gastrointestinal tract of the normal fetus will also contain the liposoluble contrast medium.

DETERMINATION OF FETAL DEATH

Clinically, the subjective diagnosis of fetal death often is suspected when the patient ceases to feel fetal movements. Objectively, cessation of uterine growth or perhaps even regression suggests fetal death. Absence of fetal heart tones may be noted, nonetheless; unless the area of the heart is localized by B-scan ultrasound and then the Doppler ultrasonic instrument directed to that precise point, an absent fetal heartbeat cannot be determined with certainty. Biologic tests are of little value because the placenta may continue to function for a time. X-ray signs of fetal death include overlapping of the fetal cranial bones in a patient not in labor (Spaulding's sign), demonstration of gas in the fetal heart or large vessels, and abnormal angulation of the fetal spine.

SELECTED REFERENCES

Borrelli, A. P., Woodrow, P., Pinck, R. L., and Freedman, H.: Amniography: useful radiographic procedure, N. Y. State J. Med. 67:1395, 1967.

Brosnes, J., and Gordon, H.: The estimation of maturity by cytological examination of the liquor amnii, J. Obstet. Gynaecol. Br. Commonw. 73: 88, 1966.

Browne, A. D. H., and Brennan, R. K.: The application value and limitation of amnioscopy, J. Obstet. Gynaecol. Br. Commonw. 75:616, 1968.

Clements, J. A., Platzker, A. C. G., and Tierney, D. F.: Assessment of the risk of the respiratory and distress syndrome by a rapid test for surfactant in amniotic fluid, N. Engl. J. Med. 286: 1077, 1972.

Donald, I.: Sonar in obstetrics and gynecology. In Greenhill, J. B., editor: The year book of obstetrics and gynecology, 1967-1968, Chicago, 1968, Year Book Medical Publishers, Inc.

Donald, I.: Ultrasonics in diagnosis (sonar), Proc. Roy. Soc. Med. 62:442, 1969.

Dorfman, A., editor: Antenatal diagnosis, Chicago, 1972, The University of Chicago Press.

Droegemueller, W., Jackson, C., Makowski, E. L., and Battaglia, F. C.: Amniotic fluid examination as an aid in the assessment of gestational age, Am. J. Obstet. Gynecol. **104**:424, 1969.

Farr, V., and Mitchell, R. G.: Estimation of gestational age in the newborn infant, comparison between birth weight and maturity scoring in infants premature by birth, Am. J. Obstet. Gynecol. **103**:380, 1969.

Gluck, L., Kulovich, M. V., Borer, R. C., Jr., Brenner, P. H., Anderson, G. G., and Spellacy, W. N.: Diagnosis of the respiratory distress syndrome by amniocentesis, Am. J. Obstet. Gynecol. **109**:440, 1971.

Gruenwald, P.: Growth of the human fetus, Am. J. Obstet. Gynecol. **94**:1112, 1966.

Gruenwald, P., Funakawa, H., Mitani, S., Nishimura, T., and Takeuchi, S.: Influence of environmental factors on foetal growth in man, Lancet **1**:1026, 1967.

Gutenberg, J.: The bilirubin concentration of amniotic fluid as an indicator of fetal maturity, J. Am. Osteopath. Assoc. **68**:285, 1968.

Hellman, L. M., Kobayashi, M., Fillisti, L., and Lavenhar, M. P. H.: Growth and development of the human fetus prior to the twentieth week of gestation, Am. J. Obstet. Gynecol. **103**:789, 1969.

Huntingford, P. J., Brunello, L. P., and Dunstan, M.: The technique and significance of amnioscopy, J. Obstet. Gynaec. Br. Commonw. **75**:610, 1968.

Keniston, R. C., Pernoll, M. L., Buist, N. R. M., Lyon, M., and Swanson, J. R.: A prospective evaluation of the lecithin/sphingomyelin ratio and the rapid surfactant test in relation to fetal pulmonary maturity, Am. J. Obstet. Gynecol. **121**:324, 1975.

Loeffler, F. E.: Clinical fetal weight prediction, J. Obstet. Gynaecol. Br. Commonw. **74**:675, 1967.

Mandelbaum, B., LaCroix, G. C., and Robinson, A. R.: Determination of fetal maturity by spectrophotometric analysis of amniotic fluid, Obstet. Gynecol. **29**:471, 1967.

Margolis, A. J.: A method for radiologic detection of fetal maturity, Am. J. Obstet. Gynecol. **101**:383, 1968.

Michie, E. A.: Urinary estriol excretion in pregnancies complicated by suspected retarded intrauterine growth, toxemia, or essential hypertension, J. Obstet. Gynaecol. Br. Commonw. **74**:896, 1967.

Miles, P. A., and Pearson, J. W.: Amniotic fluid osmolality in assessing fetal maturity, Obstet. Gynecol. **34**:701, 1969.

Milunsky, A.: The prenatal diagnosis of hereditary disorders, Springfield, Ill., 1973, Charles C Thomas, Publisher.

Pernoll, M. L., Prescott, G. H., Hecht, F., Olson, C. L.: Prenatal diagnosis: practice, pitfalls and progress, Obstet. Gynecol. **44**:773, 1974.

Pitkins, R. M.: Prenatal estimation of fetal maturity, Int. J. Gynecol. Obstet. **7**:199, 1969.

Prescott, G. H., Pernoll, M. L., and Hecht, F.: A prenatal diagnosis clinic: an initial report, Am. J. Obstet. Gynecol. **116**:942, 1973.

Usher, R., and McLean, F.: Intrauterine growth of live-born Caucasian infants at sea level: standards obtained from measurements of infants born between 25 and 44 weeks of gestation, J. Pediatr. **74**:901, 1969.

4

Assessment of fetal health in high-risk labor

CLINICAL PARAMETERS
General assessment

On admission to the labor and delivery area, every patient must be reevaluated for maternal and/or fetal jeopardy.

1. Review history, physical examinations, laboratory data, course of pregnancy, and nutritional and hydration states.
2. Ascertain
   a. Time of the onset of labor
   b. Presence or absence of a bloody show or other vaginal bleeding
   c. Status of the fetal membranes (approximately 10% of membranes rupture prematurely)
   d. Temperature, pulse, and blood pressure
   e. Time last food or fluid was taken
   f. Any allergies to medication
   g. Maternal and paternal emotional states
3. Perform
   a. Brief general physical examination
   b. Palpation of the uterus for fetal lie, presenting part, engagement
   c. Assessment of fetal size (Chapter 3)
   d. Pelvic examination (if not contraindicated by abnormality of any of the above) for cervical dilatation, cervical effacement, consistency and position of the cervix, fetal presenting part (including station), and position of presenting part

   e. Assessment of pelvic capacity
   Clinical pelvimetry is notoriously inaccurate; however, it is useful as a screening device for those patients who will need more accurate evaluation of their pelvic capacity. One of the most important indications for radiographic pelvimetry will be the progress in labor. (See Table 4-1.) Other indications for radiographic pelvimetry are as follows:
   1. Fetopelvic disproportion occurring in a previous pregnancy
   2. If physical examination indicates
      a. A diagonal conjugate of 11.5 cm or less
      b. A narrow midpelvis (prominent spines and converging sides walls)
      c. A narrow intertuberous (less than 9 cm) or decreased sum of the intertuberous and posterior sagittal (less than 15 cm)
   3. Lack of engagement of the fetal head with labor to 5 cm of cervical dilatation (in the presence of empty bowel and bladder)
   4. A primigravida presenting at term with
      a. Breech presentation
      b. Nonengagement of the fetal head
   f. Auscultation of the fetal heart rate

(FHR) and the point of maximum intensity identified for monitoring

g. Evaluation of the amniotic fluid for meconium

4. Institute
   a. Clean-catch urine for protein and glucose
   b. Periodic evaluation of maternal vital signs (never less than every hour, but frequency will depend on the situation)
   c. Intake and output
   d. Intravenous fluids through a large needle
   e. Fetal monitoring (electronic) for fetal heart rate and uterine contractions
   f. Other (scalp sampling, ultrasonography, x-ray pelvimetry, etc., as indicated)
   g. Prepare and cleanse the pudendum
   h. Enema (optional)
   i. Nothing by mouth (Stomach empty-

ing time is delayed in pregnancy; therefore should anesthesia be administered or any complication ensue, the hazard of aspiration is greatly enhanced.)

   j. Lateral positioning if at bed rest (The cardiac output is markedly influenced by the uterus' compressing of the inferior vena cava in the supine position; the extreme is the supine hypotensive syndrome.)

Assessment of progress in labor

Labor is defined as the process by which the products of conception are normally delivered. It implies progressive effacement and dilatation of the cervix.

1. Differentiation of false labor from true labor (Table 4-2)
   Braxton Hicks' contractions, or prodromal labor, may be mistaken for true labor. Not infrequently the discomfort is as great with false labor as it is with true labor, and the differential diagnosis is exceedingly important.
2. Cervical dilatation
   a. For fetal reference, labor is divided into two stages
      1. The first stage of labor begins with demonstrable progressive dilatation and effacement of the cervix in response to uterine contractions and ends with complete (10 cm) dilatation of the cervix.
      2. The second stage of labor begins

Table 4-1. Minimal values acceptable for radiographic pelvimetry if the fetus is of average or greater size

Planes	Anteroposterior (cm)	Transverse (cm)	Posterosagittal (cm)
Inlet	10.0	12.0	—
Midplane	11.5	9.5	4.0
Outlet	11.5	10.0	7.5

Table 4-2. Differentiation of false labor from true labor

	True labor	False labor
Contraction interval	Regular (gradually shortens)	Irregular (remains irregular)
Contraction duration	Regular	Irregular
Contraction intensity	Gradually increases	Remains same
Discomfort location	Generally in back and abdomen, spreading from back to front in a girdlelike distribution	Located primarily in lower abdomen; however, may be fundal but rarely in back
Effect of exercise	Intensifies by walking	Not intensified by walking
Effect of mild sedation	Not affected	Usually relieved

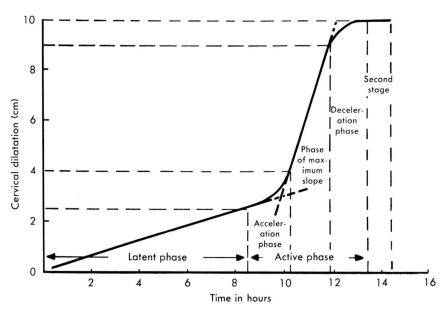

Fig. 4-1. Composite of the patterns of the cervical dilatation-time function based on a study of 500 nearly consecutive nulliparas. (From Friedman, E. A.: Obstet. Gynecol. 6:569, 1955.)

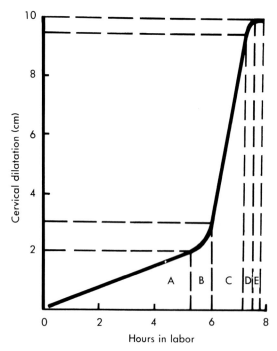

Fig. 4-2. Mean multiparous labor pattern based on a study of a series of 500 multiparas. **A,** Latent phase. **B,** Acceleration phase. **C,** Phase of maximum slope. **D,** Deceleration phase. **E,** Second stage. **B** to **D** is the active phase. (From Friedman, E. A.: Obstet. Gynecol. 8:692, 1956.)

Table 4-3. Mean nulliparous labor*

	Mean	Mode	Median	SD†	SE$_m$‡	Range	Statistical limit§
Latent phase (hr)	8.6	6.0	7.5	6.0	0.27	1.0-44	20.6
Active phase (hr)	4.9	3.0	4.0	3.4	0.15	0.8-34	11.7
Deceleration (hr)	0.9 (54 min)	0.5	0.8	1.2	0.05	0.0-14	3.3
Maximum slope (cm/hr)	3.0	1.5	2.7	1.9	0.08	12.0-0.4	1.2
Second stage (hr)	0.95 (57 min)	0.6	0.8	0.8	0.04	0.0-5.5	2.5

*From Friedman, E. A.: Primigravid labor, a graphicostatistical analysis, Obstet. Gynecol. 6:567, 1955.
†Standard deviation, SD = $\sqrt{\Sigma d/N}$; d = deviation from mean.
‡Standard error of mean, SE$_m$ = SD/$\sqrt{N}$.
§Deviation twice standard deviation greater than mean, p = 0.05, except maximum slope, which because of its skew distribution has a lower limit 95 percentile points below the median.

Table 4-4. Mean multiparous labor*

	Mean	Mode	Median	SD	SE$_m$	Range	Statistical limit
Latent phase (hr)	5.3	3.5	4.5	4.1	0.19	0.4-36	13.6
Active phase (hr)	2.2	1.5	1.8	1.5	0.07	0.3-15	5.2
Deceleration (hr)	0.23 (14 min)	0.1	0.2	0.33	0.01	0.0-3.5	0.88 (53 min)
Maximum slope (cm/hr)	5.7	4.5	5.2	3.6	0.16	2.4-0.7	1.5
Second stage (hr)	0.24 (14 min)	0.1	0.2	0.30	0.01	0.0-3.0	0.83 (50 min)

*From Friedman, E. A.: Labor in multiparas, a graphicostatistical analysis, Obstet. Gynecol. 8:691, 1956.

when the cervix is completely dilated and ends with complete birth of the baby.

b. For obstetric purposes there is also a third, or placental, stage of labor, from the birth of the infant to the delivery of the placenta. Evaluation of cervical dilatation allows the determination of relative progress in labor. Friedman's data for the mean nulliparous labor and mean multiparous labor are shown in Figs. 4-1 and 4-2. The hours and limits are included in Tables 4-3 and 4-4. Every laboring patient should be evaluated by means of the data. Fig. 4-3 illustrates a management program for the secondary arrest of dilatation-time patterns.

3. Descent of presenting part

Friedman's data for descent of the fetal presenting part are correlated to cervical dilatation and time in Figs. 4-4 and 4-5. Again, these correlative data are extremely important for assessment of the progress in labor. From Friedman's data it is demonstrated that the presenting part must be below the level of ischial spines at the onset of the second stage (in both multiparous and nulliparous labor) to fall within two standard deviations of normal.

Assessment of amniotic fluid

Meconium staining of amniotic fluid in late pregnancy may be an early sign of fetal distress. Fetal death before the onset of labor most often is accompanied by the passage of meconium. The few exceptions are probably due to very acute compression

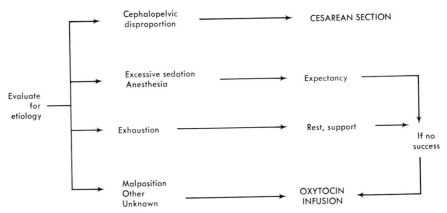

Fig. 4-3. Recommended program of management of the patient with secondary arrest of dilatation-time patterns. (From Friedman, E. A.: Bull. Sloane Hosp. Women 9:20, 1963.)

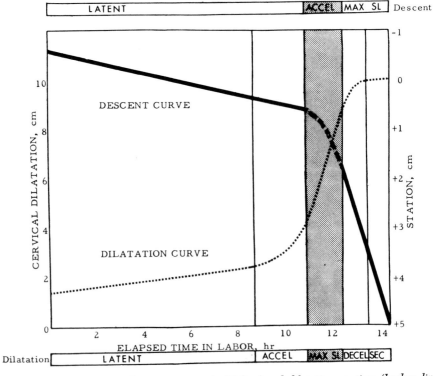

Fig. 4-4. Composites of mean descent vs. time *(solid line)* and dilatation vs. time *(broken line)* curves for a series of 421 unselected nulliparas. (From Friedman, E. A.: Am. J. Obstet. Gynecol. 93:525, 1965.)

of the umbilical cord. Meconium passage before the middle of the last trimester or staining of the premature infant is infrequent and perhaps due to the immaturity of the fetal autonomic nervous system in its influence on gastrointestinal activity.

When the amniotic fluid is clear at the onset of labor, the perinatal mortality is low (less than 1%); when amniotic fluid is stained by meconium, perinatal mortality rises to about 6%. The Apgar scores are significantly lower in the latter group.

Amniotic fluid staining in the last trimester is of such concern that continuous observation of the pregnancy is necessary, with the inclusion of fetal monitoring, measurement of estriol excretion, assessment of fetal age and size, etc. to best determine the timing and method of delivery. Meconium passage before and even during labor, particularly prolonged labor, should alert the obstetrician to a possible emergency and need for a reassessment of management.

1. Incidence of meconium passage (green- or yellow-stained amniotic fluid) in late pregnancy, taken from various sources
   a. In a general pregnant population— 5% to 10%

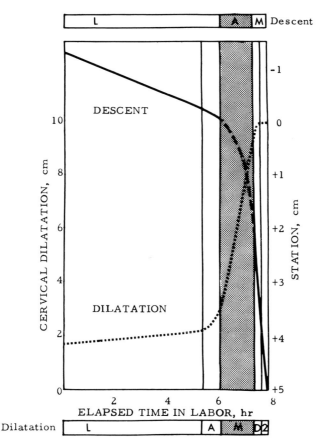

Fig. 4-5. Composite mean curves for descent *(solid line)* and dilatation *(broken line)* for 389 unselected multiparas. Intervals: **L**, latent; **A**, acceleration; **M**, maximum slope; **D**, deceleration; **2**, second stage. (From Friedman, E. A., and Sachtleben, M. R.: Am. J. Obstet. Gynecol. 93:522, 1965.)

b. In women with no adverse factors—
1% to 2%

c. In selected groups of high-risk patients—up to 35%

2. Indications for screening amniotic fluid for meconium passage

a. Maternal disease, for example, toxemia, diabetes, hypertension—usually screened at 36 to 37 weeks

b. Prolonged pregnancy—42 weeks or more

c. Impaired fetal growth or change in fetal activity

d. Late or prolonged variable FHR deceleration

3. Methods of evaluating amniotic fluid

a. Amnioscopy—widely used in Europe Requires practice for reasonable accuracy when minor color changes in amniotic fluid have occurred. If there is doubt, amniocentesis should be performed.

1. Technique

a. Slip tubular or cone-shaped amnioscope into the slightly dilated cervix against the membranes.

b. Focus a light source on the membranes (avoid fiberoptics because of greenish tinge to the light).

c. Observe for color, meconium, and blood within the amniotic sac.

2. Complications

a. Rupture of the membranes occurs in approximately 3% of patients.

b. Occasional minor bleeding may develop—rarely placental separation.

c. Maternal or fetal sepsis is rare.

b. Amniocentesis

This procedure is also important when the fetus is rhesus sensitized or when insufficient fluid escapes from a membrane rupture to determine the color of the amniotic fluid.

1. Technique (p. 30)
Fluid obtained is evaluated against a white background.

2. Complications

a. Injury to placental vessels with possible fetal exsanguination

b. Injury to fetus itself

Overactivity of the fetus

Threshing or tumultous movements of the fetus have been time-honored signs of fetal distress. Carbon dioxide retention stimulates the fetal respiratory center, and hyperreflexia follows. Brief overactivity of the fetus has been reported in cord compression and abruptio placentae. Nevertheless, with progressive hypoxia, fetal depression follows rapidly. Hence the value of this largely subjective sign of fetal danger is minimal.

FETAL HEART RATE PATTERNS AND FETAL DISTRESS

Fetal distress is a symptom complex indicative of a critical response to stress. Fetal distress implies metabolic derangements, including hypoxia and acidosis, that affect essential body functions to the point of temporary or permanent injury or death. Fetal distress may be acute, chronic, or "additive" (e.g., narcosis plus asphyxia). An immature or compromised fetus has a lower reserve; hence fetal distress and its consequences are more likely. Meaningful fetal monitoring will diagnose fetal distress—perinatal jeopardy—in at least 20% of all obstetric patients, many of whom have serious medical or obstetric complications (Table 4-5).

The influence of labor on the fetus already at high risk adds to the likelihood of asphyxial insult. This is particularly true of the low birth weight infant who has delicate structures, enzyme immaturity, and limited fat stores and glucose reserves. With asphyxia, respiratory gas exchange across the placenta falls, accompanied by hypoxia ($P_{O_2}\downarrow$) and hypercapnia ($HCO_2\uparrow$)

Table 4-5. Fetal distress—associated disorders

Maternal problems	Fetal problems
Acute fetal distress	
A. Marked reduction of placental perfusion or fetal circulation	
1. Hypertonic uterine contractions	1. Umbilical cord compression
2. Hypotension	a. Tight or short cord
3. Decreased uterine blood flow	b. True knots
4. Abruptio placentae	c. Prolapsed cord
B. Inadequate systemic circulation	
1. Shock (hemorrhagic, septic, anaphylactic)	1. Cardiac failure (hydrops fetalis, myocarditis)
2. Sudden cardiac failure	2. Congenital anomaly (cardiac, cord)
3. Normovolemic hypotension secondary to conduction anesthesia	3. Hemorrhage (velamentous insertion of the cord, other)
4. Placenta previa	
C. Insufficient blood oxygenation	
1. Severe anemia, hemorrhage	1. Acute hemolytic crisis (erythroblastosis)
2. Hypoxia and/or hypercarbia (as with poorly controlled anesthesia)	
3. Impaired respiratory efforts (acute poliomyelitis, tetanus, bronchospasm)	
4. Methemoglobinemia	
Chronic fetal distress	
A. Moderate reduction of placental perfusion or fetal circulation	
1. Toxemia of pregnancy	1. Multiple pregnancy (twin-to-twin) transfusion, competition for circulation)
2. Diabetes mellitus	
3. Hypertensive cardiovascular disease	2. Dysmaturity
4. Dysmaturity (postmaturity)	3. Partial cord compression
5. Elderly or grand multipara	
6. Premature placental aging, intervillous fibrin deposition, etc.	
B. Inadequate systemic circulation	
1. Cardiovascular disease (congenital, acquired)	1. Congenital cardiovascular disease
	2. Maternal-fetal transfusion syndrome
C. Insufficient blood oxygenation	
1. Extensive tuberculosis (emphysema)	1. Accidental injection of anesthetic into fetoplacental circulation (paracervical or caudal accident)
2. Impaired respiratory efforts (kyphoscoliosis, chronic)	
3. Low oxygen tension (high altitude)	2. Dystocia (shoulder, breech)
	3. Prolonged labor
"Additive," or combined, fetal distress	
A. Drug overdosage (narcosis)	
B. Labor and fetopelvic disproportion	

in the fetus. The result is a combination of respiratory and metabolic acidosis. The latter is enhanced by the accumulation of organic acids, which are dependent on anaerobic metabolism and the utilization of carbohydrates. Acidosis is identified by a falling blood pH. It has been amply demonstrated that considerable reduction of oxygen to the fetus may cause a significant rise in basal fetal heart rate (FHR) initially; severe oxygen lack invariably results in bradycardia and/or arrhythmia and, finally, fetal death.

Fetal distress is an everyday obstetric

challenge; however, with the advent of earlier and more precise detection of fetal distress and its more definitive management, the specter of a "continuum of reproductive wastage" from death through varying degrees of disability has now been lessened. The recognition of specific pathophysiologic events (fetal heart rate changes and fetal acidosis) that occur in fetal distress will now be discussed.

Diagnostic aids

1. Indirect monitoring of fetal heart rate
   a. Auscultation with traditional stethoscope
   Although electronic recording of the fetal heart rate has demonstrated the limitations of the stethoscope, nurses and aides must be trained in its more effective use. An important detail for using it more advantageously is counting the fetal heartbeat throughout and just after a contraction, rather than waiting until the uterus is well relaxed.
   The following method is useful for the observation of the fetus during labor, particularly when an increased risk to the fetus is present (Whitfield):
   1. Count heartbeats for successive 5-second periods during and after contractions.
   2. The lowest 5-second count times 12 gives the approximate depth of bradycardia in beats/min.
   3. The number of 5-second periods from the end of contraction to the first count of more than 10 beats, that is, a rate of over 120 beats/min, gives a simple measure of the delay in recovery of a uteroplacental insufficiency pattern or the duration of an episode of late deceleration (type II dip).
   4. Any beat-to-beat arrhythmia must be noted.
   5. The intervals of observations are shortened if any bradycardia or irregularity is observed.

   b. Electronic FHR monitoring by indirect methods
   The indirect forms of electronic monitoring are external means of gathering data concerning uterine contractions and FHR patterns. Their interpretation is basically the same as that of the direct methods. The indirect methods have, however, two important limitations: the uterine activity is indicated in a qualitative manner and cannot be interpreted as being quantitative and the indirect methods all produce FHR patterns that appear to have normal beat-to-beat variation, but this phenomena is an inherent artifact and does not actually reflect the beat-to-beat variation seen with direct monitoring.
   1. Phonocardiography utilizing an electronic pickup, amplifier, and speaker system
   2. Ultrasonic monitoring (Doppler principle)

2. Direct monitoring of fetal heart rate
   The clinical criteria for fetal distress have been poorly defined. Hence, until recently, only unusual fetal responses have been related to serious stress. Tumultuous or prolonged uterine contractions and fetal cord compression are prime examples of acute situations that are likely to cause marked FHR changes, which may be recognized only when occasional auscultation is affected. In contrast, with continuous monitoring, major and minor changes of significance that may escape the periodic check are noted. A normal FHR pattern almost invariably presages the delivery of a neonate with a good Apgar score (over 7). Conversely, gravely abnormal FHR patterns may predicate a severely compromised fetus (Apgar score under 4).
   a. Electronic monitoring with fetal scalp electrode and simultaneous intrauterine pressure recording (p. 52)

b. Biochemical monitoring by fetal-scalp blood sampling

In complications of the fetus that impair gaseous exchange (most often of placental and/or maternal origin), any hypoxia leading to fetal acidosis will threaten cellular metabolism after a variable latent period. The circulation, muscle tone, motility, and respiratory functions may all suffer as a result. The latent period between the onset of hypoxia and the adverse effect on the fetus depends on whether the hypoxia is acute or chronic, considering the condition of the fetus at the time the complication occurs,* and the duration of the metabolic disturbance.

The determination of the fetal blood pH value in a complicated pregnancy after established labor gives the obstetrician an accurate method for assessment of impending catastrophe. A fall in pH value to 7.15 or below is an indication to perform rapid delivery by the best means possible.

Although fetal heart changes and meconium passage have a correlation with fetal asphyxia, they do not indicate the degree of distress as accurately as the fetal blood pH determination does, and in addition, meconium is not easily passed by the immature fetus.

Through the innovative work of Erich Saling, the development of fetal blood sampling has added an important parameter to the recognition of the fetus in distress. It is now agreed that the pH and blood gas measurements taken under defined conditions truly represent the arterial circulation, particularly in the first part of labor.

1. Indications for fetal blood sampling
   a. Acute problems
      1. Meconium present (vertex or breech presentation)
      2. Fetal heart rate over 160 or under 100/min

3. Bradycardia that continues for more than 30 seconds after the end of a contraction (late deceleration)
4. Severe variable deceleration or combination of late and variable deceleration

If the first fetal blood sample done at the appearance of these signs is pH = less than 7.25, repeat the test immediately.

   b. Chronic problems include

Moderate or marked eclamptogenic toxemia, diabetes mellitus, severe Rh sensitization, and amnionitis, as well as postterm births, dysmaturity, and dystocia; borderline cephalopelvic disproportion, uterine dyskinesia, prolonged labor, oxytocin stimulation, and a history of unexplained prior stillbirth.

The first fetal blood sample obtained at the onset of labor should be repeated if signs of fetal distress develop.

Deliver the fetus at once if pH is less than 7.20 on two successive samples, in the absence of maternal acidosis.

2. Method for obtaining fetal blood
   a. Pass amnioscope and wipe scalp or buttock with antiseptic on gauze.
   b. Apply silicone to allow a drop of blood to remain at the incision site.
   c. Nick skin, no more than 2 mm.
   d. Aspirate blood into the capillary tube.
   e. Do not remove amnioscope until bleeding has ceased. Determine pH without delay.

3. Advantages of this technique
   a. An operative delivery indicated by the usual signs of fetal distress may be avoided if the acid-base balance of the fetus is satisfactory.
   b. Fetal asphyxia of a mild type (pH 7.20 to 7.24) that is only slowly progressive (a substantial majority) can be followed serially every half hour, and if operative intervention

---

*For example, a fetus that has suffered growth retardation or wasting has reduced glycogen resources for the support of anaerobic metabolism.

becomes necessary, it can be performed under optimum conditions.

c. Acute and severe reductions in fetal acid-base balance demand immediate cesarean section.

d. Fetal distress, for example, in erythroblastosis, may not be evident by clinical signs of meconium passage or FHR changes.

e. Recognition of fetal acidosis will allow early correction at birth by the injection of buffer solution through an umbilical vessel (p. 102). This procedure prevents an aggravated peak of metabolic acidosis, which usually occurs 5 to 10 minutes after delivery and if untreated may intensify the already depressed function of vital centers and contribute to cerebral hemorrhage.

4. Reasons for discrepancies between the level of fetal acidosis as measured by pH and the vigor of the newborn at birth include the following:

a. The development of acidosis may have been too recent to affect the infant even though he was threatened.

b. The fetus may have recovered from acidosis if the complication, for example, uterine tetany or compression of the cord, has been relieved.

c. Conversely, the newborn may be depressed without the demonstration of fetal acidosis. Examples are excessive anesthesia and intrauterine infection without hypoxia.

d. Fetal acidosis may reflect the transfer of excess organic acids as a contribution from the mother. Although this increment may be harmless, it should be estimated whether maternal acidosis is present.*

---

*Values of pH of less than 0.05 between mother and fetus indicate a maternal contribution and are of no great concern as long as the fetal pH is above 7.15 in these instances.

5. Risks in fetal scalp sampling
   The risks to the fetus have been infrequent infection and bleeding. In the latter, pressure alone will suffice, but a suture in the scalp rarely may be necessary.

Appraisal of FHR patterns

The interpretation of fetal well-being is determined primarily by heart rate patterns at the present time. To understand the patterns it is necessary to differentiate between the FHR pattern during the uterine contraction (transitory changes) and the FHR pattern during the interim between contractions (base line). Thus the major diagnostic criteria currently applicable are as follows:

1. Base line changes
   a. Beat-to-beat variation (irregularity)
   b. Tachycardia
   c. Bradycardia
2. Transitory changes
   a. Accelerations
   b. Decelerations
      1. Early
      2. Late
      3. Variable
3. Combination patterns

All FHR pattern interpretation depends on ensemble characteristics. The diagnosis of a given pattern cannot be made on the basis of a single contraction. Fig. 4-6 demonstrates direct electronic FHR methodology. A full discussion of FHR pattern interpretation is beyond the scope of this book; however, a brief introduction may be useful. Fig. 4-7 schematically illustrates the terminology of FHR pattern interpretation.

1. Base line changes (FHR pattern not under the influence of uterine contraction)
   a. Beat-to-beat variation (irregularity)
      Fluctuations in the basal FHR of 1 to 8 beats/min and a frequency of 3 to 10 cycles/min are nearly always obtained in normal mature fetuses.

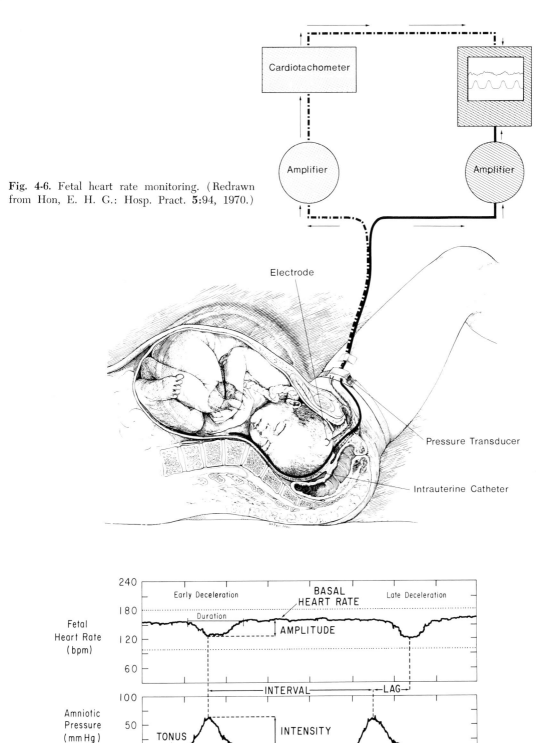

Fig. 4-6. Fetal heart rate monitoring. (Redrawn from Hon, E. H. G.: Hosp. Pract. 5:94, 1970.)

Fig. 4-7. Some of the variables measured in the tracings of the fetal heart rate and amniotic fluid pressure (uterine contractions) and their chronologic relationships.

It is believed that this irregularity is created by the asynchronous attempts of the two portions of the autonomic nervous system (sympathetic and parasympathetic) to regulate the fetal heart rate. Beat-to-beat variation is not seen in immature fetuses or in those without an intact nervous control of the heart. Absence of beat-to-beat variation may be ominous in the term or near-term fetus, implying altered nervous control of the heart because of anoxia, acidosis, or drug effects. Hon has suggested classification of irregularity on the basis of the peak-to-peak amplitude of the fluctuations, thus:

1. No irregularity—0 to 2 beats/min
2. Minimal—3 to 5 beats/min
3. Average—6 to 10 beats/min
4. Moderate—11 to 25 beats/min
5. Marked—greater than 25 beats/min

b. *Tachycardia*—sustained elevations of FHR above 160 beats/min
Clinically established FHR categories in beats/min for at least 10 minutes have been suggested (Hon) as follows:

1. Normal rate—120 to 160 beats/min
2. Moderate tachycardia—161 to 180 beats/min
3. Marked tachycardia—181 beats/min or more

Tachycardia is frequently associated with immaturity, maternal fever, and minimal fetal hypoxia. It is more ominous as a predictor of fetal distress if there is absence of beat-to-beat variation, when it is associated

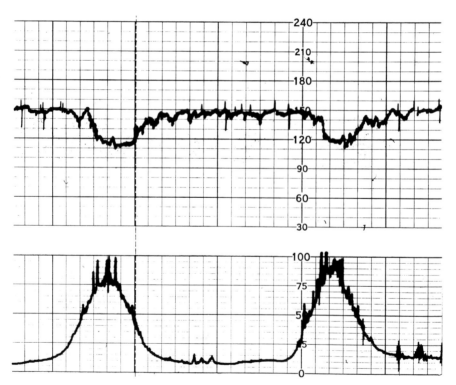

Fig. 4-8. Early deceleration (head compression). Note the early onset of bradycardia, its recovery by the end of the contractions, and the proportionate relationship between the individual patterns and the associated contractions.

with late or prolongd variable deceleration, or when it is associated with FHR irregularity late in the contracting phase of the uterus.

c. *Bradycardia*—sustained depressions of FHR below 120 beats/min
  1. Moderate bradycardia—100 to 119 beats/min
  2. Marked bradycardia—99 beats/min or less

Unless persistent bradycardia is associated with marked FHR decelerations, it has not been associated with neonatal depression. It may, however, be associated with congenital heart lesions.

2. Transitory changes (FHR patterns in relation to a uterine contraction)
  a. *Accelerations* are transient increases of the FHR concomitant with uterine contractions. They may be the earliest indicators of possible fetal compromise, although, in Hon's experience, the presence of accelerations, without other abnormalities of FHR pattern, has not been associated with poor clinical outcome or significant changes in fetal acid-base status.
  b. *Decelerations* are transient decreases of the FHR in response to a uterine contraction. As noted previously there are three "pure" types currently known: early, late, and variable.
    1. *Early deceleration* is a transient decrease in FHR in response to a uterine contraction. The deceleration is of uniform shape, reflecting the intrauterine pressure curve (Fig. 4-8). It is believed to be due to fetal head compression. The amplitude of the deceleration

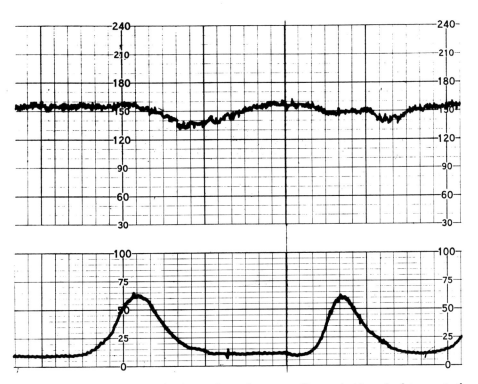

Fig. 4-9. Late deceleration (uteroplacental circulatory insufficiency). Note the late onset, the lag, the delay in recovery, and the proportionate relationship between the individual patterns and the associated contractions *(bottom)*.

does not exceed 40 beats/min and it normally occurs between 140 and 100 beats/min. An important differentiating characteristic is that recovery of the FHR to the base line rate occurs at or before the end of the contraction. This FHR pattern has not been associated with depressed newborns, and therefore it appears to be innocuous.

2. *Late deceleration* is a transient fall in FHR occurring after the uterus has begun to contract. It has a uniform shape but has a later onset than early deceleration and may not cease immediately with the contraction (Fig. 4-9). It is believed to be caused by uteroplacental insufficiency and is an ominous sign of fetal distress. An important differential between early and late deceleration is that late deceleration has its onset late in the uterine contracting phase and the FHR does not return to base line until after cessation of the uterine contraction. It usually occurs between 180 and 120 beats/min but if severe may be 60 or less beats/min. It is frequently associated with high-risk pregnancy and with maternal hypotension or uterine hyperactivity. It is critical to note that this most ominous indicator of fetal distress occurs in the normal FHR range.

3. *Variable deceleration* is a transient decrease in FHR that may occur at varying times in relationship to

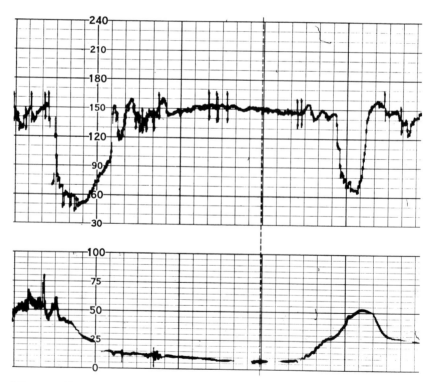

Fig. 4-10. Variable deceleraion (cord compression). Note the marked variability in onset, depth, shape, and recovery in relation to the uterine contractions.

the uterine contraction. The pattern is not of uniform shape and varies in intensity (Fig. 4-10). It usually occurs in the range of 140 to 160 beats/min and is thought to be associated with umbilical cord compression. It may be associated with depressed newborns if prolonged and severe but is usually alleviated by maternal position change.

3. Combined patterns
The full significance of combined patterns is not yet known. Suffice it to note, however, that combinations of those patterns which are indicative of fetal distress are probably an ominous sign.

TREATMENT OF FETAL DISTRESS FROM INTERPRETATION OF FHR SIGNS

Currently the most readily available data concerning fetal status are from FHR patterns obtained by one of the means just outlined. The treatment of fetal distress will therefore be discussed in relationship to FHR pattern interpretation.

1. No fetal distress
   Short-term early deceleration of the FHR usually indicates innocuous fetal head compression (Fig. 4-8). No therapy is indicated. The consequences of long-term FHR deceleration are unknown.
2. Possible fetal distress
   Variable FHR deceleration may be seconds to a minute long; it is a warning

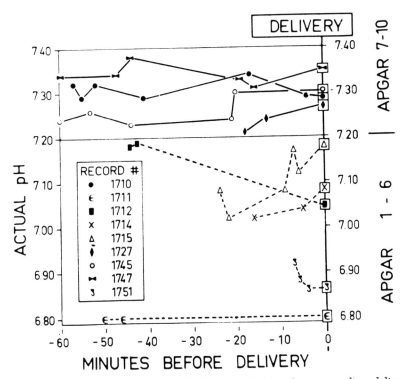

Fig. 4-11. Actual pH of fetal capillary blood during the last hour preceding delivery. The values corresponding to each case are identified by different symbols. The fetuses having a pH lower than 7.20 were depressed at birth (first-minute Apgar score 1 to 6). Fetuses with a pH between 7.20 and 7.40 were not depressed at birth (first-minute Apgar score 7 to 10). (From Mendez-Bauer, C., Arnt, I. C., Gulin, L., Escarcena, L., and Caldeyro-Barcia, R.: Am. J. Obstet. Gynecol. 97:530, 1967.)

that may indicate cord compression (Fig. 4-10), especially with tachycardia of more than 160 beats/min. The FHR does not mirror the uterine contraction curve or the strength of the contractions. If the variable FHR acceleration is confined to the period of uterine contraction, even if associated with marked temporary bradycardia, it probably is reflex in nature and not serious.

Reposition the patient to one side or the other. Treat as fetal distress if improvement does not follow change of position.

3. Definite fetal distress
   a. Prolonged or worsening *variable FHR deceleration* (more than 1 minute) with bradycardia of under 100 beats/min indicates possible cord compression.

1. Give oxygen, 6 to 7 L/min by mask. Reposition the patient.
2. Begin administration of 10% glucose intravenously.

b. *Late FHR deceleration* (with or without tachycardia) generally identifies uteroplacental circulatory insufficiency and fetal hypoxia (Fig. 4-9). The problem may be critical also if tachycardia and a relatively smooth FHR base line are present.

1. Give oxygen as just indicated. Avoid supine position. Alleviate problems that lead to reduced uteroplacental circulation.
2. Correct maternal hypotension (drugs).
3. Give intravenous fluids.
4. Change the patient's position or

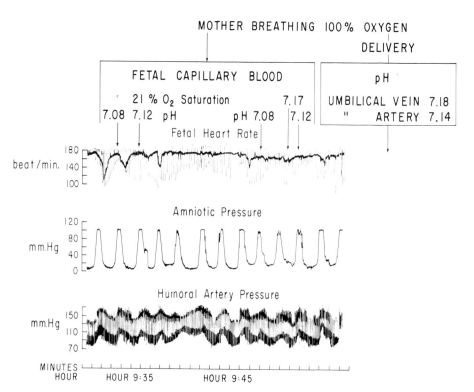

Fig. 4-12. Fetal-maternal relationships during labor. (Redrawn from Mendez-Bauer, C., Arnt, I. C., Gulin, L., Escarcena, L., and Caldeyro-Barcia, R.: Am. J. Obstet. Gynecol. **97**:540, 1967.)

elevate her legs during conduction anesthesia.

5. Reduce high intrauterine tension by rupture of the membranes.
6. Alert the operating room to possible cesarean section.
7. Discontinue oxytocin.
8. Consider fetal scalp blood for pH determination (Fig. 4-11).

4. **Critical fetal distress**

When the therapy just suggested yields no improvement in FHR patterns indicative of definite fetal distress, the condition may be termed critical fetal distress. Delivery should be effected immediately. An example (Fig. 4-12) demonstrates marked tachycardia in relation to severe acidosis, indicating the necessity for prompt delivery.

If one records the FHR continuously and does fetal scalp blood pH determinations when problems arise, a good correlation between these indices and the Apgar score will be noted.

FETAL NURSING

Intensive nursing care for women in labor must also include the zealous guarding of the fetus. Although this may seem entirely logical, the product of pregnancy is too often treated as a casual by-product.

Nursing has always been patient oriented, but when one considers the parturient, a double responsibility must be assumed, particularly during labor and delivery, when the needs and problems of the fetus become especially demanding. Assessment of fetal well-being now demands special training and experience in the quest for a successful conclusion of pregnancy.

The first objective of fetal nursing is maternal homeostasis. Proper physical and psychological support is most important. Information regarding the gravida's past and present health is particularly pertinent because, as in hypothyroidism or eclamptogenic toxemia, fetal growth and development may be compromised. Specific ther-

apy may have to be initiated, continued, or changed. The nurse must also appreciate the character of labor because dystocia may add another, often cumulative, dimension to other problems.

The change in fetal environment before, during, and after parturition is extreme. The offspring's environment is totally altered. The stresses of labor and delivery induce complex, often critical variations in maternal and fetal physiology. The number of alterations and the degree of change may vary even from minute to minute.

Fetal nursing has always been limited, but new approaches are now feasible, particularly with the general availability of practical, accurate monitoring equipment. Nevertheless the nurse still cannot visualize the fetus as being pink or blue, sleeping or critically irresponsive, or bathed in clear or meconium-stained amniotic fluid. Even with its life at stake, the fetus cannot plead its case.

The nurse can do much, however, to establish safety or jeopardy, observing and reporting (1) emotional maternal symptomatology and (2) signs of fetal embarrassment. The nurse is a vital member of the medical team, even though it is the physician who must decide ultimately whether obstetric management must be continued or altered.

The accuracy and completeness of the nurse's observations invariably will strengthen the physician's judgment. Grave responsibility is carried by the nurse who may be the only professionally trained person with the obstetric patient, and on whose decisions the life or health of the fetus may depend.

Fetal distress requires special vigilance, particularly in high-risk cases. Moreover, one cannot anticipate crises like cord compression or predict accidents such as concealed partial separation of the placenta. The nurse who is knowledgeable, attentive, and concerned may in fact be a lifesaver.

Prompt detection and reporting of abnormal fetal heart signs often mark the initial steps in fetal rescue. This is especially important because about 50% of perinatal deaths are preventable. Fenton and Steer have stated, "Fetal survival is directly correlated with the time interval between the discovery of the signs of fetal distress and delivery. Thirty minutes is the critical time."

Matousek has suggested the following excellent routine for fetal nursing:

1. Complete observation
   a. Note any unusual fetal activity. Record findings.
   b. Identify and record the presence of meconium when the membranes rupture. Repeat each time the patient is examined.
   c. Auscultate and record the fetal heart rate every 10 to 15 minutes in the pregnancy at risk, more often in the second stage of labor, and immediately after rupture of the membranes.
   d. Note particularly the duration of any tachycardia or bradycardia continuing after a contraction.
2. Prompt reporting
   Promptly describe unusual signs (hyperactivity, bradycardia, passage of meconium, etc.) to the physician.
3. Complete reporting
   Relate the current fetal signs, as well as the former pattern, to the following conditions of the fetal environment:
   a. Maternal vital signs
   b. Medications administered: amount and time given
   c. Frequency, type, and duration of uterine contractions
   d. Intactness of the membranes and the presence or absence of meconium
   e. Bleeding: amount, if any

f. Other significant changes in the mother's condition that occur at or near the time of altered fetal signs

SELECTED REFERENCES

Althabe, O., Jr., Schwarcz, R. L., Pose, S. V., Escarcena, L., and Caldeyro-Barcia, R.: Effects on fetal heart rate and fetal pO_2 of oxygen administration to the mother, Am. J. Obstet. Gynecol. **98**:858, 1967.

Beard, R. W., Filshie, G. M., Knight, C. A., and Roberts, G. M.: The significance of the changes in the continuous fetal heart rate in the first stage of labour, J. Obstet. Gynaecol. Br. Commonw. **78**:865, 1971.

Fenton, A. N., and Steer, C. M.: Fetal distress, Am. J. Obstet. Gynecol. **83**:354, 1962.

Figueroa-Longo, J. G., Poseiro, J. J., Alvarez, L. O., and Caldeyro-Barcia, R.: Fetal electrocardiogram at term labor obtained with subcutaneous fetal electrodes, Am. J. Obstet. Gynecol. **96**:556, 1966.

Hon, E. H.: An atlas of fetal heart rate patterns, New Haven, 1968, Harty Press.

Hon, E. H.: Direct monitoring of the fetal heart, Hosp. Pract. **5**:91, Sept., 1970.

Huntingford, P. J., Hüter, K. A., and Saling, E., editors: Perinatal medicine, First European Congress, Berlin, Stuttgart, 1969, Georg Thieme Verlag.

Matousek, I.: Fetal nursing during labor, Nurs. Clin. North Am. **3**:307, 1968.

Mendez-Bauer, C., Arnt, I. C., Gulin, L., Escarcena, L., and Caldeyro-Barcia, R.: Relationship between pH and heart rate in the human fetus during labor, Am. J. Obstet. Gynecol. **97**:530, 1967.

Perinatal factors affecting human development, Washington, D. C., 1969, Scientific Pub. No. 185, Pan American Health Organization, Pan American Sanitary Bureau, Regional Office of the World Health Organization.

Saling, E.: Foetal and neonatal hypoxia in relation to clinical obstetric practice, Baltimore, 1968, The Williams & Wilkins Co.

Shnider, S. M.: Obstetric anesthesia, Baltimore, 1970, The Williams & Wilkins Co.

Whitfield, C. R.: Clinical significance of electronic methods for monitoring the fetal heart. In Huntingford, P. J., Hüter, K. G., and Saling, E., editors: Perinatal medicine, Stuttgart, 1969, Georg Thieme Verlag.

5

Delivery of the high-risk fetus

SPECIAL CONSIDERATIONS IN HIGH-RISK DELIVERY

Birth may be an individual's most traumatic experience. Certainly this is true for the undersized fetus. Immature and defenseless, the offspring is impelled by waves of stormy uterine contractions, buffeted against bony promontories, and squeezed through pelvic straits. Rescue is often more trying than Fate—the offspring may be literally dragged from the watery depths, scarcely gasping, more dead than alive.

Assistance by the well-intentioned but unskilled may be worse than no help at all. Errors of omission as well as mistakes of commission may compound misadventures in premature parturition.

Spontaneous premature rupture of the membranes occurs approximately four times as often in premature labor as in the control group. Spontaneous labor generally is shorter, but abnormal presentations are much more frequent. Placenta previa, accidental hemorrhage, and prolapse of the cord are encountered more often in premature labor. In most cases premature birth is probably not preventable once labor has become established. The best hope for salvage of the premature fetus is choosing the obstetric technique that allows delivery of the offspring in the best possible condition.

Operative measures, chiefly relating to breech extraction, internal podalic version, and manual removal of the placenta, are considerably increased in premature delivery. Serious complications occur in more than 12% of premature deliveries, as compared with 3% of deliveries at term. Maternal fever is present at least twice as often, with about one fifth of the total number of patients having fever on admission; two thirds of these are likely to have a later septic complication. Vaginal and perineal lacerations occur with unexpected frequency (more than 10%), but when a local anesthetic is used, tears are less common.

INDUCTION OF LABOR

Induction of labor is the initiation of effectual uterine contractions by medical or surgical means. In contrast with the need for extension of pregnancy in conditions where intervention would lead to premature delivery, there are other disorders that may seriously affect the fetus and lead to death in utero. For example, the obstetrician must not stand idly by while the undersized fetus is being starved or jeopardized by a disease process. The physician must be prepared to rescue the fetus to protect it. Thus, despite what has been said about preventing early birth (Chapter 16), purposeful premature delivery may be required to save the life of an offspring when an incubator would seem to offer a better environment than the uterus does. Answers to the questions of *when?* and

61

how? often require considerable knowledge, skill, and experience, however.

The conditions that hazard the fetus, and in which early delivery may provide an increase in the perinatal survival include diabetes mellitus, eclamptogenic toxemia, erythroblastosis, and partial premature separation of the placenta. Naturally, decisions as to the optimum times for induction of labor and delivery must be individualized. Maternal or fetal jeopardy requires the conclusion of pregnancy in between 5% and 10% of patients. Many of the offspring are premature. Termination of gestation may also be elective (more than 20% of deliveries in some hospitals in the United States) for social, economic, or other nonmedical reasons. Supposedly, the neonates in this category are at term, but all too often they are avoidably preterm.

The success of induction is not a linear function of fetal age but relates to the maturity of the labor mechanism. Moreover, the "end point" of pregnancy is difficult to predict, even with reasonably good "dates" and careful fetal observations. Scheduling delivery by the calendar is a questionable, risky practice. The incidence of prematurity after induced labor and delivery is at least 5%. Moreover, many of these babies develop respiratory disorders or may show signs of central nervous system abnormality postnatally—an appreciably higher frequency than after an uncomplicated vaginal delivery at term.

Induced labor may be shorter than natural labor but is often the result of stimulation pushed to dangerous levels. Elective induction often adds an element of risk, however, particularly for the premature infant. Whenever labor is induced, especially when oxytocin is employed, the fetus should be electronically monitored and observed for evidence of fetal distress so that cesarean section can be substituted, if necessary.

1. Indications
   a. Fetus
      1. Severe degrees of isoimmunization
      2. Fetal death
      3. Anencephaly or other critical anomaly
      4. Prolonged gestation
   b. Mother
      1. Complications of pregnancy unresponsive to accepted medical therapy
         a. Pyelonephritis
         b. Diverticulitis
         c. Diabetes mellitus
      2. Obstetric problems unresolved by the usual measures
         a. Progressive preeclampsia, partial placental separation, or minor degrees of placenta previa
         b. Premature prolonged rupture of the membranes
         c. Previous precipitate delivery for a gravida far from a hospital
2. Prerequisites
   a. A mature fetus
   b. Legitimate indication (preferably vertex presentations)
   c. Cervix "ripe" (soft, anteriors more than 35% effaced, more than 2 cm dilated)
   d. Absence of disproportion (successful depression of the presenting part to or below the level of the ischial spines)
   e. Gravida willing and able to withstand procedure
3. Contraindications (by any method)
   Because a value judgment is required, deterrents must also be considered. These include
   a. Fetopelvic disproportion
   b. A firm, closed, uneffaced posterior cervix (Do a vaginal examination before induction of labor to determine the "ripeness" of the cervix.)
   c. An unfavorable presentation (for example, transverse lie)
   d. Previous cesarean section or extensive myomectomy (Uterine rupture may occur.)

e. Grand multiparity
f. Placenta previa
g. Serious maternal illness (for example, cardiac functional class 3 or 4 condition; acute manic-depressive state or schizophrenia)
h. Hypertonic or dystonic early labor pattern in which constriction ring or rupture of the uterus may ensue
i. Poor facilities for stimulation or inadequate supervision of induction, as with home delivery and delivery without a physician in attendance, sometimes permitting a fetomaternal complication

4. Dangers
   a. Fetus
      1. Hypoxia, acidosis, and fetal distress
      2. Premature birth when estimated date of confinement has been grossly miscalculated
      3. Prolapse of the cord or cord compression
      4. Infection, for example, fetal pneumonia, septicemia, or omphalitis after amnionitis
   b. Mother
      1. Violent labor—premature separation of the placenta, uterine rupture, cervical laceration, tetanic contraction
      2. Uterine inertia, prolonged labor
      3. Intrapartum infection
      4. Postpartum hemorrhage
      5. Hypofibrinogenemia
      6. Amniotic fluid embolization
      7. Emotional crisis—fear or anxiety

5. Methods
   a. Medical induction
      1. Intravenous drip of oxytocin, 5 units/1,000 ml in 5% dextrose in water, with initial flow set at 10 drops/30 min until the patient is in labor or the rate of flow is 60 drops/min.
      2. Check and record the fetal heart rate frequently, preferably by continuous electronic monitoring.

If fetal distress develops, oxytocin must be discontinued *immediately.*
      3. Constant observation of maternal patient is essential.
      4. Intramuscular oxytocin is more dangerous and is no longer recommended because
         a. Some patients show an unexpected, marked cumulative response even to small doses of the drug.
         b. Once a concentrated intramuscular dose is given, it cannot be withdrawn or stopped.
      5. Nasal and buccal forms of oxytocin are less predictable and controllable than is intravenous or intramuscular oxytocin.
         a. There is a longer lag period.
         b. They are more difficult to titer to the patient's needs.
         c. They may cause sudden, unexpected uterine tetany.
      6. Sparteine sulfate, a capricious, potentially dangerous oxytocic, should never be used.
   b. Surgical induction
      1. Amniotomy
         a. Check the fetal heart tone to be certain of normal rate and rhythm.
         b. Apply gentle pressure to the fundus to encourage engagement of the presenting part.
         c. Introduce the forefinger through the cervix to guide a hook or other sharp instrument to the membranes. Rupture the membranes. Put the patient in a low Fowler's position. Allow the fluid to drain without displacing the presenting part, or the cord may prolapse. Stripping of the membranes is of doubtful value and may be traumatic.
      2. Amniocentesis and injection of prostaglandins or hypertonic saline solution is appropriate only after fetal death.

c. Combined induction
Medical induction followed by amniotomy may indicate sensitivity of the uterus to stimulation and initiate contractions and a reduction in uterine volume that may speed labor.

6. Prognosis
   a. If the cervix is "ripe," labor begins within 48 hours in the great majority of patients. If repeated, intensive efforts toward induction are unsuccessful, especially after rupture of the membranes, consider a cesarean section.
   b. Amniotomy is the most effective single means of induction of labor, but the chance of infection is increased. Medical induction, combined with amniotomy, is even more likely to terminate pregnancy. (Amniotomy may not be necessary and should often be avoided if the patient goes into labor promptly with oxytocic stimulation.)
   c. Induction of labor, including elective induction, carries definitely increased risks for both the mother (principally rupture of the uterus, hemorrhage, infection) and the fetus (prematurity, infection, hypoxia, precipitous labor and delivery, injury of the central nervous system, trauma). *The physician must decide whether the hazards of allowing pregnancy to continue will exceed those of induction while considering the possible advantage of cesarean section.*

ANALGESIA AND ANESTHESIA

The use of analgesia and anesthesia for the high-risk patient, especially in premature labor, poses very special problems. Medication poorly chosen or too liberally administered will be seriously depressing, particularly for the fetus that is not mature or is otherwise jeopardized. All the procedures and agents used to relieve the discomforts of labor and delivery have some advantage or desirable characteristic, but none is perfect. Almost universally, the safety factor is deficient, particularly for the premature infant.

Methods preferred for the fetus at risk in premature labor

1. Prepared childbirth or psychoanalgesia
   a. Familiarize the patient before labor (if possible) with relaxing techniques (Lamaze or Read) and the use of her delivery powers to reduce tension and pain (psychoprophylaxis).
   b. Establish rapport and provide emotional support.
   c. Employ reassurance and kindly direction.
   d. Use suggestion and reinforcement when possible.
2. Regional anesthesia
   Conduction analgesia and anesthesia usually are more desirable than inhalation or parenteral anesthesia. The safest, simplest, and most satisfactory anesthesia is paracervical combined with pudendal block anesthesia.

   All regional blocking agents are rapidly absorbed. These anesthetics may intoxicate the fetus when overdosage occurs, with resultant apnea and vascular collapse from medullary depression, bradycardia because of the quinidine-like effect on the myocardium, and convulsions because of cortical excitation. Those with the amide molecular linkage (lidocaine, mepivacaine, and prilocaine) have a stability that resists enzymatic splitting and rapidly cross the placental barrier intact. In contrast, local anesthetics with an ester bond (procaine, 2-chloroprocaine, and tetracaine) are metabolized in the plasma and placenta with only minor transfer to the fetus, if the total dose of procaine is less than 8 mg/kg. With larger doses, procaine is found in the fetal circulation in concentrations 40% to 60% lower than in the maternal circulation. Hence it is a safer obstetric agent despite a shorter duration of action.

3. Paracervical anesthesia
   a. Rapid dilatation follows when the cervix is dilated more than 4 or 5 cm. Earlier labor is slowed–other injections may be necessary.
   b. Almost immediate, complete relief of pain is achieved until the presenting part distends the lower birth canal,

when a pudendal block or other procedure is indicated.

1. Prepare the mucosal site 2 cm lateral to the cervix, in the vaginal fornix, with antiseptic solution.
2. Insert a 6-inch 20-gauge needle 0.3 to 0.5 cm into the lateral fornix, using an "Iowa trumpet" (Fig. 5-1). Slowly inject 5 ml of

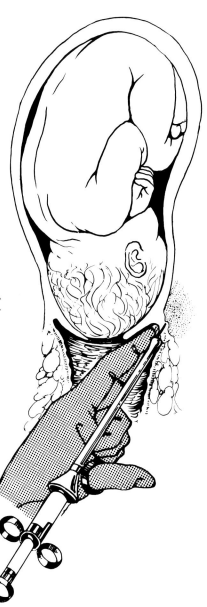

Fig. 5-1. Paracervical block. (From Benson, R. C.: Handbook of obstetrics and gynecology, ed. 4, Los Altos, Calif., 1971, Lange Medical Publications.)

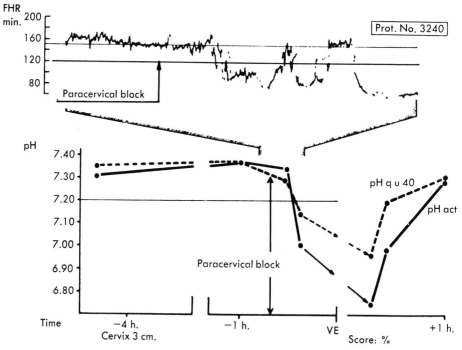

Fig. 5-2. Acute acidosis after paracervical block. (Modified from Käser, O.: Fetal blood sampling. In Huntingford, P. J., Hüter, K. A., and Saling, E., editors: Perinatal medicine, Stuttgart, 1969, Georg Thieme Verlag.)

1% procaine *just beneath the mucosa.* Observe the fetal heart rate for bradycardia, or wait for several uterine contractions to avoid an anesthetic reaction; then inject the other side.

3. When the presenting part is deeply engaged and the fornices are blocked, inject the drug high in the lateral vaginal walls and again just beneath the mucosa (to retard absorption).

c. Ideally, the anesthetic lasts about 60 minutes, and only a minority of patients will require subsequent paracervical blocks. "Cervical dystocia" is often overcome, but a temporary reduction in the intensity and duration of contractions may occur.

d. Avoid paracervical block when
   1. Excessive uterine bleeding occurs

2. Vaginal or cervical sepsis is present

e. Complications (exceptions)
   1. Hematoma formation
   2. Infection
   3. Faintness, syncope, or vascular collapse from inadvertent intravenous administration, too rapid absorption, or sensitivity to the anesthetic agent
   4. Chemical lumbosacral neuritis
   5. Fetal bradycardia, acidosis (Fig. 5-2), and rarely cardiac arrest because of rapid absorption of the drug, toxic effect
   Paracervical block probably is associated witn more rapid drug absorption than most other blocks because of marked cervicouterine vascularity. Therefore precautions must be taken with its use:

a. Avoid injection of an anesthetic drug directly into the maternal circulation or into fetal tissues by limiting the volume of the anesthetic agent to 5 ml to each side of the cervix and placing the drug just beneath the mucosa as a "blister."

b. Avoid paracervical block when the fetus may already be hypoxic and acidotic, as in maternal toxemia, diabetes, and possibly postmaturity.

c. Deny paracervical anesthesia in cases of fetal heart irregularity or after meconium passage in vertex presentations.

d. Employ constant fetal heart rate monitoring in all complicated cases, especially when bradycardia occurs.

4. Pudendal nerve block

a. The nerves supplying the lower birth canal are anesthetized by blocking the pudendal nerve at the ischial spines.

b. A transvaginal injection is preferred. Only a spinal type of needle is required, and the procedure can be carried out without assistance.

1. Identify the ischial spines on each side by digital examination through the elastic vagina. Then note the sacrospinous ligament across the sacrospinous notch above and posterior to the spines. The pudendal nerve lies just below the ligament, approximately 1.5 cm medial to the spine.

2. Apply an antiseptic solution to the mucosa of the lateral vaginal wall for about 2 cm inside the introitus. Inject a small amount of 1% procaine or its equivalent at the site of penetration. Advance the needle until the sacrospinous ligament is pierced slightly medial to the ischial spines.

3. Aspirate. If no blood returns, slowly inject 10 ml of anesthetic solution in the vicinity of each pudendal nerve.

c. A satisfactory block will usually anesthetize the entire vaginal canal, relax the musculature of the introitus, and persist for about 45 minutes. After a 5-minute "take," the introitus should gape, and the anus cannot be contracted.

d. *Note:* The inferior pudendal nerve may have an independent origin from the sacral plexus, or it may take off unusually high from the pudendal nerve. Also, the dorsal clitoral nerve may have an anomalous origin. Under these circumstances, additional infiltration of the perirectal and anterior labial regions may be necessary to supplement the pudendal block for satisfactory control of pain at delivery.

5. Lumbar epidural block
Continuous lumbar epidural block, properly carried out in centers with well-trained personnel, is a very safe method of anesthesia in the delivery of a jeopardized fetus. It may be selected in certain maternal complications such as congenital or acquired heart disease, pulmonary disorders, some endocrine dysfunctions (diabetes, toxemia, hypertension), and renal or hepatic disease. It may be the best technique for preterm or postterm labor, prolonged labor, or cervical dystocia. The low dosage technique can be augmented to produce anesthesia for cesarean section, if it becomes necessary.

6. Caudal block
Epidural placement of an anethetic solution in the caudal canal (caudal block), although it has less risk of dural puncture, requires more medication (with attendant fetal risks), and the procedure blocks a larger nerve distribution with the hazard of hypotension. The anes-

thetic also may lead to a failure of spontaneous internal rotation. Nevertheless, in experienced hands it is a useful technique.

7. Spinal block

Maternal hypotension with decreased uterine blood flow is the greatest risk to the fetus when subarachnoid (spinal) block is employed. It is useful for the alleviation of maternal discomfort only during delivery because it often arrests labor.

8. General anesthetics

General anesthetics may be useful adjuncts in certain high-risk cases. It should be recalled, however, that all the agents are transferred across the placenta and can depress the fetus. General anesthetics may be selected if regional anesthetics are contraindicated, if deep utrine relaxation is necessary, for alleviation of constriction rings, for relief of tetanic uterine contractions, or when prompt deep anesthesia is necessary.

Medications to be used with caution in high-risk pregnancy

1. Analgesics
   a. The commonly employed analgesics are either narcotic drugs (opiates or synthetic opiates) or inhalants.
   b. Injectable narcotics relieve pain by
      1. Elevation of the pain threshold by more than 50% with usual doses
      2. Creation of a relaxed, indifferent, or euphoric state
      3. Induction of lethargy or somnolence
   c. The fetus is adversely affected by analgesics because of central nervous system depression, particularly of the respiratory center. A lack of fetal maturity and any maternal medical complications, as well as difficulty during labor and delivery, increase the undesirable side effects for the offspring.
   d. A shorter-acting agent such as alpha-

prodine (Nisentil), 30 mg administered intravenously, or 60 mg subcutaneously, that is readily reversible by narcotic antagonists is the best narcotic choice in high-risk pregnancy for analgesia. (Do not exceed 240 mg/24 hr; usual dosage is 0.4 to 0.6 mg/kg administered intravenously, or 0.4 to 1.2 mg/kg subcutaneously.)
   e. *Caution:* Should the delivery occur during the maximal effect of the narcotic, respiratory depression may be present. This condition should be reversed by levallorphan (Lorfan) or nalorphine (Nalline).

2. Sedatives (hypnotics)
   a. These drugs are poor analgesics because they
      1. Reduce reception to suggestion in small, moderate doses
      2. Slow mentation and reduce discrimination in large doses
      3. Fail to raise pain threshold
      4. Do not produce amnesia
      5. May slow labor, particularly in large doses, if given too early
   b. The likelihood of critical central nervous system depression in the preterm fetus contraindicates all sedatives in early termination of labor. These drugs cause periodic apnea or even abolition of all movement in the offspring and do not respond to antagonists.

3. Amnesics (scopolamine and paraldehyde)
   a. Eliminate recent memory
   b. Produce little analgesic effect
   c. Subdue fetal central nervous system (paraldehyde only)
   d. Often cause delusions or hallucinations (patients must be restrained, and operative delivery is usually necessary)
   e. Should be used rarely, if at all, in premature labor

4. Ataractics
   a. Promazine (Sparine), propiomazine

maleate (Largon), or hydroxyzine pamoate (Vistaril) may be administered in the usual dosage to patients in premature labor.

  b. They have the following effects:
1. Reduce maternal anxiety
2. Suppress nausea and vomiting
3. Potentiate analgesics

5. Inhalation anesthetics
  a. Ethyl ether causes deep, prolonged narcosis of the neonate—contraindicated for delivery of the premature or immature fetus.
  b. Cyclopropane, halothane, ethylene—acceptable in premature labor, when given by skilled anesthetist for short period of time.
  c. Nitrous oxide or trichloroethylene may be self-administered as an analgesic, *not* as a surgical anesthetic.

6. Parenteral anesthetics, thiopental sodium (Pentothal sodium) and thiamylal sodium (Surital), cross the placenta quickly in anesthetic doses. Even 3 to 4 minutes after the start of administration, a premature fetus may have already received so much of the drug that resuscitation may be difficult.

Anesthesia for cesarean section

A light general anesthetic usually has minimal effect on the baby and at the same time is likely to be safe and comfortable for the mother. A combination of nitrous oxide and a muscle relaxant is an excellent choice for a rapid cesarean section, provided an individual experienced in anesthesiology is available. Following is a successful, light general anesthetic combination:

1. Give up to 300 mg of thiopental for induction of anesthetic but less than 4 mg/kg of body weight shortly before the skin incision.
2. Start nitrous oxide–oxygen (75%:25%), with reduction in the concentration after about 3 to 4 minutes to a 50%:50% mixture.
3. Administer succinylcholine, 2.5 mg/

min in 2 mg/ml dextrose solution (10%), up to 100 mg total.

If delay is hazardous or the fetus' or mother's condition is critical and no anesthesiologist is available, local anesthesia by direct infiltration of 0.5% or 1% procaine, or its equivalent, is a safe and effective approach to cesarean section. Procedures that will reduce the fetal hazard are as follows:

1. Leave patients in lateral position until skin preparation.
2. Elevate left hip slightly throughout procedure to lessen possibility of vena-caval syndrome.
3. Give 100% oxygen to the mother by mask when fetal heart tones are decreased or irregular and for 5 minutes before delivery.
4. Make an ample uterine incision.
5. Lift the fetus out through the incision promptly, avoiding aspiration of bloody fluid, and clamp the cord.
6. Transfer the neonate to a waiting physician or a nurse experienced in resuscitation and supportive therapy.

Anesthesia for the patient in shock

An obstetric patient in shock or threatened with collapse requires a special choice of anesthesia. The physiology involved in hypovolemic shock (hemorrhage), for example, and supportive measures and drugs required in therapy are important to the success of delivery. The patient should be responsive to antishock therapy prior to surgery, but in critical cases a calculated risk must be accepted.

As preoperative medication, atropine sulfate, 0.4 mg, well diluted in normal saline solution, should be given slowly intravenously. Regardless of the anesthetic used, the supine gravida should have the right hip slightly elevated to avoid vascular (caval) obstruction by the pregnant uterus.

Although the choice of anesthetic method may depend on the skill and experience of the anesthesiologist, as well as availability of drugs and equipment, the following have considerable advantages:

1. *Hypovolemic shock.* Inhalation anesthesia with maximum oxygen concentration, when nitrous oxide or ethylene is used, causes no serious electrolyte or metabolic alterations. Certain anesthetics carry serious disadvantages in hypovolemic shock. Hypercarbia (retention of CO_2) is likely when there is inadequate pulmonary ventilation during the use of halothane, cyclopropane, or fluroxene. Moreover, halothane, which causes uterine relaxation, may increase hemorrhage. Spinal or epidural anesthesia often is followed by serious irreversible hypotension.

2. *Septic shock.* Cyclopropane or thiopental (Pentothal), nitrous oxide, oxygen, and succinylcholine are good choices because fever, vascular collapse, and renal failure complicate the problem. Although succinylcholine is well hydrolized, it does intensify oliguria, which may prolong the metabolism of the drug.

3. *Neurogenic shock.* Shock that follows acute uterine inversion requires an anesthetic such as halothane or cyclopropane, which has very rapid induction time.

4. *Anaphylactic shock.* Oxygen, vasopressor drugs, and corticosteroids are of value preoperatively. Epinephrine by injection or inhalation (spray) is beneficial for the relief of bronchospasm. Infiltration anesthesia should be used, assuming no sensitivity to local anesthetics.

5. *Cardiogenic shock.* Place the patient in Fowler's position with slight elevation of the left hip and use local infiltration for delivery.

MANAGEMENT OF DELIVERY OF THE HIGH-RISK FETUS
General considerations

1. Monitor fetal heart rate constantly, observing for fetal distress.
2. Obtain frequent maternal pulse and blood pressure.
3. Avoid maternal hypotension.

    a. Increase intravenous fluids (administer blood if indicated).
    b. Try positional changes to remove the uterus from the inferior vena cava. Maintain the lateral recruitment positions until delivery.
    c. Push the uterus off the inferior vena cava.
    d. Elevate (Trendelenburg) or wrap the legs with elastic supports.
    e. Consider alternative positions for delivery if the supine hypotensive syndrome is severe (e.g., Sims).
4. Administer maternal oxygen if there is any evidence of fetal distress.
5. Have an intravenous catheter (18 gauge or larger) in place and working. Consider central nervous system pressure monitor if there is any possibility of hemorrhage.
6. Have type-specific blood and fibrinogen available for the mother.
7. Have a perinatal team ready to assist in the delivery
    a. Obstetrician
    b. Obstetric assistant
    c. Scrub nurse
    d. Circulating nurse
    e. Anesthesiologist and/or anesthetist
    f. Neonatologist or neonatally trained pediatrician
    g. Neonatal assistant
8. In addition, the following should have been accomplished while the patient was in labor:
    a. Abdomen shaved and scrubbed with povidone-iodine (Betadine) (in preparation for possible cesarean)
    b. Elastic (antiembolic) support hose
9. A retention catheter and prep set should be open and ready for immediate insertion should cesarean section become necessary.
10. Plan for the most atraumatic delivery possible.

Cesarean section delivery

A cesarean section is often done on an urgent indication when the offspring is not mature or is severely stressed. Regional anesthesia is one of the few methods that will not contribute to the depression of the neonate—provided the maternal blood pressure is kept stable, reasonable amounts are used, and toxic reactions (i.e., convulsions) are avoided. Regional anesthesia will minimize the possibility of maternal aspiration. Unfortunately, maternal complications such as extreme hypertension or hypotension and the time required for "fixation" of the anesthetic agent may mitigate against spinal or epidural anesthesia.

The indications for cesarean section are classified as fetal or maternal.

1. Fetal indications

The fetal indications for cesarean section occasionally are urgent.

a. Fetal distress often is recorded. The problem may be one of hypoxia because of cord compression, premature separation of the placenta, placental insufficiency, etc.

b. Diabetes mellitus—early cesarean section has reduced the high incidence of intrapartal and postnatal death in diabetes. However, it may be unnecessary in many cases if labor is properly monitored.

c. Isoimmunization—cesarean section may avoid irreparable damage to the infant or fetal exodus from icterus gravis or hydrops fetalis in Rh sensitization of the mother when induction is unsuccessful.

d. Prolapse of the cord in early labor.

e. Herpes labialis or vaginalis complicating labor.

2. Maternal indications

a. Fetopelvic disproportion, the most common indication for cesarean section

b. Weakness of the uterine scar after a myomectomy, unification operation, or previous cesarean section; the occurrence of dehiscence of a prior uterine incision site (partial or complete)

c. Placenta previa that covers more than 30% of the internal cervical os

d. Abruptio placentae with serious hemorrhage

e. Ruptured uterus—an abdominal emergency

f. Obstructive pelvic tumors

g. Abnormal presentation, that is, transverse, shoulder, posterior face, and many breeches°

h. Fulminating eclamptogenic toxemia

i. Maternal complications such as previous vesicovaginal fistula or invasive cervical carcinoma

An emergency cesarean section obviously is a lifesaving measure for mother and/or fetus. Technically, operative delivery of the offspring is most desirable within a 5- to 10-minute period. This may not be possible, but expedition is vital. In any event, the surgery must be a successful blend of haste and safety.

3. General considerations

a. Complications of pregnancy requiring abdominal removal of a known premature infant occur in 1% to 2% of gravidas.

b. About 15% of premature infants are subjected to the hazard of cesarean section to avoid the greater risk of remaining in utero until the time of natural delivery.

c. Between 5% and 10% of elective, repeat cesarean sections are timed inappropriately, and the neonates actually are preterm.

4. Analgesia, anesthesia (p. 69)

5. Precautions

a. Inaccuracy in the estimation of fetal size or gestational age is the most important single factor in neonatal wastage after elective cesarean section because maturity largely deter-

°Many centers, including our own, are tending toward the delivery of all "breeches" by cesarean section, regardless of gestation or gravidity. Certainty of maturity (other than those in labor) and an expert team in attendance are prerequisites.

mines survival and normality. More than ten times as many of these newborn infants in the low birth weight category are lost, as compared with term neonates. Morbidity also is much higher in the former group. When in doubt regarding the expected date of confinement, repeat cesarean section had best be done at the onset of labor.

  b. Even for "normal," apparently healthy women, elective cesarean section carries a slight but definite fetal hazard, as contrasted with vaginal birth. We suspect that some of the problems relate to analgesia-anesthesia, but trauma, atelectasis, and respiratory distress syndrome are also serious complications.

Forceps delivery

In the delivery of a premature baby, instrumentation generally should be avoided. Nevertheless, a skilled physician can assist the delivery of a vertex or aftercoming head with proper forceps, achieving an appreciable reduction in perinatal (and maternal) morbidity and neonatal mortality.

1. Obstetric forceps, in the hands of a physician experienced in their use, are effective for
   a. Guidance of the fetus and protection of the offspring and mother
   b. Rotation—usually occiput transverse to occiput anterior
   c. Traction in the pelvic curve
2. The concept of prophylactic (low) forceps delivery embodies prevention of damage to
   a. The fetal central nervous system (from marked or extended compression)
   b. The maternal pelvic floor structure (laceration and overstretching during the second stage of delivery procedure)
3. The fetus is eased out (a shoehorn, in

comparison, is used to direct the foot into a shoe, not to force the heel in).
4. Prophylactic (low) forceps delivery of a premature infant requires
   a. The complete dilatation of the cervix with vertex on the perineum dilating the introitus
   b. A generous episiotomy
   c. The application of small or light forceps (deep cephalic curve, narrow-shank instruments preferred—Elliott or Tucker-McLean forceps) and slow delivery with minimal traction
5. Delivery of the aftercoming head can be accomplished with Piper or similar forceps while an assistant supports the baby.

Internal podalic version and extraction

Internal podalic version and extraction is the most dangerous obstetric operation for the undersized (and even mature) infant. This procedure should be abandoned.

Emergency delivery in the home

Home delivery, never recommended for premature birth or high-risk pregnancy, may be unavoidable; disaster or hostilities may prevent hospitalization. Premature delivery in the home, then, is generally an emergency. The gravida not infrequently goes into labor much before her expected date of confinement, without warning, and she may deliver abruptly. The woman usually gives birth unattended by professional personnel, and the infant is thoroughly contaminated. Hence definitive care of both the mother and neonate is delayed. If medical personnel can be present at the delivery, the usual precautions in the management of premature labor are observed, even though improvisation is invariably required.

Medical attendants may have equipment and supplies for home delivery with them. In most instances one must use mainly what is at hand: soap and water, a few towels, sheets, kitchen stove heat, kitchen table, and some form of light.

1. Attention to the neonate (Chapter 6)
   a. Ensure an airway with postural drainage; gently wipe away any pharyngeal materials if suction is not handy.
   b. Use mouth-to-mouth resuscitation if the infant continues to be apneic and has not responded to gentle skin stimulation.
   c. Tie the cord with available twine or string and cut it with any cutting edge previously wiped with an antiseptic.
   d. Wrap the infant in a clean towel or blanket and place him in a convenient container, with his mouth to the side.
   e. Place covered hot-water bottles near the infant but not against him.
2. Attention to the mother
   a. Examine the mother for complications such as abnormal bleeding or lacerations.
   b. Transfer the mother to a hospital if any serious medical problems exist.
   c. Determine whether the placenta is intact or abnormal.
   d. Send an unusual placenta to the hospital for study.

SELECTED REFERENCES

Benson, R. C., Shubeck, F., Clark, W. M., Weiss, W., and Deutschberger, J.: Fetal compromise during elective cesarean section, Am. J. Obstet. Gynecol. 91:645, 1965.

Bradford, W. P., and Gordon, G.: Induction of labor by amniotomy and simultaneous Syntocinon infusion, J. Obstet. Gynaecol. Br. Commonw. 75:698, 1968.

Brown, A. A., Hamlett, J. D., Hibbard, B. M., and Howe, P. D.: Induction of labor by amniotomy and intravenous infusions of oxytocic drugs: comparison between prostaglandins and oxytocin, J. Obstet. Gynaecol. Br. Commonw. 80:111, 1973.

Busby, T.: Local anesthesia for cesarean section, Am. J. Obstet. Gynecol. 87:399, 1963.

Case, B. D., Corcoran, R., Jeffcoate, N., and Randee, G. H.: Cesarean section and its place in modern obstetric practice, J. Obstet. Gynaecol. Br. Commonw. 78:203, 1971.

Craig, C. J. T.: Eclampsia and the anesthetist, S. Afr. Med. J. 46:248, 1972.

Crawford, S.: Maternal mortality associated with anesthesia, Lancet 2:918, 1972.

Johnson, W. L., Winter, W. W., Eng, M., Bonica, J. J., and Hunter, C. A.: Effect of pudendal, spinal and peridural block anesthesia on the second stage of labor, Am. J. Obstet. Gynecol. 113:166, 1972.

Lamaze, F., and Vellay, P.: Psychologic analgesia in obstetrics, New York, 1957, Pergamon Press, Inc.

Laros, R. K., Jr., Work, B. A., Jr., and Whitting, W. C.: Amniotomy during the active phase of labor, Obstet. Gynecol. 39:702, 1972.

Lee, B. O., Major, F. J., and Weingold, A. B.: Ultrasonic determination of fetal maturity at repeat cesarean section, Obstet. Gynecol. 38:294, 1971.

Lettew, W. L.: Paracervical block in obstetrics, Am. J. Obstet. Gynecol. 113:1079, 1972.

Lilienthal, C. M., and Ward, J. P.: Medical induction of labor, J. Obstet. Gynaecol. Br. Commonw. 78:317, 1971.

Normington, E. A. M.: A simplified method of Syntocinon infusion following amniotomy, J. Obstet. Gynaecol. Br. Commonw. 79:1108, 1972.

Read, G. D.: Childbirth without fear, New York, 1944, Harper & Row, Publishers.

Rosofsky, J. B., and Petersicl, M. E.: Prenatal deaths associated with mepivacaine paracervical block anesthesia in labor, N. Engl. J. Med. 278:530, 1968.

Rutter, P.: Domiciliary midwifery: is it justifiable? A review of over 1,000 cases in general practice, Lancet 2:7371, 1964.

Schifria, B. S.: Fetal heart rate patterns following epidural anesthesia and oxytocin infusion during labor, J. Obstet. Gynaecol. Br. Commonw. 79:332, 1972.

Schokman, F. C. M., and Correy, J. F.: Pudendal block: assessment of efficacy and area of analgesia, Aust. N.Z. J. Obstet. Gynaecol. 11:91, 1971.

Shnider, S. M., deLorimier, A. A., Holl, J. W., Chapler, F. K., and Moreshima, H. O.: Vasopressors in obstetrics. I. Correction of fetal acidosis with ephedrine during spinal hypotension, Am. J. Obstet. Gynecol. 102:911, 1968.

Turnbull, A. C., and Anderson, A. B. M.: Induction of labor, J. Obstet. Gynaecol. Br. Commonw. 74:849, 1967.

Usubiaga, J. E., La Iuppa, M., Moya, F., Wikinski, J. A., and Velazco, R.: Passage of procaine hydrochloride and para-aminobenzoic acid across the human placenta, Am. J. Obstet. Gynecol. **100**:918, 1968.

Utting, J. E., and Gray, T. C.: Obstetric anesthesia and analgesia, Br. Med. Bull. **24**:80, 1968.

Vasicka, A., Robertazzi, R., Raji, M., Scheffs, J., and Kasmowski, J.: Fetal bradycardia after paracervical block, Obstet. Gynecol. **38**:500, 1971.

Webb, M. J., and Fogarty, A. J.: The timing and dosage of oxytocin in the induction of labor, Aust. N.Z. J. Obstet. Gynaecol. **12**:43, 1972.

Wiese, J.: Induction of labor using small transbuccal doses of Syntocinon, Acta Obstet. Gynecol. Scand. **47**:333, 1968.

Witting, W. C.: A graphic record for monitoring labor induction or stimulation, Obstet. Gynecol. **39**:948, 1972.

Wollman, S. B., and Marx, G. F.: Acute hydration for prevention of hypotension of spinal anesthesia in parturients, Anesthesiology **29**:374, 1968.

6

Care of the high-risk infant at birth

Since up to 40% of potential neonatal problems are still unidentified before birth, all hospitals in which infants are delivered must have sufficient facilities and personnel available for care of any distressed infant until the infant is stabilized or placed in the hands of an experienced transport team. These requirements are especially necessary for hospitals where babies with known prenatal hazards are delivered. Such hospitals should now be set up with on-call members of a perinatal team prepared to give intensive care to the fetus and neonate.

CARDIOVASCULAR AND RESPIRATORY CHANGES AT BIRTH
Circulation of the blood before and after birth (Fig. 6-1)

Oxygenated blood is carried by the umbilical vein from the placenta to the inferior vena cava through the liver and ductus venosus. This blood mixes in the inferior vena cava with blood returning from the lower extremities and abdominal viscera, enters the right atrium, and passes through the foramen ovale into the left atrium, where it joins a small amount of blood returning from the lungs by the pulmonary veins. It then flows into the left ventricle and the ascending aorta to supply the head and upper extremities. Blood returns to the right atrium by the superior vena cava and then passes into the right ventricle and into the pulmonary artery.

Most of the pulmonary arterial blood flows through the ductus arteriosus; from there part of it supplies the lower extremities and the abdominopelvic viscera through the aorta, and a larger part returns to the placenta by the umbilical arteries.

With the first breath and lung expansion, pulmonary blood flow suddenly increases. Returning blood from the pulmonary veins increases the pressure in the left atrium, resulting in functional closure of the foramen ovale. With increased oxygenation of the blood perfusing it, the ductus gradually constricts, limiting and finally obliterating this second pulmonary bypass, or right-to-left shunt. Decreasing pulmonary vascular resistance lowers the pulmonary artery pressure below the aortic pressure, causing a reversal of flow through the ductus as long as it remains open (left-to-right shunt). The ductus arteriosus is usually obliterated in the early neonatal period, resulting in the normal, or adult, type of circulation.

Reduced ventilation may, by producing hypoxia and hypercapnea, result in a combined respiratory and metabolic acidosis (augmented by anaerobic metabolism). The combination of acidosis and hypoxia is a powerful vasoconstrictive force in the newborn. Pulmonary vasoconstriction leads to an increase in vascular resistance that may on occasion exceed the systemic pressures; under these circumstances a right-to-left shunting through a patent ductus

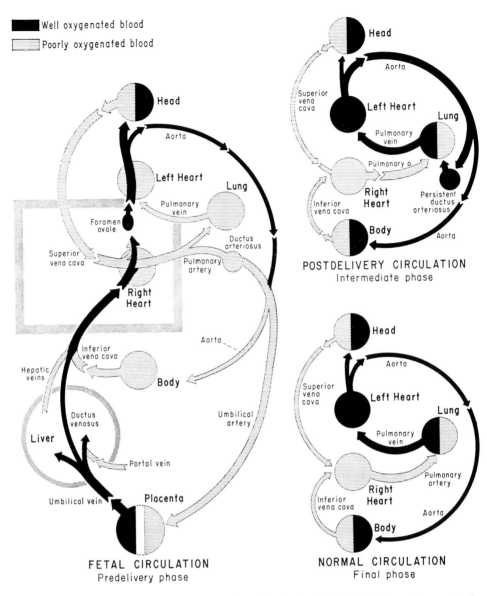

■ Well oxygenated blood

▨ Poorly oxygenated blood

FETAL CIRCULATION
Predelivery phase

POSTDELIVERY CIRCULATION
Intermediate phase

NORMAL CIRCULATION
Final phase

Fig. 6-1. Diagrams of blood circulation before and after birth. (Modified from Benson, R. C., and Griswold, H. E.: Spectrum **10:**80, 1962; courtesy Chas. Pfizer & Co., Inc.)

and/or a patent foramen ovale may occur.

Onset of respiration

The most important adjustment to the extrauterine environment for the infant is the onset of respiration. Air must replace the fluid that fills the airways and alveoli until birth. The process of a vaginal vertex delivery usually squeezes out as much as 20 ml of fluid from the infant's lungs. The remaining fluid probably is absorbed into the vascular and lymphatic bed of the lung through the decrease of pulmonary vascular resistance with the onset of respiration. Delayed onset or inefficient ventilation can delay this process and hinder the development of normal pulmonary function of the infant.

During the first breath the infant develops a negative intrathoracic pressure of 20 to 70 cm of water, drawing in about 40 to 70 cc of air, approximately 20 to 30 cc of which will remain as residual volume. This first breath frequently is followed by a vigorous cry in the undepressed infant as he expires against the closed glottis. After the first few breaths the lungs are almost completely expanded and the pressures lower than at the onset of respiration. The stimuli that provoke the onset of respiration at birth are numerous. Because the interval between birth and the first breath usually is only a few seconds, it is likely that excitation of the respiratory center follows through neurally transmitted impulses from peripherally located receptors. Thermal stimuli seem to be of particular importance here; tactile stimuli and the rise of blood pressure on cord clamping probably play secondary roles.

A significant change of blood gases at birth is another important factor governing the onset of respiration. This stimulus is particularly important for the depressed infant whose respiratory center is less sensitive to peripheral stimuli.

Physiologic aspects of oxygenation

Oxygen is carried in blood in chemical combination with hemoglobin, as well as in physical solution.

At ambient pressures most oxygen is bound to hemoglobin. The quantity is dependent on the partial pressure of oxygen and the hemoglobin-oxygen dissociation curve. This curve for fetal hemoglobin is shifted to the left (as compared with adult hemoglobin). Therefore fetal hemoglobin binds more oxygen at lower pressures, but it also releases less to the tissues.

The oxygen tension in arterial blood not only is dependent on pulmonary function but is influenced by the degree of venous admixture through shunts. Prolonged breathing of 100% oxygen will correct desaturation secondary to ventilation or diffusion abnormalities and therefore can be useful in differentiating the above causes from significant right-to-left shunts.

The oxygen tension in arterial blood at birth rises rapidly to 60 to 90 mm Hg (premature infants somewhat less). Because during the first days of life 20% of cardiac output is shunted right to left, the $P_{a_{O_2}}$ in 100% oxygen will be approximately 440 mm Hg, and not 600 as in adults. A 50% right-to-left shunt in an infant will prevent the $P_{a_{O_2}}$ from rising above 67 mm Hg even with 100% oxygen.

Placental transfusion

The blood volume of an infant at birth is dependent on the amount of blood received by placental transfusion. The blood volume in utero at term averages 66 ml/kg (approximately 78 ml at birth and between 75 to 107 ml at 72 hours, depending on time of cord clamping). As the fetus is born, a redistribution of blood takes place between the fetus and the placenta. Blood flow through the umbilical arteries stops approximately 45 seconds after birth, whereas the umbilical vein remains patent longer. The onset of uterine contractions enhances transfer of blood to the infant. Gravity significantly influences transfer of blood between neonate and placenta; elevation of the infant 50 to 60 cm above the level of the placenta for 3 minutes will prevent the otherwise normally occurring placental transfusion. If one places the neonate below the level of the placenta, the process will be accelerated, however.

The timing of clamping the cord in relation to the above-mentioned factors influences the infant's blood volume and symptomatology.

Infants whose cords have been clamped early often have hypovolemia, a lower hematocrit reading, lower initial blood pressure, peripheral vasoconstriction, and better lung compliance as compared to late-clamped infants. Late clamping of the cord tends to cause greater blood volumes, a higher hematocrit reading, and higher initial blood pressures, as well as occasional expiratory grunting due to reduced lung compliance.

During perinatal asphyxia, a redistribution of blood from the placenta to the fetus seems to take place. It explains the higher plasma and red blood cell volumes of infants with perinatal asphyxia whose cords were clamped early, as compared with nonstressed neonates.

INITIAL CARE OF THE INFANT

1. Establish and maintain a clear airway.
   a. Suction the oropharynx and nostrils with a rubber bulb syringe as soon as the head is delivered.
   b. To avoid aspiration by the neonate, aspirate the pharynx first, and then the nose.
   c. Avoid nasal suctioning with a catheter, if possible, because it may cause reflex bradycardia and laryngospasm.
2. Place the infant below level of the placenta. At cesarean section, clamp cord before lifting infant above uterus, to prevent backflow of blood into placenta.
3. Clamp the cord after the first breath, or approximately 30 seconds after delivery.
4. Dry infant's skin with a warm towel and place him under radiant heat to prevent cold stress (p. 93).
   The scoring method (Table 6-1) introduced by Virginia Apgar in 1952 is still the simplest and most practical method of appraising the condition of the newborn at birth. It permits a rapid and semiquantitative assessment of five signs of an infant's physiologic state: heart rate by auscultation,* respiration from observation of movement of chest wall, color (pallid, cyanotic, or pink), muscle tone from movement of extremities, and reflex activity from slap on soles of feet.

1. Assessment at 1 minute.
   a. A score of 7 to 10 (10 indicates best possible condition) requires no resuscitation and should apply to more than 80% of infants.
   b. Scores of 4 to 6 (approximately 15% of babies) will identify those neonates who are cyanotic and who have irregular respirations and diminished muscle tone; reflex irritability and heart rate (over 100 beats/min) may still be maintained.
   c. Scores of 0 to 3 (1% to 3% of infants) will reveal severely asphyxiated infants who should be recognized at birth as needing immediate resuscitation. Invariably, the heart rate will be under 80 beats/min or inaudible.
2. Assessment at 5 minutes.

---

*For the depressed infant, we recommend the immediate application of needle electrodes to chest wall attached to a heart-rate monitor. The battery-powered, compact, portable Parks No. 510, with visible and audible heart rate, is ideal for the delivery room as well as for transport.

Table 6-1. Evaluation by Apgar score*

Sign	Score 0	Score 1	Score 2
Heart rate	Absent	Below 100/min	Over 100/min
Respiratory effort	Absent	Gasping, irregular	Good
Muscle tone	Limp	Some flexion	Active motion
Reflex irritability (slap to feet)	No response	Grimace	Cry
Color	Body pale or blue	Body pink, extremities blue	Completely pink

*From Apgar, V.: The role of the anesthesiologist in reducing neonatal mortality, N. Y. State J. Med. **55**:2365, 1955.

Assessment at 1 minute (or before) should identify newborns who require immediate attention. The 5-minute score correlates with neonatal mortality and morbidity.

RESUSCITATION OF THE DEPRESSED INFANT

The life of an infant depends on early and adequate pulmonary ventilation at birth. Most neonates will breathe spontaneously within a minute. If they do not, they may be suffering from asphyxia acquired in utero or from respiratory depression due to maternal analgesia or anesthesia. Further delay in establishing adequate extrauterine exchange in the infant may increase the likelihood of permanent neurologic deficiency. Therefore at every delivery the attending physician or nurse assistant should be experienced in resuscitation techniques to properly treat the occasional unexpectedly depressed newborn. In the delivery of an infant who may have been asphyxiated, a specially trained physician-nurse team is needed in addition to the accoucheur for complete care.

Equipment and drugs needed for the infant at birth

1. A "resuscitation island" in the delivery room should provide
   a. Table of sufficient height to allow easy intubation
   b. Heat lamp or radiant heat for the prevention of cold stress
   c. Oxygen, compressed air, and vacuum outlets
   d. Adequate lighting for procedures
   e. Battery-powered heart rate monitor
   f. Stethoscope
   g. Bag and infant masks of varying sizes
   h. Pharyngeal airways (Nos. 00, 0, and 1)
   i. Infant laryngoscope with Nos. 1 and 0 blades, and spare battery and bulb
   j. Endotracheal tubes attached to adapters
   k. Umbilical vessel catheterization equipment
2. Drugs that should be available (for dosage, see Appendix E)
   a. Sodium bicarbonate solution (1 ml = 0.9 mEq)
   b. 10% and 50% glucose solutions
   c. Distilled water
   d. Epinephrine (1:1,000 in 1 ml ampules)
   e. 10% calcium gluconate
   f. Isoproterenol (Isuprel)
   g. Digoxin (0.1 mg/ml)
   h. Phenobarbital
   i. Nalorphine or levallorphan
   j. Dexamethasone
   k. Plasma protein fraction (human) (Plasmanate)
   l. Furosemide (Lasix)

Mildly depressed infants

Infants with an Apgar score of 7 or 8 may have cyanosis, irregular respirations, and diminished muscle tone. They probably will not require vigorous treatment and should respond to the following:
1. Stimulation by rubbing the chest or slapping the soles of the feet
2. Oxygen blown from mask or funnel into infant's face (thermal stimulation)

Moderately depressed infants

A newborn with a score of 4 to 6 will be cyanotic or pale and will have irregular or absent respirations, diminished muscle tone, and reflex irritability. The heart rate usually will not be decreased. Peripheral stimulation alone may not cause the infant to breathe regularly, however.
1. Administer oxygen by mask ventilation.
2. If the neonate does not breathe spontaneously after a few insufflations of the lungs, or if the heart rate begins to fall, visualize larynx by laryngoscopy and suction airway if needed.
3. Intubate infant if spontaneous respi-

rations have not been established after above-mentioned procedures, and treat like a severely depressed infant.

Severely depressed infants

Severely depressed infants present a medical emergency and require immediate resuscitation. They usually are flaccid, pale, and apneic and will respond slightly or not at all to stimulation. The heart rate usually is less than 80 beats/min. There will be hypoxia and significant acidosis. Absolutely no time must be wasted in this instance.

1. Place skin electrodes and connect the infant to a heart rate monitor.
2. Visualize larynx with laryngoscope and suction airway (especially if meconium is present); intubate and ventilate infant.
3. If heart rate is less than 80 beats/min, begin external cardiac massage to improve circulation; compress midsternum with two fingers at a rate of 100 to 125/min; interrupt massage every 5 to 7 seconds to allow 2 or 3 expansions of the lung.
4. Treat acidosis by administering sodium bicarbonate solution slowly through an umbilical vessel catheter in doses of 2 to 4 mEq/kg after dilution with equal amounts of sterile distilled water.
5. Support glucose metabolism by starting a constant infusion of 10% dextrose with a 3 ml 10% calcium gluconate added per 100 ml $D_{10}W$. Infuse at a rate of 3 to 4 ml/kg/hr. (More rapid infusion or administration of more than 20% dextrose by rapid injection may cause hyperglycemia.)
6. If infant deteriorates and heart rate falls below 50 beats/min, administer 1 to 2 ml of a 1:10,000 dilution of epinephrine through umbilical catheter. However, if heartbeat is barely audible, inject the drug into the heart with a 25-gauge needle (perpendicular to skin surface at fourth costal interspace left of the sternum).
7. If infant shows signs of poor peripheral perfusion or remains pale, hypovolemic, and/or anemic, manage according to p. 234.
8. If depression of infant is caused by narcotics given to the mother during labor, inject levallorphan (Lorfan), 0.05 mg/kg, or nalorphine (Nalline), 0.1 to 0.5 mg/kg, intramuscularly or intravenously.
9. For infants continuing in respiratory difficulty and/or cyanosis, obtain chest x-ray studies while continuing ventilatory support. Rule out diaphragmatic hernia, choanal atresia, esophageal atresia, etc., and treat according to Chapters 19 and 20.

Technique of intubation (Fig. 6-2)

1. Place infant on flat surface and gently elevate shoulders with folded towel.
2. With left hand introduce laryngoscope through right angle of infant's mouth.
3. Gently advance blade, bringing it to midline and pushing tongue toward left.
4. Visualize pharynx and epiglottis, and by lifting tip of blade, expose vocal cords.
5. Suction trachea if needed.
6. Insert endotracheal tube (Cole Fr 14 or 16 for term infants, and smaller size for preterm infants or Portex size 2.5 to 3.5 mm), advancing its tip 1.5 cm beyond vocal cords. (Stylets can be used but may be traumatic.)
7. Withdraw laryngoscope and give few short inflations to the lungs while auscultating chest to assure proper tube placement.

Methods of artificial ventilation

1. Positive-pressure breathing devices
   A number of manual positive-pressure

breathing devices are on the market, for example, Penlon, Ambu, Hope, Kreiselman. Each has advantages as well as disadvantages. To perform satisfactorily, a good infant bag should

a. Deliver up to 100% oxygen
b. Create variable pressures
c. Be equipped with masks of variant sizes that fit comfortably over infant's nose and mouth

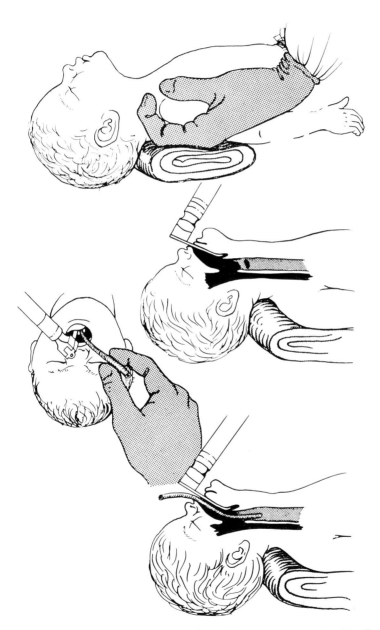

Fig. 6-2. Technique of resuscitation of the newborn. (From Benson, R. C.: Handbook of obstetrics and gynecology, ed. 4, Los Altos, Calif., 1971, Lange Medical Publications.)

d. Adapt to endotracheal tubes
   Technique of use
   1. If infant is intubated, connect the endotracheal tube to a bag and ventilate the infant in this manner.
   2. When applying bag-to-mask ventilation, cover infant's nose and mouth snugly with mask, and lift mandible upward to prevent airway obstruction.
   3. Initially apply one or two inflations at pressures of 30 to 40 cm of water, holding pressure for 0.5 to 1 second to expand infant's lungs.
   4. Continue to ventilate with lower pressures (10 to 20 cm of water) at a rate of 40 to 50/min.
   5. Gastric distention may occur during mask ventilation; decompress stomach by placing orogastric tube.

2. Mouth-to-tube ventilation
   a. To minimize danger from overexpansion of lung, use cheek muscles only when blowing into tube.
   b. Deliver oxygen by placing a tube connected to an oxygen source into operator's mouth while the operator is applying mouth-to-tube ventilation.

3. Mouth-to-mouth ventilation
   This technique can be used by persons inexperienced with other methods and requires no equipment. Therefore it can be applied in almost any situation.
   a. Place airway into infant's mouth.
   b. Place operator's mouth firmly over infant's nose and mouth and inflate infant's lungs gently by blowing from cheeks.
   c. Remove operator's mouth from infant to let infant's lungs recoil.
   d. Repeat maneuver at a rate of 40 to 50/min.
   e. Oxygen, if available, can be given as above.

EXAMINATION IN THE BIRTH ROOM*

The infant who has been assessed by the Apgar score may be placed briefly at the mother's breast if all is well after drying and warmly wrapping. Nonetheless, if signs of continued depression, respiratory difficulty, cyanosis, or pallor become evident, continued emergency care must be offered, preferably in an intensive care unit (Chapter 7).

The placenta should be inspected for staining, infarction, infection, etc. and put aside for weighing. The cord should also be observed for the number of vessels and for its thickness, length, and insertion. Unusual appearance, as in the case of multiple birth, or evidence of disease requires pathologic study.

Minimal physical examination, including assessment of maturity

1. External
   a. Note skin color, staining, peeling, and evidence of wasting (dysmaturity).
   b. Observe length of nails and extent of creasing on soles of feet.
   c. Palpate for presence or absence of breast tissue.
   d. Note testicular descent, scrotal rugae, and labial development.
   e. Check nasal patency by occluding one nostril at a time and observing the infant's respiration and color.
2. Chest
   a. Auscultate the heart for rate and quality of sounds and palpate for position of maximum impulse.
   b. Listen with a stethoscope in each axilla for comparison and efficiency of respiratory exchange, including the presence of rhonchi and rales.

---

*This brief examination may be performed on admission to the nursery, but wherever it is performed, it should be accomplished quickly and under a radiant warmer to prevent heat loss.

c. Percuss each lung posteriorly with the index finger for comparison of resonance.

3. Abdomen

Palpate the liver for consistency and enlargement (3 cm or more below costal margin). Enlargement of the liver (and spleen) may indicate

   a. Infection—viremia, bacteremia, or sepsis
   b. A depressed diaphragm from emphysema or pneumothorax
   c. Cardiac failure
   d. Erythroblastosis fetalis

4. Neurologic examination

   a. Note muscle tone and reflex behavior.
   b. Test the Moro reflex.
   c. Feel the fontanel for fullness or bulging.
   d. Palpate the sagittal sutures for approximation of parietal bone edges.

5. Supplemental observations

At least 2% of all infants have important malformations recognizable at birth. The following checks are suggested in all infants and particularly when oligohydramnios or polyhydramnios is present, placental abnormalies including two-vessel cord are noted, or the neonate is small-for-dates.

   a. Inspect for such external defects as misshapen or low-set ears, lymphedema, macroglossia, palatal abnormalities, umbilical defects, variations in the size or shape of the head, spinal column defects, and opacity of the lens or cornea.
   b. Pass a rubber catheter (Fr 10) attached to a DeLee trap through the mouth to establish esophageal patency and perform gastric aspiration for excessive fluid (over 20 ml) and/or green color, suggestive of intestinal obstruction.
   c. Note a protuberant, or scaphoid, abdomen (diaphragmatic hernia) and organ enlargements or displacements.

d. Check the patency of the anus and rectum with a catheter and note the consistency and color of rectal contents (normally black, sticky meconium).
   e. Observe the genitalia for sexual ambiguity.
   f. Consider multiple anomalies. One major anomaly is often associated with another (25%). Three or more anomalies suggest a chromosomal defect.

ASSESSMENT BY WEIGHT AND GESTATION

The division of infants into term and "premature" on the basis of weight above and below 2,500 gm has little biologic significance. Many term infants (40% in some countries) weigh less, and in some areas, more preterm infants weigh 2,500 gm or more.

Yet both weight and gestational age are important in classifying infants at birth so that morbidity and mortality risks can be anticipated to ensure optimal care. An accurate weight on admission to the nursery is necessary for statistical requirements, as well as for drug dosage. A careful menstrual history is an important method of estimating gestational age but should not supplant a clinical estimate of gestational age as part of the physical examination, particularly when the history is inexact or a discrepancy between birth weight and gestational age exists. Prenatal estimation of gestational age is discussed in Chapter 3. Table 6-2 presents a guide for the combined estimation of gestational age by measurement, appearance, and neuromuscular behavior.

The classification by gestational age and growth pattern proposed by Battaglia and Lubchenco has been modified to conform with the expected mortality and pattern of fetal growth in 40,000 single, white infants born to a middle-class population in Portland, Oregon. These data are shown in

Table 6-2. Postnatal estimation of fetal age on the basis of maturity (assuming normal growth)

	27 weeks	28 to 33 weeks	34 to 37 weeks	38 to 41 weeks	42 weeks or more
Anatomic maturity					
Sole creases	None	Minimal—one or two creases	Anterior third	Extend to heel	Deep creases over entire sole
Scrotum	Testes undescended	Testes high in scrotum; few rugae	Testes above raphe; more rugae	Testes bulge below raphe; rugae complete	Pendulous, deep rugae, well pigmented
Labia	Labia majora undeveloped	Minora prominent	Labia of equal prominence	Majora covers minora	Same
Ear cartilage	Pinna soft and folded	Still folded	Returns from folded position	Erect, with sharp ridges	Same
Breast tissue	None	None	Up to 4 mm	5 mm or more	Usually more than 10 mm; areolae very prominent
Skin	Translucent and edematous	Red	Pink to red	Pinkish white	Thicker and white; often desquamated
Nails	Visible; soft and small	Soft and extending to fingertips	Soft and extending to fingertips	Extending to just beyond fingertips; not as soft	Hard in consistency and extending well beyond fingertips
Eyes	Closed	Closed	Eyes opening	Open eyes that fixate	Open, good fixation
Neuromuscular maturity					
Body flexion	None	Flexes legs—froglike	Flexes arms. Knees under abdomen	Same	Same
Moro reflex	Aimless	Lateral extension	Beginning embrace	Embrace	Same
Neck tone	Limp	Limp	Head control on arm flexion (36 to 37 weeks)	Raises head in prone position	Raises head in prone position; turns head from side to side
Sucking and deglutition	Not synchronized	Insufficient for total nipple feeding	Adequate for normal intake	Same	Perfect
Glabella tap (blink)	No response	Develops (32 to 33 weeks)	Good response	Same	Same
Pupil to light	No response	Gradual contraction	Good response	Same–begins to follow	Same
Measurements					
Weight (gm ± 1 SD)	$1,000 \pm 350$	$1,150\text{-}2,000 \pm 450$	$2,200\text{-}2,950 \pm 450$	$3,150\text{-}3,600 \pm 500$	$3,300\text{-}4,100 \pm 500$
Length (cm ± 1 SD)	37.5 ± 1.5	$38.5\text{-}44.0 \pm 1.5$	$45.0\text{-}47.5 \pm 1.5$	$48.5\text{-}53 \pm 2.0$	$50\text{-}54 \pm 2$
Head circumference (cm ± 1 SD)	25.5 ± 1.0	$26.0\text{-}30.0 \pm 1.0$	$31.0\text{-}33.5 \pm 1.0$	$34.0\text{-}36.5 \pm 1.5$	$35\text{-}37.5 \pm 1.5$

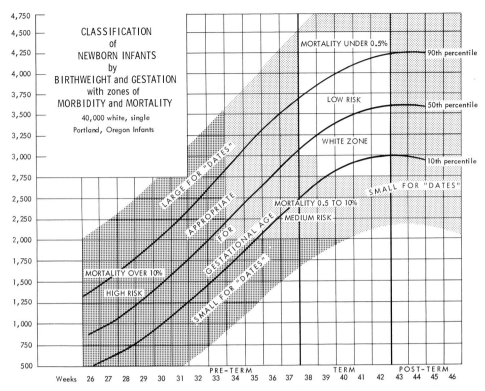

Fig. 6-3. Zones of mortality and morbidity in relation to both weight and gestation (Behrman and Babson).*

Fig. 6-3, which presents zones of neonatal mortality and morbidity on the basis of weight and gestational age, which may apply to many similar populations. The infants at high risk, with a mortality over 10%, are grouped together in the heavily shaded zone. They represent 2% to 3% of all infants, including those born before 33 weeks of gestational age and those weighing under 2,000 gm, regardless of gestation. Several times this number may be added to this high-risk group because of complications of pregnancy or delivery. Infants falling into the white zone have a perinatal mortality of less than 0.5%. They have a weight range from 2,750 to 4,500 gm (usually between the 10th and 90th percentiles) and a gestational age of 38 through 42 weeks and seldom present difficulty in the delivery room. All the remaining newborn infants, numbering about 15% to 20% of all deliveries, are placed in the medium-risk category (lightly shaded zone); they have a mortality of 0.5% to 10%. This zone of infants includes the postterm baby (often clinically dysmature), the undergrown infant with or without loss of subcutaneous tissue, and the otherwise normal "large-for-dates" infants, including a sizable group of preterm infants who weigh over 2,500 gm but are 33 weeks or more of gestational age. Thus small- and large-for-gestational-age infants (SGA and LGA) should be designated, as well as those who are preterm and postterm, so that they receive extra vigilance in the first days of life.

*Copies of this graph (8 × 11 inches) in color may be obtained from the printing department at the University of Oregon Medical School, Portland, Ore.

TRANSITIONAL CARE OF THE INFANT

All infants should be admitted to an area near the nurses' station for a period of close observation—particularly infants at medium risk. In view of the fluctuations in physiologic behavior and the ease with which airway obstruction can occur in the weak or depressed newborn, babies should be observed according to this general plan.

Observational and minimum nursery care necessary for all infants during transitional period after birth

1. Place the undressed neonate on side or stomach in a prewarmed incubator or under radiant heat to maintain skin or axillary temperature between 96° to 98° F (35.5° to 36.5° C).
2. Have adequate illumination available for longitudinal observation, for example, 100 footcandles of white fluorescent light at infant level.
3. Observe every 15 minutes (for a minimum of 4 hours) for color, respiration, and activity and report variation from the usual.
4. Record respiration rate every 30 minutes for at least 4 hours and then every hour until rate has stabilized (40 to 60 minutes).
5. Offer feedings (Chapter 8) by 6 to 8 hours of age, and sooner if infant seems hungry. Report regurgitation, choking, or distention.
6. Dress after 6 to 12 hours only if condition is good and infant has successfully accepted an initial water feeding. An infant whose condition is not satisfactory should remain in the admitting nursery area or be transferred to a special care nursery.

Special attention for infants in the following categories (medium-risk care)

1. Neonates with tachypnea (over 60 beats/min) and those likely to develop respiratory distress syndrome, such as preterm infants who have suffered asphyxia or have low levels of pulmonary surfactants (Any developing or continuing respiratory distress demands an emergency chest x-ray examination.)
   a. Start 10% glucose by intravenous drip—80 ml/kg/24 hr, with appropriate electrolytes. (See Chapter 8.)
   b. Monitor heart rate and/or heart and respiratory rate.
   c. Record serial vital signs.
   d. Obtain hematocrit and blood pressure readings.
   e. Administer sufficient oxygen* (warmed and humidified) to prevent cyanosis; then gradually decrease as condition improves. Increase concentration to cover central cyanosis.
   f. Obtain blood gas levels.
2. Dysmature and small-for-dates infants
   a. Begin with 20-calorie/30 ml milk formula by 2 to 4 hours of age after a successful water feeding. If feedings are not tolerated, give parenteral glucose infusion.
   b. Screen for hypoglycemia, using a Dextrostix test at least every 4 to 6 hours for 48 hours or until blood glucose levels are over 50 mg/100 ml.
   c. Check carefully for congenital disease.
3. Large-for-dates infants
   a. Observe for hypoglycemia, using a Dextrostix test every 2 hours for 12 hours.
   b. Anticipate hyperbilirubinemia and respiratory distress if preterm.
4. Preterm babies (34 to 37 weeks' gestation) who suck well

*Continuing concentrations of oxygen above 25% for the very immature infant require oxygen tension measurements to warn of excessive levels (over 70 mm Hg from central artery—over 45 mm Hg by arterialized capillary blood).

a. Monitor heart rate and observe closely until feedings are taken well.
b. Offer 20-calorie/30 ml formula at 6 hours after a successful water feeding.
c. Keep in transitional nursery area until weight gain is established. (For discharge, see p. 98.)

5. Babies with early jaundice
   a. Jaundice in first 24 hours or a bilirubin level over 10 mg/100 ml by 36 hours requires screening for erythroblastosis fetalis, etc. (Chapter 23).
   b. Place under phototherapy while appropriate tests are awaited.
   c. Consider transfer if bilirubin level rises above 15 mg/100 ml in term or 12 mg/100 ml in preterm infants, if facilities for exchange transfusions are wanting.

Infants with early cyanosis or an increase in respiratory rate, expiratory grunting, or rib retraction who do not improve after 3 hours of life should have consultation with a regional center. Very immature infants and those distressed at birth should have received earlier consideration of transport to a regional center.

Summary of the transitional period

Effectiveness of the perinatal programs in hospitals has traditionally been evaluated on the basis of mortality rates. Prevention, detection, and treatment of less-than-lethal conditions have become more important in the assurance of maximum quality of life. Desmond and associates have reported nursery morbidity during the early days of life to be present in one of five infants weighing over 2,500 gm and two of three infants of low birth weight. Morbidity-to-death ratios were 37:1 in "term" infants and 5:1 in low birth weight infants. In the past we have offered care

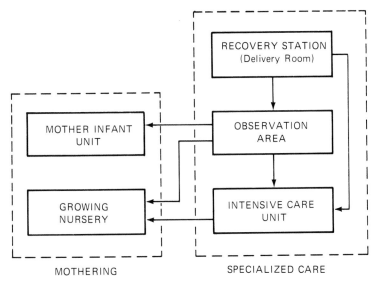

Fig. 6-4. Method for division of care of the newborn. Such a system allows special consideration of infants during their early hours in an observation nursery, an intensive care nursery when necessary, and a "mothering" nursery for full development of the maternal-infant relationship so important in the first days of life. In small maternity areas, the observation area may also serve as a combined nursery for growing infants and those who require very specialized care. (Modified from Silverman, W. H.: Clin. Obstet. Gynecol. 13:87, 1970.)

on the assumption that newborn infants are healthy until proved ill, but today, by placing all of them in an observational or transitional nursery, *infants are considered potentially ill until good health is demonstrated.*

Fig. 6-4 demonstrates the functional arrangements of a modern nursery in which fluctuations in physiologic behavior as well as early manifestations in breathing difficulty, or cyanosis, may be more easily noted. During the first 6 to 24 hours, constant observation and appropriate treatment by nursery personnel may be necessary.

Special note should be made of respiration, which may be the most reliable early sign of physiologic well-being. In the premature infant a persistent respiratory rate between 40 and 60/min without dyspnea is favorable. An initial tachypnea that reverts to normal usually is an indication of physiologic improvement. A sustained rapid respiratory rate or a rising respiratory rate is an indication of some form of respiratory distress and requires investigation. A rate below 40/min in the premature infant suggests respiratory depression and demands attention. (See Chapter 19.)

Infants requiring continuing intensive care not available in the hospital of birth should be transported to a regional center (Chapter 11).

SELECTED REFERENCES

Abramson, H., editor: Resuscitation of the newborn infant and related emergency procedures in the perinatal center special care nursery, ed. 3, St. Louis, 1973, The C. V. Mosby Co.

American Academy of Pediatrics, Committee on Fetus and Newborn: Nomenclature for duration of gestation, birthweight and intrauterine growth, Pediatrics **39**:935, 1967.

American College of Obstetricians and Gynecologists, Committee on Terminology: Nomenclature—dissenting views, Pediatrics **39**:942, 1967.

Amiel-tison, C.: Neurological evaluation of the maturity of newborn infants, Arch. Dis. Child. **43**:89, 1968.

Avery, M. E., and Fletcher, B. D.: The lung and its disorders in the newborn infant, ed. 3, Philadelphia, 1974, W. B. Saunders Co.

Babson, S. G., Osterud, H. T., and Thompson, H.: The congenitally malformed, Northwest Med. **65**:729, 1966.

Battaglia, F. C., and Lubchenco, L. O.: A practical classification of newborn infants by weight and gestational age, J. Pediatr. **71**:159, 1967.

Behrman, R. E., James, L. S., Klaus, M., Nelson, N., and Oliver, T.: Treatment of the asphyxiated infant, J. Pediatr. **74**:981, 1969.

Cordero, L., and Hon, E. H.: Neonatal bradycardia following nasopharyngeal stimulation, J. Pediatr. **78**:441, 1971.

Dahm, L. S., and James, L. S.: Newborn temperature and calculated heat loss in the delivery room, Pediatrics **49**:504, 1972.

Delivoria-Papadeopoulos, M., Roncevic, N. P., and Oski, F. A.: Postnatal changes in oxygen transport of term, premature and sick infants: the role of red cell 2, 3-diphosphoglycerate and adult hemoglobin, Pediatr. Res. **5**:235, 1971.

Desmond, M. M., Rudolph, A. J., and Phitaksphraiwan, P.: The transitional nursery care, Pediatr. Clin. North Am. **13**:651, 1966.

Desmond, M. M., Rudolph, A. J., and Pineda, R. G.: Neonatal morbidity and nursery function, J.A.M.A. **212**:281, 1970.

Dubowitz, L. M. S., Dubowitz, V., and Goldberg, C.: Clinical assessment of gestational age in the newborn infant, J. Pediatr. **77**:1, 1970.

Engel, R., and Benson, R. C.: Estimate of conceptional age by evoked response activity, Biol. Neonate **12**:201, 1968.

Gruenwald, P.: Infants of low birth weight among 5,000 deliveries, Pediatrics **34**:157, 1964.

James, L. S., and Adamsons, K.: Respiratory physiology of the fetus and newborn infant, N. Engl. J. Med. **271**:1352, 1954.

Karlberg, P.: The adaptive changes in the immediate postnatal period, with particular reference to respiration, J. Pediatr. **56**:585, 1960.

Koenigsberger, M. R.: Judgment of fetal age. I. Neurologic evaluation, Pediatr. Clin. North Am. **13**:823, 1966.

Lind, J. E., Tahti, E., and Hirvensalo, M.: Roentgenologic studies of the size of the lungs of the newborn baby before and after aeration, Ann. Paediatr. Fenn. **12**:20, 1966.

Moss, A. J., and Monset-Couchard, M.: Placental transfusion: Early versus late clamping of the umbilical cord, Pediatrics **40**:109, 1967.

North, A. F.: Nomenclature—dissenting views, Pediatrics **39**:941, 1967.

Oh, W., Wallgren, G., Hannson, J. S., and Third, J.: The effects of placental transfusion on respiratory mechanics of normal term newborn infants, Pediatrics **40**:6, 1967.

Prod'hom, L. S., Levison, H., Cherry, R. B., Drorbaugh, J. E., Hubbell, J. P., Jr., and Smith, C. A.: Adjustment of ventilation, intrapulmonary gas exchange and acid-base balance during the first day of life, Pediatrics **33**:682, 1964.

Saigal, S., O'Neill, A., Surainder, Y., Chua, L., and Usher, R.: Placental transfusion and hyperbilirubinemia in the premature, Pediatrics **49**:406, 1972.

Saint-Anne Dargassies, S.: La maturation neurologique du premature, Etud. Neo-natal **4**:71, 1955.

Sjostedt, S., Engleson, G., and Rooth, G.: Dysmaturity, Arch. Dis. Child. **33**:123, 1958.

Strang, L. B.: Uptake of liquid from the lungs at the start of breathing. Development of the lung, Ciba Foundation Symposium, London, 1967, J. & A. Churchill, Ltd.

Usher, R., McLean, F., and Scott, K. E.: Judgment of fetal age. II. Clinical significance of gestational age and an objective method for its assessment, Pediatr. Clin. North Am. **13**:835, 1966.

World Health Organization, Expert Committee on Maternal and Child Health: Public health aspects of low birth weight, WHO Techn. Rep. Ser. **217**, 1961.

Yao, A. C., and Lind, J.: Placental transfusion, Am. J. Dis. Child. **127**:128, 1974.

7

Intensive care of high-risk infants

NURSERY FACILITIES*

Improved knowledge and greater emphasis on protection of the fetus during labor and the infant at delivery have resulted in an increased number of living, immature infants who require nursery care. The larger general hospital is geared to intensive care in units for the severely ill and postoperative adult patients. Such an institution has a similar responsibility for ensuring optimal treatment for newborns with critical problems.

The very small premature infants are too often the recipients of substandard care in the expectation that they will die. They may be deposited in incubators of uncertain efficiency, and if they show signs of survival after a period of neglect, consultation may be sought. Then, if they do live, the delay in metabolic and nutritional support may have impaired their chance for normal development.

The smaller premature infants, as well as infants with recognizable problems, should be transferred to a medical center if facilities and skills for appropriate care are not available. General nursery facilities for intensive newborn care should include the following:

1. Scrub facilities at the entrance with hot and cold water, knee or arm

controls, orange sticks, and an organic iodine solution, for example, Virac

2. Open radiant warmers or incubators with controlled air environments and bacterial filters over the air intake for all high-risk neonates (Fig. 7-1 demonstrates a basic intensive care module.) (Radiant warmers have the advantage of easy access for providing critical care, but their use increases the chance of bacterial contamination.)

3. Accurate monitoring equipment for oxygen concentration, heart rate, respirations, and blood pressure

4. Facilities to provide phototherapy

5. An accurate scale, preferably of the automatic beam type, such as Toledo Baby Weigh scales

6. Approximately 60 square feet for each infant (Critical care in an open warmer will require more space, whereas a recovering infant is an isolette will need less.)

7. Effective illumination for vision (A daylight fluorescent light source, placed at 7 to 8 feet from the floor, will improve observation of the infant and should supply approximately 75 to 100 footcandles at the incubator level.)

8. Eight to twelve electrical outlets available for each infant, with ade-

*See also the discussion of regionalization of perinatal care and requirements for personnel and services in Chapter 12.

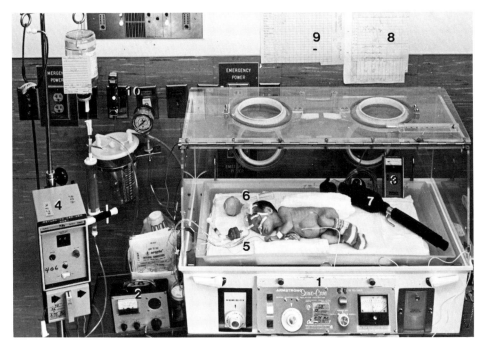

Fig. 7-1. Simplified intensive care module for the high-risk neonate. **1,** Intensive care incubator to regulate automatically environmental temperature to maintain the infant's temperature at a preset level by means of a skin sensor attached to the infant's abdominal skin (Ohio Armstrong). **2,** Battery-powered heart rate monitor with audible and visual beat and a low alarm signal; monitor cable attached to the skin with Grass needle electrodes (Parks Electronics, Grass Instruments Co.). **3,** Oxygen continuous analyzer (BMI). **4,** Infusion pump to regulate parenteral fluid administration (IVAC). **5,** Millipore filter to screen out bacteria and particulate matter from parenteral solution (Millipore). **6,** Suction bulb and DeLee trap. **7,** Bag and mask used for resuscitation (Penlon). **8,** Graphic record to portray the longitudinal physiologic state of an infant. (See Fig. 7-3.) **9,** Flow sheet for recording of sequential blood gas and other laboratory data of an infant. **10,** Utilities providing outlets for electricity, oxygen, air, and vacuum.

quate grounding and half of the outlets on an emergency power circuit

9. Two oxygen outlets and at least one each for vacuum and compressed air for each infant

10. Temperature of the nursery maintained at 75° F (24° C)

11. Air conditioning under positive-pressure ventilation (twelve changes per hour), with neutral humidity in the range of 50%, desirable in all new units

12. An area for preparation of formula and intravenous solutions

13. Diaper and soiled linen receptacles in each nursery division, with foot-controlled covers (Disposable diapers are recommended.)

14. Demonstration room for mothers to be instructed in the care of their infants

15. Rocking chairs for the comfort of nurse and infant during feeding periods

16. Soiled clothing specially autoclaved separately from the regular hospital laundry

17. An area for special segregation of infants requiring isolation technique

NURSERY REGULATIONS FOR CONTROL OF INFECTIONS

Nursery infections are spread to healthy infants from other babies who are infected, from contaminated equipment and incubators, or from insufficient handwashing, poorly treated laundry, and infected personnel.

The head nurse of any nursery must have the responsibility of "policing" the nursery and firmly but gently enforcing the rules of cleanliness. Regulations have become less restrictive since many nurseries (including our own) now allow nurses to wear regular short-sleeved uniforms in the nursery, but they must cover with scrub gowns to pick up infants. Caps and masks are considered unnecessary. Emphasis continues to be on hand-washing. This easing of regulations has increased the participation of physicians in the care of the patient and opened up the "off limits" to students and parents under supervision.

1. Technique to be used before entering the nursery
   a. Remove watch and ornamental rings and wash hands.
   b. Scrub hands and arms to elbows for one minute with soap containing hexachlorophene or an organic iodine solution.
   c. Clean fingernails with an orange stick and repeat b.
   d. Dry hands with a paper towel.
   e. Physicians and visitors should don short-sleeved gowns if they handle infants.
2. Technique in nursery
   a. Wash hands just before and after handling any infant or one's own face, handkerchief, etc.
   b. Consider the incubator's tops, sides, controls, and handles as part of the baby's environment.
   c. Consider pencils, tape measures, thermometers, bulb syringes, etc. as not interchangeable and as part of each baby's environment.
3. Responsibilities of the charge nurse
   a. Limit entry to the nursery to only those who are responsible for care, those who would benefit from observation of the infants, or parent(s).
   b. Exclude from the nursery any person with infection, that is, open draining skin lesions or herpes, viral, bacterial, respiratory, or gastrointestinal infections.
   c. Orient and supervise all new personnel, students, and parents in the routines for infection control.
   d. Maintain strict protective techniques.
4. Equipment and cleaning
   a. Sterilize all equipment at the time of discharge by autoclaving or gas sterilization if possible; otherwise, clean with 0.25% acetic acid or commercial antiseptic, for example, Microphene (1:1,000).
   b. Clean humidity tanks if they are to be used, and replace sterile water daily.
   c. Wet-mop floors daily with 0.25% acetic acid or commercial antiseptic, for example, Microphene (1:1,000).
   d. Clean inside and outside surfaces of occupied incubators and cribs with 0.25% acetic acid solution.
   e. Wipe stethoscopes and other equipment between use with Virac or a similar antiseptic solution.
   f. Sterilize thermometer bottles, cotton ball jars, etc. once weekly.

TEMPERATURE CONTROL

Temperature homeostasis after birth is impaired in the premature infant because of his relatively large surface area, the paucity of subcutaneous tissues (including "brown fat"), lessened muscular activity, decreased metabolic response to cooling, and limited ability to sweat or shiver. A temperature that seems warm to adults is cool for babies.

To maintain the skin or axillary temperature of the unclothed, depressed, prematurely born neonate at 97° F (36° C) for minimal oxygen consumption, a surrounding temperature between 90° and 97° F (32° and 36° C) will be required, depending on the infant's maturity, size, and metabolic activity.

This neutral zone of temperature should apply from the period of birth, during transfer to the nursery, and throughout any procedure.

Hazards from excessive temperature

1. Obligatory increase in metabolic rate and O₂ requirement
2. Increase in apneic attacks
3. Danger of shock from vasodilatation

Hazards from cooling

1. Obligatory increase in metabolic rate and O₂ requirement
2. Vasoconstriction with increase in acidosis and hypoxia
3. Rise in free fatty acid level of the blood, with reduction in glucose and interference with bilirubin binding
4. Increase in apneic attacks
5. Increase in mortality rate (may intensify hyaline membrane disease)

If an incubator offers insufficient heat to maintain skin temperature, particularly in the very small infant, the use of a heat shield or, temporarily, a 150-watt Sylvania or G.E. spotlamp focused on the baby through the incubator top from a distance of about 1 M (3 feet) will maintain his body temperature.

1. Techniques of temperature regulation
   a. Clinical thermometer capable of registering to 84° F (29° C)
      1. Hold the thermometer firmly in the infant's axilla* for 90 seconds.
      2. Take the infant's temperature every hour until it is stabilized at

97° ± 1° F (36° ± 0.5° C) by adjustment of the incubator control dial; then take and record the temperature every 4 to 8 hours.
   b. Servo-Control—an automatic sensing device used in the modern incubator for maintaining the infant's temperature at a prescribed level through a thermistor attachment to the skin
      1. Attach the thermistor at the infant's abdomen with nonirritating plastic tape (Hy-tape) between the navel and xiphoid process, while the infant is kept on his back; the attachment to the side of the infant's abdomen allows the baby to be on his abdomen as well as on his back.
      2. Record the infant's and the incubator temperature every 2 to 4 hours, except when the temperature is low or high.
   c. Automatic temperature control similar to that mentioned under b. but used with open warmers utilizing radiant heat
2. Problems in temperature regulation
   a. Check the infant's temperature if his body or extremities are cool to the touch.
   b. Report a temperature drop of more than 1° to 2° suspect
      1. An unadjusted or disconnected incubator
      2. Radiation loss to a cold window, wall, or cool environment (The use of a plastic shield placed over the infant will minimize this radiant heat loss.)
      3. Air-oxygen mixtures entering a plastic hood and not warmed to the required environmental temperature of the infant, thereby cooling him
      4. Impending sepsis
   c. Note and report the infant's temperature if it is over 99° F. Identify
      1. An overwarm incubator

---

*We do not recommend rectal temperature measurement because of hand contamination, possible injury to the infant, and delayed response of core temperature to sudden thermal changes.

2. The heat effect of direct sunlight
3. Abnormally high temperature of air-oxygen mixture entering plastic hood
4. Developing illness

3. *Technique of rewarming* the hypothermic infant (skin temperature less than 96° F, or 35.5° C)

Gradual rewarming of the infant may be achieved by keeping the isolette temperature 1 to 1½° F above his skin temperature. Intermittent readjustments of the incubator temperature may be necessary as the skin temperature reaches a normal level (97° F or 36° C). Limiting the temperature difference between infant and environment assures minimal metabolic demands.

Rapid rewarming should be tolerated as long as attention is paid to the possibility of vasodilation of the skin by the heat. Administration of volume expander may be necessary to prevent shock.

HUMIDIFICATION

Humidity* should be maintained in the neutral range of 40% to 60%, allowing no visible mist or moisture to form on incubator walls. This level usually is produced without adding water to humidity trays. Controlled studies have failed to demonstrate any favorable influence of high humidity, nebulized water, or detergent mist in the treatment or prevention of idiopathic respiratory distress. When high humidity is desired, ultrasonic nebulization may be preferable to standard techniques because of the smaller droplet size.

Increased humidity (nebulization) may be desirable in the following situations:
1. High-oxygen environments, since oxygen dries mucous membranes
2. Meconium aspiration syndromes with signs of respiratory obstruction

3. Excessive or thickened mucous secretions such as occur in tracheoesophageal fistulas, although humidity is no substitute for proper hydration
4. Extended intubation
5. Postanesthesia per intubation

MONITORING FOR APNEA

Recurring apnea is the most serious problem in any nursery caring for preterm and sick infants, since apnea usually is followed by bradycardia and frequently by cyanosis. Early detection and appropriate management is essential in avoiding CNS damage or death.

Thus all infants at medium to high risk (i.e., small preterm infants, infants with respiratory distress syndrome, etc.) should be monitored in all hospitals.

Types of monitors

1. Heart rate and respiration monitors. These monitors measure the impedance across the chest throughout respiratory movements, in addition to monitoring the heart rate.

2. Heart rate monitors. We prefer the inexpensive Parks* unit for routine monitoring of most infants. This small battery-powered monitor is especially useful in the delivery room, during transport, and for prolonged monitoring periods. It also offers protection from severe electrical shock. *Exceptions:* Occasionally infants become cyanotic with a minimal fall or no fall in heart rate. In the former case, the alarm should be set at a higher rate; in the latter case, apnea monitors must be used.

Use of heart rate monitors

1. Application of electrodes
   With the Parks model, two electrodes are placed over the anterior chest (right upper and left lower sternal area). Other models frequently require an additional electrode on the left leg.

---

*A wet and dry bulb hygrometer is necessary for occasional checks of the nursery and incubators.

*Parks Electronics, Beaverton, Ore.

a. Surface "stick-on" electrodes—apply to clean dry skin in previously mentioned areas.

b. Needle electrodes*
Clean skin with organic iodine followed by alcohol; let dry. Insert needle parallel to skin surface just beneath skin; cover needle with clear tape to keep in place. Connect electrodes to monitor cables.

2. Alarm settings
Set low alarm at 80 beats/min (higher if needed); set high alarm at 200 and turn switch to "on" position.

Use of respiration-apnea monitor

1. Application of electrodes (exception for the mattress type of apnea monitor)
Movement of the chest wall usually is detected adequately when electrodes are placed in the positions used for heart rate monitors. Occasionally they may have to be placed slightly farther apart.

2. Alarm settings
a. Either by rate of respiration, that is, low setting at 20/min or
b. By duration of apnea—usually at 10 to 15 seconds

3. When an alarm is sounded
a. Rule out false alarm (infant shows respiration and usual color), caused by
1. Lead failure—faulty placement, detached leads, etc.
2. Monitor failure or wrong alarm settings
b. If infant is found apneic, treat as suggested on pp. 224 and 225.

DETAILS OF CARE
Admission care

1. Check identification and eye prophylaxis.
2. Weigh the infant and obtain length and head circumference; these values are necessary for base line observa-

---

*Grass Instrument Co., Quincy, Mass. 02169.

tions, precise medication, and collection of vital statistics.

3. Note and record color, rate and type of breathing, activity, state of nutrition, signs of bleeding or infection, and abnormality. Infants with purulent skin infections or watery diarrhea should be admitted only after consultation with the physician in charge.

4. Administer 0.5 to 1 mg of vitamin K_1, for example, AquaMephyton, if not given previously.

5. Label the incubator with the name, race, and sex of the infant, date and hour of birth, birth weight and gestational age, age at admission (hours under 72 hours of age), and admission weight. The depressed and premature infant should be handled minimally, and cold exposure is to be avoided. Any bathing is postponed.

6. Attach monitoring equipment.

Positioning

1. Place the infant in a position of comfort, such as on abdomen with the head to the side, on side with a blanket roll at the back, or on back with some elevation of the shoulders (may be useful in respiratory distress).

2. Change the infant's position at feeding times.

Clothing and crib transfer for the premature infant

1. Use no clothing on infants weighing under 1,500 gm during the first week.

2. Then diaper infants over 1,250 gm who are in good condition.

3. Dress infants weighing around 2,000 gm and transfer them to open cribs when they are sufficiently mature to maintain their own temperatures in a surrounding nursery environment of 75° F (24° C) and their conditions require no special observations and treatments.

Nursing notes

Any variation in appearance or behavior may be extremely important and an early warning of disease or physiologic imbalance. Personnel on each nursery shift should record and report these changes.

The intensive nursing graphic is shown in Fig. 7-2 and presents a longitudinal record for the high-risk infant. This form is used to record the infant's and the incubator temperature, heart and respiratory rate per minute, oxygen concentration, stool and

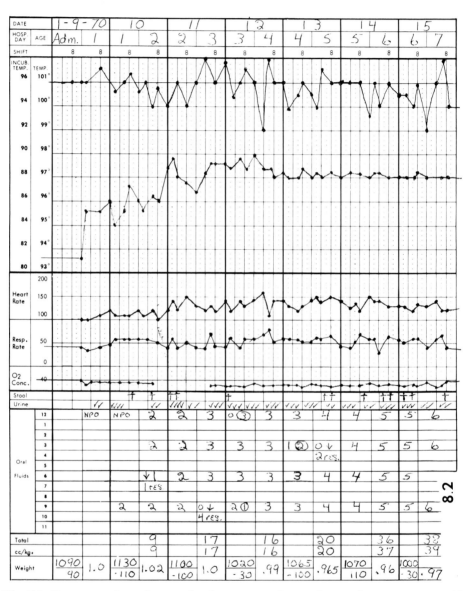

Fig. 7-2. Nursery graph to show vital information at the incubator side. Note unacceptable temperature of infant on admission, which jeopardizes his survival. Also the relatively high incubator temperature necessary to maintain a skin or axillary temperature of 97° F is an indication of extreme prematurity. Weight loss was minimal because of parenteral fluid administration while oral feedings were cautiously increased.

urine passages, feeding record, and the infant's weight. Nursing notes are minimized by using this record, and basic information is available to the physician and nurse from its inspection.

Miscellaneous care

1. Skin
   a. Dry skin care is recommended, except for cleansing of contaminated areas, such as buttocks, with plain water. Bathing with dilute pHisoHex (less than 3%), followed by thorough rinsing of the skin, may be indicated for an infant with skin lesions culturing *Staphylococcus aureus* or for all cohorts of a nursery

during a *Staphylococcus* epidemic. pHisoHex is potentially harmful when not thoroughly washed off, and its use in preterm infants under 1,500 gm may best be avoided because of the chance of neurotoxicity.
   b. Omit specific cord care. Nevertheless, a moist stump may be treated with 70% alcohol three times a day and exposure to air.
2. Nose, eyes, and mouth
   a. Aspirate any nasal secretions gently with a bulb syringe.
   b. Flush any eye debris or discharge with cotton dipped in sterile water (smear and culture recurring material).

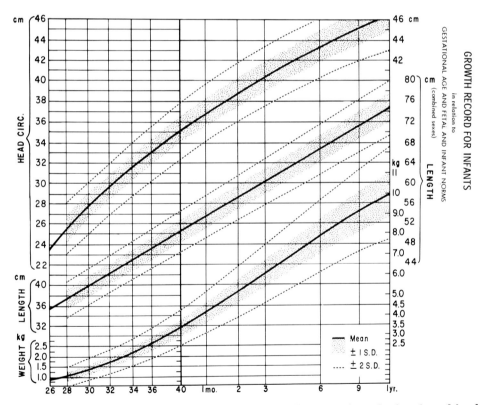

Fig. 7-3. Fetal infant growth graph, which shows growth curves of weight, length, and head circumference from 26 weeks of gestational age through 1 year of life after "term" has been reached. The curves have been smoothed through the usual transitional period of growth. Any disproportion among the three measurements, as well as deviations from the normal, can be easily recognized for evaluation. (Modified from Babson, S. G.: J. Pediatr. 77:11, 1970.)

c. Inspect the mouth daily for the white patches of thrush.
3. Urine and stool
   a. Expect urine to be passed in the first 24 hours. Time the first voiding and note the adequacy of the stream (especially in males).
   b. Observe for the time, color, and consistency of the first stool passage. There may be a delay of several days in the immature infant. Any distention should be reported to the physician.
4. Weighing and measuring
   a. Weigh the infant daily (sometimes more often) to gauge excessive weight changes. Any weight change of 2% or more daily after the initial weight loss (usually 5% to 10% of body weight) is an indication for clinical assessment.
   b. Weekly measurement of head circumference and body length allows a comparison of growth of each infant with self as well as with fetal-infant norms (Fig. 7-3).
5. Intramuscular injections
   a. Use a tuberculin syringe with a 25-gauge needle attached.
   b. Pick up thigh tissues between the thumb and forefinger.
   c. Aspirate and inject material at right angles into the mid anterolateral area. This technique avoids injury to the sciatic nerve and major leg vessels.

PARENT-INFANT RELATIONSHIPS

One very important yet easily neglected aspect of the care of a critically ill neonate, or even a "well" premature infant, is the role of parents. Their emotional shock over the advent of premature birth or the delivery of an infant with a major cardiac or surgical problem may be magnified as the infant is admitted to an intensive care unit.

It is the responsibility of the medical team to minimize the emotional stress of the parents and to encourage a mother-father-infant relationship in the following ways:

1. Preparing the parents antenatally for the problems their baby might have and the type of care their infant will probably receive
2. Explaining the purpose of equipment used for the care of their infant before entering the intensive care unit
3. Exhibiting empathy and tact in outlining the prognosis
4. Keeping parents informed at regular intervals about the progress of their infant or calling them promptly should the child's condition change drastically
5. Encouraging the parents to see and touch their baby as soon and as often as possible even if the infant is still critically ill or in an isolette
6. Having the parents share in the care of their baby whenever possible
7. Letting the mother feed her baby as soon as the infant can suck adequately on a soft nipple
8. Encouraging breast feeding once the infant is vigorous enough
9. Offering information the parents might desire about high-risk infants in general
10. Being frank and honest with them about their infant

By strengthening parent-infant ties during the hospitalization of their infant, the confidence of parents in caring for their baby after discharge will be supported and emotional stability of that family unit fostered.

CRITERIA FOR DISCHARGE FROM THE INTENSIVE CARE UNIT

Discharge is not dependent on weight but on the maturity and general health of the infant and the efficiency of the mother. A thorough physical examination is required, with neurologic assessment and visualization of the retina. Response to auditory and visual stimuli should be ascertained. Measurements of the head circumference and length are useful. The following are prerequisites to discharge from the nursery:

1. The assurance of at least 36 weeks of postmenstrual age, as determined by the infant's developmental state from longitudinal observations (growth and development, Chapter 26)
2. The conclusion of treatment for disease or congenital anomalies
3. Adequate oral intake and satisfactory gain in weight
4. A hematocrit over 25% (8 gm of hemoglobin), or if it is less, a reticulocyte count of 3% or more
5. An adequate home environment, as determined by the visiting public health nurse or personally by the private physician, and freedom from infectious diseases in the home
6. Ability of the mother to care for her infant

RESPONSIBILITIES OF THE PUBLIC HEALTH NURSE

A visit to the home by a public health nurse should be scheduled as soon as the infant's survival is reasonably ensured. This nurse may note environmental problems of which even the physician is unaware. Home visits are for the following purposes:

1. Establishing a meaningful relationship with the parents to be able to give effective help in readying the home to receive the baby and to provide ongoing supervision if needed
2. Determining the capabilities of the mother and recognizing and working on special needs and problems
3. Reporting observations and plans to the physician and hospital staff
4. Supporting the family through the period of separation while the baby is hospitalized

5. Reassuring the parents as they become acquainted with parenthood and the new baby
6. Demonstrating procedures such as formula preparation, feeding, bathing, and dressing the baby
7. Supplying information that will increase parental understanding of the child's behavior
8. Observing the growth and development of the child
9. Emphasizing the need for good medical supervision

Many emotionally immature parents are not ready to assume the responsibility of raising an infant. By design or through ignorance some infants are neglected. Recognition of this fact by the alert nurse or physician is important for the child's welfare.

Because of the circumstances surrounding the baby's birth, the mother has been identified as at high risk. An important aspect of the nursing visits will be to ensure interpregnancy health supervision in an effort to prevent subsequent high-risk infants.

RESPONSIBILITIES OF THE SOCIAL WORKER

The hospital social worker is part of the ward team and participates in planning at discharge to be aware of the needs of the family and any special requirement deemed advisable by the physician. The social worker is a supportive person as well as a sympathetic listener; most high-risk infants are a source of anxiety to the parents.

Social service does not duplicate the services of public health nursing or other disciplines. It implements team recommendations for optimum care and personal adjustment of the patient and family.

Discharge planning is a process that begins with the patient's admission to the hospital. The social worker's role is to (1) interview the family regarding social health, attitudes toward the infant's problems, and acceptance of the infant by both father and mother; (2) provide the health team with information on social, economic, or family problems; (3) contact resources in the community for the provision of health care needed by the family in total care of the infant; and (4) give support directly to the family by providing a relationship of trust, setting the stage for the alleviation of anxieties.

SPECIAL ADVICE FOR THE MOTHER

When discharged, low birth weight infants may be as sturdy as full-term newborn infants. Therefore they should be handled in the same easy way and with the same loving attention.

1. General instructions
   a. Protection against illness
      All babies are susceptible to illness. We therefore recommend the following specific care:
      1. Wash the hands before feeding or handling and after diapering the baby.
      2. Keep everyone who has the "flu," a cold, a sore throat, a cough, diarrhea, or a skin infection away from the baby during the first year.
      3. Restrict handling of the infant by friends and relatives during the first few months.
   b. Control of room temperature
      1. Maintain the temperature at about 70° to 72° F (22° C) during the day.
      2. Prevent a drop in temperature below 60° F (16° C) at night until the infant is 6 months of age.
   c. Clothing
      1. Clothe the child according to the temperature, always lightly enough to avoid perspiration or heat rash.

   2. Avoid rubber or plastic pants, which promote diaper rash.
   3. Do not restrict the infant's activity.
   d. Bathing (two or three baths a week are sufficient)
      1. Use a warmer room (75° to 78° F, 25° C). The water should be comfortable to the elbow.
      2. Apply a mild antiseptic soap such as Dial, and use it sparingly. Oils and lotions are best avoided.
   e. First outing
      1. Delay outings until after the first visits to the physician or clinic.
      2. Avoid crowds during the first year.
2. Feeding
   Directions for making formula are given at the time of discharge. The following points will be helpful to the mother in feeding her baby:
   a. Hold the baby in the arms in a comfortable, relaxed way.
   b. Tilt the bottle so that the milk fills the nipple to help prevent the sucking in of air.
   c. Rest the baby for a few minutes during the feeding.
   d. Burp the baby by gentle patting of the back while in an upright position. This should be done at least once during the feeding and again at the end to allow the air out that has been swallowed with the milk. Placing the infant on the stomach will often help in the release of this air. Failure to burp the baby well may cause discomfort later.
   e. See that nipple holes are of adequate size.
      1. They should be large enough to permit the milk, when cooled a little, to drop about as fast as it can without running in a stream.
      2. If the holes are too small, the baby may get tired and stop before having enough to eat. *This*

is the most common reason for feeding problems.

   3. Holes may be enlarged by inserting the point of a red-hot needle held in a cork, in a raw vegetable, or with pliers.

   f. Ignore the spitting up of small amounts of milk unless choking occurs.

   g. Do not give the baby more milk than desired. The amount may vary from feeding to feeding. The baby is the best judge of the amount, if the nipple hole is large enough.

   h. Allow the baby to set feeding intervals (between 3 and 5 hours). The night feeding may be skipped if the infant does not wake for it.

3. Special supplements

   a. Iron medication is to be given daily for the first year of life unless it is contained in the formula. It will be added to the milk according to the nurse's directions.

   b. Vitamin mixtures are to be given daily for at least the first year of life.

4. Medical care for premature infants

   a. Have the mother report any variation in behavior such as the following to the physician or clinic responsible for the infant's care:

     1. Repeated vomiting or diarrhea
     2. Difficulty with breathing
     3. Change in color
     4. Refusal of milk
     5. Overly quiet or "too fussy" behavior

   b. Suggest an appointment between the first and fourth week after discharge, depending on the physician's decision.

THE SPECIALIZED NEONATAL NURSE

As in other intensive care units, the neonatal nurse specialist works with the physician as a team member. Because such nurses have more contact with the infant, they are likely to be the first to recognize a significant change in an infant's clinical state and to offer appropriate care, often as an emergency. Therefore they must be trained and knowledgeable in the diagnosis and management of conditions encountered in neonates in an intensive care unit. Other responsibilities of the neonatal nurse in a specialized center include the following:

1. Maintenance of parenteral infusions
2. Drawing of blood gases and recognizing numerical deviations in their measurements
3. Application of monitoring equipment
4. Familiarity with oxygen administration on the basis of hypoxia
5. Performance of Dextrostix and Clinistix tests and understanding their significance
6. Passage of orogastric tube, performance of suctioning and maintenance of tube in situ when indicated
7. Understanding correct drug dosages and methods of intravenous and intramuscular administration
8. Measurement of blood pressure and familiarity with its variations
9. Initiation of rewarming as well as maintenance of the infant's thermoneutrality
10. Adept at suction and positive pressure ventilation with bag and mask in extended apnea
11. Ready contact with physicians in charge for reporting all significant variations in patient behavior
12. Encouragement and support of parent-infant binding

In the sophisticated center capable of offering continued assisted ventilation, in addition to the previous list, the specialized neonatal nurse should be trained in and capable of the following:

1. Recognizing respiratory failure and need for ventilatory support
2. Performing tracheal suction and pul-

monary physiotherapy for infants on respirators

3. Recognizing failure in ventilator support because of the following:
   a. Mechanical failure of equipment
   b. Obstruction in or displacement of endotracheal tube
   c. Pneumothorax
   d. Shock and hypotension
4. Performing emergency intubation
5. Placing umbilical artery catheter

In the transport of high-risk infants to a regional intensive care center (Chapter 11), the specially trained neonatal nurse stands out as a key figure in such a program. Its success is directly related to the degree of training and capability of the transporting team. The vast numbers of high-risk neonates requiring transport and specialized care lend importance to the development of training programs for such highly skilled nurses to assure intact survival. This goal may well be more dependent on the alert and trained nurse who has elected to make a profession of neonatal nursing than on any other member of the neonatal team.

PROCEDURES

Any procedure performed on a distressed or small infant should be accomplished in an incubator or under radiant heat and appropriate supplemental oxygen.

Peripheral vein infusion

1. Use a sharp needle (23 to 25 gauge) suitable to the vein size. The scalp vein needle set with winged tabs and plastic tubing is recommended (Abbott).
2. Prepare the skin with suitable antiseptic.
3. Distend the veins by compression proximal to the point of needle entry. An elastic band placed around the head will accomplish this distention for scalp veins.
4. Grasp the tabs between thumb and

forefinger and insert the needle, bevel up, into the skin a short distance above the selected site of venipuncture after filling the set with solution.

5. Introduce the needle into the center of the distended vein and advance it well into the vein. Blood will appear in the attached tubing.
6. Release vein compression and attach to infusion pump (Holter, Harvard, IVAC, Sigma-motor) after clearing contained air, and apply tape for needle restraint.

Umbilical vessel catheterization

Catheterization of umbilical vessels is an additional hazard to the infant, since it may result in thrombosis, necrosis, emboli, or sepsis.

1. General guidelines
   a. Observe sterile technique.
   b. Keep the infant warm.
   c. Supply oxygen if needed during procedure.
   d. Use radiopaque end hole catheters only (Argyle).
   e. Prepare infant's abdomen with organic iodine and wash with alcohol and let dry.
   f. Remove catheters immediately if
      1. Signs of arterial spasm or darkening of tips of toes occurs.
      2. Clots are visible in the catheter and cannot be aspirated.
      3. Signs of omphalitis or sepsis develop.
2. Umbilical vein
   a. Candidates for umbilical vein catheterization
      1. Asphyxiated infants in the delivery room
      2. Infants who require monitoring of cardiovascular pressure
      3. Infants who need temporary infusion of glucose and electrolyte solutions when other avenues are impossible

4. Neonates who require exchange transfusion
  b. Technique
    1. Mark catheter (part to be inserted) at a point representing 60% of the perpendicular distance from level of shoulders to the umbilicus (about 5 to 7 cm).
    2. Make fresh cut across cord about 1 cm from skin.
    3. Grab thin-walled vein with forceps; located anteriorly.
    4. Insert gently Fr 5 or 8 radiopaque catheter while exerting traction on cord stump (helps to relieve obstruction at level of abdominal wall).
    5. Withdraw tip several centimeters and rotate forward if obstruction is met in portal area.
    6. Attempt to place catheter in inferior vena cava (avoids liver damage).
    7. Check placement by x-ray examination for continued use of emergency infusions.
3. Umbilical artery
  a. Candidates for umbilical artery catheterization
    1. Infants with respiratory distress in need of frequent blood gas sampling
    2. Small premature infants who frequently develop severe apneic attacks during the first few days of life and require quite high concentrations of oxygen, making sequential blood gas determinations necessary
    3. Infants severely ill due to other causes (septic shock, etc.) for continued infusion of emergency medications
  b. Technique
    1. Take a radiopaque catheter (Fr 3½ or 5).
    2. Cut off and discard the last 9 cm of the wide end of the catheter.
    3. Insert a blunt No. 18 needle into this end to reduce dead space.
    4. Attach a sterile stopcock, fill the system with heparinized solution (1 unit of heparin per milliliter of normal saline solution), free of air bubbles, and turn stopcock to the catheter off.
    5. Mark catheter for insertion at a point from tip one third the baby's crown-heel length (12 to 17 cm).
    6. Make a fresh cut across cord.
    7. Use of a small Iris forceps for initial dilatation of the umbilical artery is helpful for insertion of a catheter into this vessel.
    8. Overcome obstruction at level of abdominal wall by gentle traction on umbilicus.
    9. Relieve obstruction at level of bladder by gentle steady pressure for 30 to 60 seconds. *Never use force.*
    10. Prevent accidental removal of catheters by suturing them to the umbilical stump.
    11. Obtain x-ray film of abdomen and chest to assure proper location.
    12. Locate tip above the diaphragm (between seventh and ninth thoracic vertebrae), or just above the aortic bifurcation (between the third and fourth lumbar vertebrae). If the catheter needs to be repositioned, do not advance it further once the sterile field has been contaminated, but reinsert a new catheter using sterile technique. However, you may withdraw the catheter to a new position if necessary.
    13. To minimize infection, change dressing and apply neomycin ointment daily to umbilical stump. Have stopcock and syringes changed every 8 hours or whenever they do not appear to

be clean or when they contain visible clots. If clots or debris are seen in a catheter and cannot be aspirated (never flush them into the infant), the catheter must be removed and replaced with a new one.

14. To prevent clotting of an umbilical catheter
    a. The catheter may be used for continuous infusion of parenteral fluids.
    b. After obtaining blood samples, flush catheter with heparinized saline solution (1 unit of heparin/ml).

Blood gas sampling

1. From arterial catheter
    a. With a clean syringe, aspirate contents of catheter (approximately 1 ml).
    b. With a tuberculin syringe—its dead space filled with heparin—slowly aspirate 0.5 ml of blood, preventing air bubbles from entering the syringe.
    c. Cap syringe, rotate it in the hands to enhance mixing, and place it entirely in ice water. Send it to the laboratory at once for processing.
    d. Inject previously aspirated catheter contents into patient to prevent unnecessary loss of blood.
    e. Flush catheter with 1 ml of heparinized saline solution.
    f. Keep a record of amounts of blood aspirated and amounts of fluid used for flushing.
2. From heel stick
    a. Warm infant's foot by immersing it in warm water (40° C) for 5 minutes or wrapping it in a warm moist towel.
    b. Rub the heel with 70% alcohol on a cotton pledget and dry.
    c. Puncture the heel with a Bard-Parker No. 11 or Redi-lance blade, sufficiently deep to obtain a free flow of blood.

d. Discard the first drop and rapidly collect the blood free of air bubbles in the proper capillary tubes.
    e. Insert metal sliver into capillary tube.
    f. Tightly seal ends of tube.
    g. Mix blood by sliding magnet over capillary tube, which will move metal sliver through the blood.
    h. Place capillary tube in ice water and take to laboratory for processing.
3. Arterial puncture
    a. Prepare the skin over the vessel.
    b. With heparin solution, fill the dead space of a tight-fitting tuberculin syringe, using a firmly attached 25-gauge needle.
    c. Insert the needle with the bevel up into the vessel.
    d. Withdraw the needle slowly with gentle suction on the syringe (a bubble-free sample of 0.5 ml is necessary).
    e. Hold a pledget of cotton firmly over the vessel to prevent hemorrhage.
    f. Seal the syringe and place it in ice water for determination of blood gases.

Spinal fluid tap

1. Technique
    a. Have the infant held firmly in a sitting or side position, with his spine flexed.
    b. Use a 22-gauge short spinal needle or a 23-gauge disposable needle.
    c. Mark the iliac crests with a skin pencil.
    d. Enter the intervertebral space opposite the crest marks.
    e. Slowly insert the needle (0.5 to 1.5 cm), directed toward the sternum.*
    f. Supply external heat to the infant.
2. Usual findings
    a. Cells less than 10/mm³ (more than five polymorphonuclear leukocytes suggests meningitis)

---

*Blood-colored fluid from trauma should clear.

b. Protein less than 100 mg/100 ml
c. Glucose more than 20 mg/100 ml (less than 50% of the blood glucose level supports a diagnosis of bacterial meningitis)
d. Xanthochromia (at 1 to 20 days of age)

Subdural tap

1. Technique
   a. Use a short-bevel, 20 to 22-gauge spinal needle.
   b. Hold the needle close to the point and insert to a depth of about 0.5 cm through the coronal suture, about 3 to 6 cm from the midline of the vertex.
   c. Direct at right angles to the surface.
   d. Feel a "pop" to signify entry.
   e. Allow backflow in place of aspiration.
2. In the normal infant only a few drops of clear to pinkish fluid are obtained.

Transillumination

Edema of the scalp from any cause will reflect light, which may give a falsely positive observation.
1. Technique
   a. Dark-adapt the eyes in a dark room.
   b. Apply a rubber-cuffed flashlight* to the cranial vault and move the flashlight over the brain areas.
   c. Maintain the flashlight in contact with the skin.
2. Usual findings in the premature infant
   a. Areas of transmitted light are seen, measuring from 2 to 4 cm, depending on maturity.
   b. Some increase in transmission of light will be noted in the more immature infants at 6 to 8 weeks of age.
   c. A gradual decrease will occur during the first year of life.

___
*Rubber bushings from Pour-O-Vac 10-gallon jugs make excellent covers for use in flashlight application.

Aspiration of tension pneumothorax

1. Attach 21-gauge needle to three-way stopcock and 30 ml syringe; turn stopcock off to needle.
2. Prepare skin over anterior thorax with organic iodine, followed by alcohol.
3. Carefully introduce needle vertically into pleural cavity through fourth or fifth costal interspace in anterior axillary line.
4. Open stopcock to syringe and aspirate air; then withdraw needle from patient, holding gentle pressure over site of entry for a few seconds.

Technique of retinal examination

1. Dilate the pupils with one drop of tropicamide (Mydriacyl) or 1% phenylephrine hydrochloride (Neo-Synephrine) 1 hour before observation.
2. Darken the room and hold the lids away from the pupils with the help of an assistant.
3. Keep a nipple in the infant's mouth to relax him.

Techniques of urine collection

Urine examinations for bacteria are of questionable value unless the collection is critically supervised. Occasionally, unsuspected pyuria may be discovered during the nursery course. A carefully collected urine specimen is particularly important when illness is considered. A few pus cells per high-power field or the presence of one or more bacteria in a stained, concentrated smear under the oil immersion lens indicates the necessity for a culture and bacterial count of urine obtained by bladder tap.
1. Urethra or penis
   a. Wash the genital area thoroughly with pHisoHex solution.
   b. Apply a plastic urine collector* to the infant after the diaper has remained dry for at least 1 hour.

___
*Two-chambered U-Bag (Hollister).

c. Observe closely for urination so that a clean, freshly voided specimen can be immediately processed.

2. Bladder tap

When positive cultures are obtained by urine collection or sepsis is considered possible, urine specimens for smear and culture are best obtained by bladder tap.

   a. Wait at least 1 hour after urine passage.
   b. Obstruct the urethra with a finger or fingers.
   c. Prepare suprapubic skin.
   d. Insert slowly a 3 cm, 22-gauge needle just above the symphysis pubis in the midline toward the vertebral column with slight negative pressure applied to the plunger.

Technique for Dextrostix screening

Longitudinal qualitative blood glucose screening is necessary for oversized infants, infants of diabetic mothers, and all small-for-dates or malnourished infants. Infants demonstrating apnea, eye-rolling, tremors, or other signs of hypoglycemia are screened in addition.

1. In Dextrostix testing, follow the manufacturer's directions (Ames).*
2. Obtain a quantitative laboratory confirmation in all screens in which a faint blue color is not seen (usually under 30 mg/100 ml).

Intubation

See p. 80.

SELECTED REFERENCES

Baker, D. H., Berdon, W. E., and James, L. S.: Proper localization of umbilical arterial and venous catheters by lateral roentgenograms, Pediatrics 43:34, 1969.

*The use of the Ames Reflectance meter is a more precise qualitative method for blood glucose screening.

Buctow, K. C., and Klein, S. W.: Effect of maintenance of "normal" skin temperature on survival of infants of low birth weight, Pediatrics 34:163, 1964.

Chernick, V., and Raber, M. B.: Electrical hazards in the newborn nursery, J. Pediatr. 77:143, 1970.

Cochran, W. D., Davis, H. T., and Smith, C. A.: Advantages and complications of umbilical artery catheterization in the newborn, Pediatrics 42:769, 1968.

Dunn, P.: Localization of the umbilical catheter by post mortem measurements, Arch. Dis. Child. 41:69, 1966.

Hey, E. N., and Mount, L. E.: Heat losses from babies in incubators, Arch. Dis. Child. 42:75, 1967.

Lucey, J., editor: Problems of neonatal care units, report of 59th Ross Conference, Columbus, Ohio, 1969, Ross Laboratories.

Neal, W. A., Reynolds, J. W., Jarvis, C. W., and Williams, H. J.: Umbilical artery catheterization: demonstration of arterial thrombosis by aortography, Pediatrics 50:6, 1972.

Silverman, W. A.: The effect of the atmospheric environment on the premature infants, J. Pediatr. 58:581, 1961.

Silverman, W. A.: Diagnosis and treatment: use and misuse of temperature and humidity in care of the newborn infant, Pediatrics 33:276, 1964.

Silverman, W. A.: Intensive care of the low birth weight and other at-risk infants, Clin. Obstet. Gynecol. 13:87, 1970.

Silverman, W. A., Agate, F. J., Jr., and Fertif, J. W.: A sequential trial of the nonthermal effect of atmospheric humidity on survival of newborn infants of low birth weight, Pediatrics 31:719, 1963.

Standards and recommendations for hospital care of newborn infants, Evanston, Ill., 1971, American Academy of Pediatrics.

Stein, B., Lucey, J. F., and Tooley, W. H.: Grounding and electrical leakage of phototherapy equipment, Pediatrics 44:614, 1969.

Vapaavuori, E. K., and Raiha, N. C. R.: Intensive care of small premature infants, Acta Paediatr. Scand. 59:353, 1970.

Wigger, H. J., Bransilner, B. R., and Blane, W. H.: Thromboses due to catheterization in infants and children, J. Pediatr. 76:1, 1970.

Williams, C. P. S., and Oliver, T. K., Jr.: Nursery routines and staphylococcal colonization of the newborn, Pediatrics 44:140, 1969.

8

Feeding the infant at risk, including supplemental and total parenteral alimentation

WATER BALANCE

Early and adequate provision of calories and water is now accepted as vital for the preterm, malnourished, or stressed infant who, in addition to exposure of asphyxia at birth, has been abruptly separated from the placental lifeline. Limited or depleted nutritional reserves, increased metabolic demands because of respiratory effort, evaporation losses under radiant heat and phototherapy, and gastrointestinal and renal immaturity, as well as the requirements for growth at a critical period, pose a challenge. Supplying a thermoneutral environment for minimal caloric expenditure and attention to the infant's nutritional and water requirements are undoubtedly major factors in decreased neonatal mortality and morbidity in the last 10 years.

Heird and associates have estimated that an infant weighing 1,000 gm, if supplied with water alone, can survive for 4 or 5 days with his calorie stores. The addition of 10% glucose (75 ml/kg/24 hr) can support life for only 10 or 11 days. The hazards of thirsting and fasting include depression of blood glucose, nitrogen loss, acidosis, rise in plasma osmolality,* and a delay in me-conium passage that intensifies bilirubinemia.

Weight loss

The large fluid component of the preterm infant (up to 85% of body weight, most of which is extracellular water) magnifies the weight loss even without delay of fluid administration or feeding.

Other factors in early weight loss include the following:
1. Insufficient fluid intake
2. Evaporation losses through the thin skin exposed directly to radiant heat (up to 4 ml/kg/hr)
3. Insensible water loss from lungs, increased by tachypnea and low humidity (15 ml/kg/24 hr)
4. Water loss by catabolism
5. Miscellaneous: osmotic diuresis, inhibition of antidiuretic hormone (ADH), passage of meconium

Acceptable weight loss limits are as follows:
1. Preterm—10% to 12%
2. Term—5% to 10%
3. Dysmature and undergrown—0% to 5%

---

*Plasma osmolality should be maintained below 300 mOsm/L and can be estimated from this simple equation:

$$2 \times Na(mEq/L) + \frac{Glucose \ (mg/100 \ ml)}{18} + \frac{BUN \ (mg/100 \ ml)}{3}$$

After the first 3 days of life, weight loss or gain should not exceed 2% of the weight on the previous day. With ample calories and protein, the preterm infant should gain 15 gm/kg/24 hr, with an accretion of as much as 360 mg/kg of nitrogen.

Kidney and water balance

In the first week after birth, the capacity of the kidney to concentrate is limited because of its low rate of excretion of urea, shortness of the loop of Henle, and diminished response to ADH. It may concentrate up to 700 mOsm/L or, in the very premature, it can be as low as 300 mOsm/L. Therefore an infant weighing 1,000 gm may not be able to excrete more than 18 mOsm in 60 ml of urine (approximate volume with fluid intake of 150 ml/kg/24 hr). Some high-solute formulas offer more solute load (Table 8-3) than can be excreted in the available urine volume, particularly when the extra renal losses are high. Each gram of tissue accreted, however, utilizes 0.9 mOsm (Sinclair and colleagues).

A satisfactory estimate of renal solute load can be determined by the Ziegler-Fomon formula:

$$\left. \begin{array}{l} \text{gm/100 ml protein} \times 4 \\ + \\ \text{mEq of Na+, K+, Cl} \times 1 \end{array} \right\} \quad \text{mOsm/100 ml}^{\circ}$$

With decreased capacity for net acid excretion in the preterm infant, development of oliguria in respiratory distress syndrome (RDS), and acute tubular necrosis (ATN) after perinatal asphyxia, frequent use of bicarbonate infusions and increased evaporation loss through the skin makes diligent and careful attention to electrolyte balance a vital priority. At times, a striking polyuria occurs, with a

---

°In Similac 24 given at 150 ml/kg 24 hr:

$$\begin{array}{rcl} 3.3 \text{ gm protein} & \times 4 = & 13.2 \\ 9.2 \text{ mEq of electrolyte} & \times 1 = & 9.1 \\ \hline & & 22.3 \text{ mOsm/kg} \end{array}$$

loss of Na+, resulting in hyponatremia with hypotonicity of serum and increased urinary osmolality. Inappropriate ADH may be an important factor. The most effective therapy is the restriction of fluids only. Administration of isotonic saline solution will cause a further dumping of Na+ in the urine.

NUTRITIONAL REQUIREMENTS
Caloric expenditure

The energy metabolism of the low birth weight infant at first is less than that of the term infant, but metabolism gradually accelerates so that by 2 weeks of age it is considerably higher. The stressed or small-for-dates infant's oxygen consumption per kilogram is even greater than that of the average preterm infant. Table 8-1 presents the daily caloric expenditure of a growing preterm infant.

Nutritional requirements for low birth weight infants

Wide variation exists in the composition of milk formulas used. For example, infant feeding experience attests to the successful outcome for premature infants who have been fed either low-protein (1.5%) milk

Table 8-1. Caloric requirements (appropriate weight for gestation—preterm infants)

Item	Calories/kg/24 hr	
Resting	40 to 50	(depending on age)
Activity	10 to 15	
Cold stress	5 to 10	(depending on environmental temperature)
Specific dynamic action	8 to 8	
Fecal loss	2* to 12	
Growth	25 to 25	
Total	90 120	

*On parenteral feedings.

formulas with a low-mineral content (0.2%) or high-protein (4%) and high-mineral (0.7%) mixtures.

Since the fetus has a growth rate nearly double that of the term infant in the last trimester, a cogent argument can be made for supplying an increased nutritional substrate to the premature infant in order for him to approach this intrauterine growth rate. However, weight gain that surpasses the fetal rate may reflect retention of water and is no advantage to the infant. Protein

in excess of 4 gm/kg/24 hr may be detrimental.

1. Possible disadvantages of a humanized milk mixture*
   a. Growth of infants receiving formulas of low-protein composition is slower when compared with the growth of infants receiving higher amounts of protein but with the same caloric intake.
   b. Time of discharge as measured by weight may be inappropriately postponed.
   c. Serum albumin is more often found to be less than 3 gm/100 ml
2. Disadvantages of high-protein and high-mineral milk mixtures
   a. The solute load may be excessive for renal excretion.
   b. Significant edema may develop.
   c. Urea nitrogen and certain amino acids, phenylalanine and tyrosine, may rise to high levels in blood serum.
   d. Metabolic acidosis—disproportion between daily net load of nonvolatile acids and the renal capacity for H^+ excretion—may occur.
3. Range in feeding requirements of low birth weight infants (Table 8-2)

Table 8-2. Range in daily feeding requirements of low birth weight infants per kilogram of body weight

Nutrient requirements		First week of life	Active growth period
Water (ml)		80-200	130-200
Calories		50-100	110-150*
Protein	(gm)	1-2	3-4
Glucose		7-12	12-15
Fat		3-4	5-8
Sodium		1-2	2-3
Potassium		1-2	2-4
Chloride	(mEq)	1-2	2-3
Calcium		1-2	3-5
Phosphorus		1-2	2-4
Magnesium		—	0.5-1.0
Iron (mg)			1.5-2.0

*Calorie requirements of over 120/kg apply to infants with perinatal undergrowth.

*Cow's milk altered to near the composition of human milk.

Table 8-3. Contents of various milks/100 ml

	Human	Cow	Enfamil With Iron	Similac With Iron	Similac 24 With Iron	PM 60/40	SMA	SMA 27
Protein (gm)	1.3	3.3	1.5	1.8	2.2	1.6	1.5	2.0
Fat (gm)	3.5	3.7	3.7	3.6	4.3	3.5	3.5	4.9
CHO (gm)	7.0	4.8	7.0	7.0	8.4	7.5	7.0	9.7
Na+ (mEq)	0.65	2.5	1.1	1.3	1.6	0.65	0.65	0.9
K+ (mEq)	1.4	3.5	1.9	2.6	2.6	1.5	1.4	1.9
Ca++ (mEq)	1.7	6.0	3.2	3.5	4.0	1.7	2.2	3.0
Po4-- (mEq)	1.0	6.2	2.9	2.9	3.5	1.2	2.1	2.8
Cl- (mEq)	1.0	2.7	1.1	1.8	1.9	1.3	1.0	1.4
Calories	67.0	67.0	67.0	67.0	80.0	67.0	67.0	90.0
Iron (mg)			1.25	1.2	1.2	0.2	1.25	1.69
Renal solute load (mOsm)	8.25	21.9	10.1	12.9	14.9	9.9	9.1	12.2

Table 8-4. Daily vitamin requirements (National Research Council)

A	1,500	IU
Thiamine	0.2	mg
Riboflavin	0.4	mg
Pyridoxine	0.2	mg
B_{12}	1.0	μg
C	35	mg
D	400	IU
E	5	IU
Niacin	6.0	mg
Panthenol	—	
Folic acid	0.05	mg
K	1.0	mg

4. For contents of various milks used in infant feedings, see Table 8-3.
5. Vitamin requirements (Table 8-4)
   a. Administer vitamin K_1, (Aqua-Mephyton), 0.5 to 1 mg, or equivalent, on the first day of life.
   b. Add multivitamin mixtures, including pyridoxine and vitamin E, daily to the formula by the third day of life.
   c. Supply parenteral vitamin mixtures when oral feedings are delayed.
6. Iron
   Add 10 to 15 mg of elemental iron daily by the age of 2 months, for example, Ferro drops. Milk products containing iron supplements are sufficient for iron requirements when a formula intake of approximately 1 L/24 hr is achieved.
7. Criteria for assessment of adequacy of feeding
   a. Plot daily growth in weight and weekly length and head circumference on fetal-infant growth chart (Fig. 7-3). Growth lines tend to parallel standard growth curves after the first week or two of life.
   b. A blood urea nitrogen (BUN) level between 10 and 25 mg/100 ml will assure an ample but not excessive protein intake.
   c. Aim at a serum albumin of over 3 gm/100 ml to avoid edema.

When to start feedings

The infant at risk requires water, glucose, and certain electrolytes from the time of birth. Feedings by mouth may be tolerated by undergrown, dysmature, and many preterm infants sufficient to prevent hypoglycemia and further catabolic stress, but often parenteral infusions are necessary to provide initial requirements. When gastric feedings must be delayed for days, and certainly beyond a week, parenteral alimentation—preferably through a peripheral vein line—can maintain most infants in positive nitrogen balance for many weeks until oral feedings can be offered safely. Some infants can accept and will benefit from indwelling catheters placed through the pylorus. We do not recommend gastric feedings until the following conditions are met:

1. Stable respirations, with no respiratory distress
2. Absence of distention, with adequate bowel sounds
3. Acceptance of feedings with minimal residual and apneic episodes

FEEDING PLANS
Very small infants (unable to suck and usually under 1,300 gm but otherwise in fair condition)

1. Start 10% glucose infusion in the first few hours of life at a rate of 100 ml/kg/24 hr.
2. Add 3 ml of 10% calcium gluconate* (1 ml = 0.45 mEq Ca^{++}) per 100 ml of solution and 1 to 2 mEq of Na^+, K^+, and Cl^- in the form of concentrate, for example, 0.5 ml of NaCl (2.5 mEq/ml) and 1 ml of K^+ lactate (2 mEq/ml).
3. Increase rate of infusion by 10 to 20 ml/kg/24 hr to a total of approximately 150 to 200 ml/kg/24 hr, de-

*Intravenous calcium prevents acute hypocalcemia ·common in low birth weight infants after interruption of the placental lifeline.

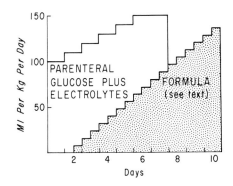

Fig. 8-1. Example of combined parenteral and oral feeding in milliliters per kilogram per day for a newborn infant weighing less than 1,500 gm at birth who is unable to suck. Increases of 2 ml/kg/24 hr of oral feeding from an initial intake of 2 to 3 ml achieve an intake of approximately 100 ml/kg/24 hr by 7 days of age. Many infants will not tolerate this volume of intake without abdominal distention, regurgitation, and risk of aspiration; continuation of parenteral fluids is advisable for these infants. (Modified from Babson, S. G.: J. Pediatr. **79**:694, 1971.)

pending on weight loss* (Fig. 8-1).

4. Check urine every 3 hours with Clinistix and if 1⁺ or more and/or if Dextrostix shows over 130 mg/100 ml, obtain blood glucose value.* If above 150/mg/100 ml, reduce glucose concentration or rate of infusion.

5. Begin oral feedings of 2 ml/kg of 20-calorie/30 ml formula by gavage every 3 hours when the condition has definitely stabilized.

6. Increase feeding by approximately 1 ml/kg/12 hr.

7. Reduce volume of infused fluids as oral feedings are increased, keeping total volume at approximately 150 ml/kg/24 hr.

8. Increase caloric concentration after several days to 24 or 27 calories/30 ml of formulas of low-solute load (Table 8-3) if condition is satisfactory and stomach residual is not over 1 ml.

9. Discontinue intravenous fluid when oral feedings have reached at least 100 ml/kg/24 hr.

10. Limit gavage feedings to 130 to 150 ml/kg/24 hr, and calories to 120/kg/24 hr. Increases above these levels are dependent on desires of infant when taking nipple, assuming 33 to 34 weeks of postmenstrual age.

11. Begin multivitamins, 0.3 ml daily, with first milk feeding.

12. Discontinue oral feedings if there is distention,* regurgitation, significant residual over 2 ml, or an increase in apneic periods. Reinstitute parenteral fluids and consider intravenous alimentation (p. 114).

Larger premature infants in good condition

1. Start with 4 to 10 ml of 20-calorie formula by 12 hours of age if condition has stabilized and offer every 3 hours if accepted by nipple. Precede with one feeding of sterile water to test feeding behavior in case of aspiration from pharyngeal incoordination.

2. Increase by 3 to 5 ml every 12 hours if accepted, to achieve an intake of 100 to 120 ml/kg of body weight by 1 week of age, and 130 to 180 ml/kg by 2 weeks. Generally, bottle-fed infants may choose their volume.

3. Gradually strengthen calorie concentration to 24 calories/30 ml in small-for-dates or hungry-acting infants.

---

*The greater volumes of fluid now used in the immature infant to compensate for evaporative skin losses have posed a problem in osmotic diuresis due to glucosuria. The glucose load must often be limited to less than 0.5 gm/kg/hr in the first days of life, which may mean reducing the glucose concentration of infused solutions.

*Distention and ileus are serious signs that may indicate infection or overfeeding, or be harbingers of necrotizing enterocolitis. Prompt discontinuation of feedings in such instances may reduce the incidence of this serious disease (Chapter 21).

4. Discontinue or reduce feeding if distention, regurgitation, diarrhea, or cyanosis occurs and supplement or substitute parenteral alimentation.
5. Give multivitamins, 0.3 ml, by the third day.
6. Breast feeding may begin at 35 to 36 weeks of postmenstrual age if the infant is vigorous.

Undersized and undernourished (small-for-dates and dysmature) infants

1. Feed 20-calorie/30 ml formula, if tolerated, to active and stable infants at 2-hour intervals, starting soon after birth. Precede with one water feeding.
2. Change to a formula of 24 to 30 calories/30 ml after a day or two.
3. Perform the Dextrostix* test every 4 to 6 hours for 48 hours until blood glucose is stabilized over 50 mg/100 ml.
4. Infuse 10% glucose if oral intake is not satisfactory, there is evidence of hypoglycemia, or weight loss exceeds 5%.
5. Continue to monitor blood glucose even after starting intravenous glucose and a few hours after its discontinuation to avoid rebound hypoglycemia.
6. Wash stomach with 5 to 10 ml of water or saline solution if there is evidence of mucus vomiting (common in the dysmature).

General precautions in oral feedings

1. Consult nurses regarding volume increases.

---

*The use of Dextrostix (Ames) offers a qualitative test for blood glucose and tends to underestimate the true level at the low end of the color range. If the test paper shows an absence of easily recognizable pale blue color, a blood level below 30 mg/100 ml is likely, and an accurate quantitative determination is necessary in this event.

2. Encourage prompt discontinuance and reporting of feeding difficulties.
3. Spitting up is a sign of excessive or too early feedings.
4. Change in feeding habits such as disinterest in sucking, delayed emptying, or distention, may indicate sepsis or necrotizing enterocolitis.
5. Do not give gastric feedings when there is tachypnea or respiratory distress (particularly with assisted ventilation). We use parenteral feedings, followed by transpyloric feedings when extended ventilation support is required.

FEEDING TECHNIQUES

No method of feeding in the neonate at risk can be satisfactory to the exclusion of other methods. Frequently, indications justify a combination of methods as well as a progression in methods, beginning with vascular infusions, moving to gavage or transpyloric feedings, and ending with the nipple. None of the recently described feeding methods has been evaluated in sufficient depth to warrant recommendation as the best way to feed low birth weight infants. Percentage of weight loss, time needed to regain birth weight, and time needed to reach discharge weight are all useful measures of success in feeding. More important are the neurologic and intellectual end points that will eventually determine the success of any method or combination of methods currently in use.

Intermittent gavage

Intermittent gavage is preferred for the smaller preterm infant in no distress until sucking is established because it is safe, simple, quick, and easily taught.

1. Place the infant on his side or back. No restraint or handling of the infant is necessary.
2. Insert a soft Fr 8 catheter through the mouth, for a distance equal to that from the bridge of the nose to the xiphoid process.

3. Observe for choking or gasping, indicative of possible tracheal entry.
4. Attach a syringe to the feeding tube and aspirate gently. If there is feeding residual of 1 to 2 ml prior to the next feeding, the amount of the feeding should be decreased by the amount of the residual. Do not discard the residual—refeed it to the infant with the new formula. Report residual of more than 2 ml and skip that feeding.
5. Pour the formula through the barrel of the syringe, allowing the milk to run slowly, with no pressure and with minimal elevation of the syringe.
6. Pinch to close the tube, and withdraw it quickly.

Bottle feeding

The bottle-feeding technique requires a good sucking and swallowing reflex and should be tried when the infant sucks the gavage tube (32 to 33 weeks of postmenstrual age). The time of feeding should not exceed 15 minutes. The procedure is accomplished by the following:

1. Using a soft, average-sized nipple with an adequate opening.
2. Applying gentle pressure on the infant's chin and touching his lip with the nipple to help him open his mouth.
3. Holding the infant semierect to facilitate nursing and "burping" when he is kept in the incubator.
4. Turning the infant on his side or abdomen when the feeding is finished. When the infant is dressed, he is removed from the incubator or bassinet and held by the nurse in a rocking chair for all feedings.

Precautions

1. Do not urge the infant to accept more than is easily taken. Be prepared to remove the nipple if he is getting milk too fast.

2. Assess clinically any infant showing reluctance to eat on two successive occasions.
3. Stop the feedings if the baby vomits, becomes cyanotic or distended, or if the stools become liquid or frequent.
4. Do not prop the bottle.

Any change in feeding habits may be the first sign of illness.

Nasogastric feeding

The newly developed smaller plastic catheters, Fr 3½ to 5, have an advantage over larger catheters for indwelling tube feedings. Many centers successfully use this method for intermittent or continuous feeding of the immature infant. The catheter is replaced every 3 days through alternate nostrils. Nevertheless, we believe that it is less safe than intermittent gavage feeding for the following reasons:

1. The tube acts as a foreign body, producing mucus that may block the airway of the weak premature infant.
2. Purulent rhinitis and conjunctivitis may develop.
3. The catheter may disturb some infants, and stabilizing tape may irritate skin.

Transpyloric feeding

Rhea and Cheek and Staub have reported on transpyloric feeding of weak or sick infants when the formula is placed through the pylorus and administered by constant infusion pump. The following infants may benefit from this method:

1. Those who exhibit repeated apnea with gavage feedings (from tube insertion as well as stomach distention)
2. Those who show continued gastric residuals without ileus
3. Those who require prolonged assisted respiration
4. Those who lack usable peripheral veins for alimentation

5. Those who have a short gut, with dumping syndrome

Technique

1. Use soft* limp silicone tubing† with a diameter of 1.4 to 1.65 mm.
2. Follow directions outlined by Rhea in placement of catheter through pylorus.
3. When bile is aspirated, tape tube in position under nose or to intubation tube.
4. Attach to infusion pump.
5. Start with a volume of 24 ml/kg/24 hr or 1 ml/kg/hr and increase by 24 ml/kg/24 hr until a volume of approximately 150 ml/kg/24 hr is reached.

Types of feedings

The possible association of hyperosmolar and excessive volume of feedings with necrotizing enterocolitis demands caution by the physician in the feeding of infants, particularly those who weigh under 1,300 gm at birth.

1. Start with an isosmolar feeding—5% dextrose for 12 hours—and then switch to 20 calories/30 ml of humanized milk or human milk (Table 8-3).
2. Consider addition of medium-chain triglycerides (MCT oil, 8.3 Kcal/gm, or safflower oil at 1 to 3 ml/24 hr), which does not increase osmolality but adds to caloric intake.

Precautions

Sufficient experience is not yet available to assess the role of transpyloric feeding in the neonate, but the evidence so far suggests that it has a definite role, particularly following, or in conjunction with, parenteral infusions. The following hazards and warning signals should be anticipated:

1. Reflux into stomach—Aspirate stomach contents every 3 to 6 hours until the amount continues under 2 ml. A volume over this amount indicates the need to reduce feedings or extend the placement of feeding tube.
2. Distention may indicate ileus, an early sign of necrotizing enterocolitis (Chapter 21).
3. Bradycardia justifies further dependence on parenteral feedings.
4. Diarrhea may indicate excessive or hyperosmolar feeding.
5. Airway obstruction may indicate rhinitis or too large a tube.
6. Pressure necrosis, laceration, and indeed perforation are unlikely with the use of a silicone tube.

PARENTERAL ALIMENTATION

Intravenous alimentation* is required for infants with severe medical or surgical problems.

Included in this category as candidates for total parenteral alimentation are infants who are in critical condition because of severe respiratory distress or complicated surgical procedures, infants who have recurrent apneic periods with feeding, or those who have distention or feeding residuals. Recovery is supported and growth is assured by maintaining a positive nitrogen balance. Because few hospitals have the expertise or sufficient personnel to justify this technique, when extended alimentation is likely, transfer to a regional neonatal center is in order.

1. Start 10% glucose intravenously in the first hours of life at the rate of 80 to 100 ml/kg/24 hr, with approximately 3 ml of calcium gluconate/ 100 ml. For infants with respiratory

---

*Polyvinyl tubes harden when left in place for several days and may perforate intestine.
†Available as Silon, American Medical & Surgical Research Corp., Wellesley Hills, Mass. 01770.

---

*Sudden discontinuation of an infusion containing high glucose concentrations, interruption due to needle infiltration, or temporary substitution by blood or blood products can promote serious hypoglycemia.

distress and metabolic acidosis see Chapter 19.

2. Add 1 to 3 mEq Na^+, K^+, and Cl^-/ 100 ml glucose solution, for example, 0.75 ml NaCl (2.5 mEq/ml) and 1 ml K lactate (2 mEq/ml).
3. Change to the alimentation infusion (Table 8-5) by 48 to 72 hours— usually HA 10.*
4. Increase the rate of infusion by 15 ml/kg/24 hr, to approximately 150 ml/kg, depending on body weight and weight loss.
5. Start with HA 6.5 solution for very immature infants whose ability to metabolize glucose is limited and who require greater volumes of fluid.
6. Move to a higher glucose concentration in the absence of significant glucosuria. More mature infants may be started on HA 13 if they tolerated 10% glucose solutions. HA 19 is solely for deep central vein infusions.
7. M.V.I.,* 1 ml, should be added daily to the infusion. Each week 1 ml of Folbesyn for vitamin B_{12} and folic acid requirements and 1 mg of vitamin K_1 (AquaMephyton) administered intramuscularly, should be given.
8. Weigh the infant daily (or more frequently) to aid in adjustment of fluid volume. Avoid a daily gain or loss of more than 2% in body weight after the first 3 days of life.
9. Check urine for glycosuria with the Clinistix test every 4 hours at first,

---

*HA and number stands for hyperalimentation and percent dextrose as used in our nursery for many years.

*Multiple vitamin infusion.

Table 8-5. Solutions for parenteral alimentation

| | | Peripheral vein | | Central catheter |
	HA 6.5	HA 10	HA 13	HA 19
Solutions				
5% Protein hydrolysate (ml)	20.0	30.0	40.0	55.0
D_5W (ml)	70.0	—	—	—
$D_{10}W$ (ml)	—	55.0	36.0	—
$D_{50}W$ (ml)	6.0	9.0	18.0	37.0
ETOH (ml)	0.5	1.0	1.0	1.0
NaCl (2.5 mEq/ml)	0.3	0.3	0.2	0.4
$KHPO_4$ (2 mEq/ml)	0.3	0.5	0.5	0.5
10% Ca gluconate (0.45 mEq/ml)	2.0	3.0	3.0	4.0
50% $MgSO_4$ (4 mEq/ml)	—	0.1	0.1	0.2
M.V.I. (ml/24 hr)	0.5	0.5	0.5	0.5
Content/100 ml				
Protein (gm)	1.0	1.5	2.0	2.8
Carbohydrate (gm)	6.5	10.0	12.5	18.5
Calories	33.0	51.0	65.0	90.0
Na^+ mEq	1.3	1.5	1.5	2.4
K^+ mEq	1.0	1.6	1.8	2.1
Ca^{++} mEq	1.0	1.5	1.6	2.1
Mg^{++} mEq	—	0.5	0.5	0.9
PO_4^{--} mEq	1.1	1.8	2.0	2.4
Cl^{--} mEq	1.1	1.3	1.2	2.0

then every 8 hours; if 2+ or more, reduce glucose to prevent osmotic diuresis and blood glucose level over 150 mg/100 ml. Sudden glycosuria may indicate infection.

10. Record summary of intake and output every 8 to 12 hours.
11. Delay oral feedings until the infant is free of distention and has active peristalsis and a stable cardiorespiratory system.
12. Replace gastric loss, including electrolytes, every 8 hours each day with an equal volume. When gastrostomy or gastrointestinal suction is employed, any gastric loss is to be measured.
13. Replace significant blood loss, chest tube drainage, etc.

The following points must be emphasized with regard to parenteral alimentation:

1. We use alcohol to provide additional calories and to limit protein for energy use.
2. Use of fatty acid (such as Intralipid, available in many countries) will allow elimination of alcohol and reduction in glucose load. Two to 4 gm/kg/24 hr can be infused over a 4-hour period simultaneously with one of the above solutions by means of a 4-way stopcock.
3. Trace elements (and fatty acids) are only partially supplied by fresh frozen plasma (10 to 15 ml/kg/wk).
4. For long-term total parenteral alimentation, trace elements of zinc 20 μg), copper (20 μg), cobalt (10 μg), and iodine (5 μg) should be added to each 150 ml of infusion.

Indications for parenteral alimentation

1. Severe respiratory distress syndrome
2. Serious gastrointestinal problems and recurrent apnea in the immature preterm or growth-retarded infant
3. Severe infections
4. Intestinal anomalies, including short gut syndrome
5. Renal failure

Methods of administration of fluids

1. *Umbilical vein.* We use this method only as a temporary and emergency avenue for infusion of glucose, bicarbonate, etc. Dangers are liver necrosis, infection, and portal vein thrombosis (occasionally portal hypertension).
2. *Umbilical artery.* We offer alimentation solutions by way of the aorta only as long as a catheter is required for obtaining serial blood gases.
3. *Peripheral veins.* We prefer this approach for most infants and have been successful in supporting growth for as long as 3 months and up to 3 kg in weight with this route as the sole source of calories.
4. *Central vein.*° We use this method only in infants who require a greater caloric load than can be given by the peripheral route or when peripheral veins have been "used up."

Preparation of alimentation solutions†

Scrupulous care by a trained team is necessary in the preparation of intravenous infusions.

1. Draw a measured volume of solution (such as protein hydrolysate or glucose solution) with the use of a disposable mixing set into a sterile evacuated container, utilizing a closed system.
2. Add small-volume additions (electrolytes, vitamins) by separate syringe.
3. Prepare sufficient solution for 12-hour period (greater volumes can be pre-

---

°For central venous catheter placement, see Filler, R. M., and Eraklis, A. J.: Care of the critically ill child: intravenous alimentation, Pediatrics **46**:456, 1970.

†Goldman, D. A., and Maki, D. G.: Infection control in total parenteral alimentation, J.A.M.A. **223**:1360, 1973.

pared if the unused portion is refrigerated and kept aseptic).

4. Attach solution to infusion pump and set for required volume per minute.
5. Place Millipore filter distal to tubing (prior to entry needle or catheter) to remove bacteria and particulate matter.

Laboratory monitoring of parenteral fluids

The following applies to extended use of glucose solutions as well as alimentation solutions.

Weight	Once or twice daily
Length	Weekly
Head circumference	Weekly
Electrolytes	Daily until stabilized; then 3 times weekly
BUN	Twice weekly
Blood glucose	(see text)
Calcium	Daily times 3; if satisfactory, weekly
Base deficit	Daily times 3; if satisfactory, weekly
Hematocrit	Weekly
SGOT	Weekly
Albumin or total protein	Weekly
Bilirubin	As indicated

Advantages of alimentation by peripheral vein

1. The danger of infection is minimal.
2. Replacement of needle after infiltration of solution is best performed by neonatal nursing staff. The 24-hour availability of nursing staff avoids rebound hypoglycemia. In addition, their facility with needle placement lessens handling of infant and preserves vein use.
3. Up to 15 microdrops/min can be given to smaller infants and up to 25 microdrops to larger more mature infants without excessive thrombosis and infiltration. Thus as much as 600 ml of a solution containing 12.5% glucose is allowed for peripheral infusion.
4. Deep central catheter placement can be avoided in most neonates.

Hazards in the use of alimentation solutions

1. Infiltration should be noted within an hour or earlier in high-volume infusion rates. Sloughs occasionally occur over the scalp—usually with a minimum of scarring. (Avoid hair-free area of forehead.) Larger infiltration in soft tissues of the extremities can produce serious sloughs. These sloughs can be substantially reduced if one is careful to avoid venous constriction.
2. Occasionally solutions become contaminated and may produce endotoxic shock, even with the use of a Millipore filter. Require bacteriologic surveillance by hospital infection control committee and a change of solutions and equipment every 12 hours.
3. Observe for glycosuria and/or hyperglycemia. Be sure to infuse solutions at a constant rate, using an infusion pump. Rate of infusion of glucose solution depends on weight loss, glycosuria (over 1+), and hyperglycemia (over 150 mg/100 ml). Many immature infants can metabolize glucose at a rate of no more than 0.4 gm/kg/hr in the first few days of postnatal life.
4. Cholestasis leading to hepatitis is not infrequent after prolonged alimentation. A temporary increase in direct bilirubin levels as well as the reduction of liver function tests may be observed. Recovery usually is complete after several weeks. The etiology is obscure.
5. Hyperammonemia, aminoacidemia, and metabolic acidosis have been reported with excessive infusion of protein hydrolysate in the range above 3 gm/kg/24 hr.

Parenteral alimentation is reserved for feeding the newborn in more serious condition; combined parenteral glucose infusion and formula feeding is appropriate for most "healthy" infants under 1,500 gm. If there is difficulty in establishing oral feedings, we change to an alimentation solution by peripheral vein.

SELECTED REFERENCES

Babson, S. F.: Feeding the low-birth-weight infant, J. Pediatr. **79**:694, 1971.

Benda, G. I. M., and Babson, S. G.: Peripheral alimentation of the small premature infant, J. Pediatr. **79**:494, 1971.

Bryan, M. H., Wei, P., Hamilton, J. R., Chance, G. W., and Swyer, P. R.: Supplemental intravenous alimentation in low birth weight infants, J. Pediatr. **82**:940, 1973.

Cheek, J. A., and Staub, G. F.: Nasojejunal alimentation for premature and full-term newborn infants, J. Pediatr. **82**:955, 1973.

Dweck, H. S., and Cassady, G.: Hyperglycemia and very low birth weight, Pediatrics **53**:189, 1974.

Heird, W. C.: Nasojejunal feeding: a commentary, J. Pediatr. **85**:111, 1974.

Heird, W. C., Driscoll, J. M., Jr., Schullinger, J. N., Grebin, B., and Winters, R. W.: Intravenous alimentation in pediatric patients, J. Pediatr. **80**:351, 1972.

Heird, W. C., and Winters, R. W.: Total parenteral nutrition, J. Pediatr. **86**:2, 1975.

Pildes, R. S., Ramamurthy, R. S., Cordero, G. V., and Wong, P. W. K.: Intravenous supplementation of L-amino acids and dextrose in low-birth-weight infants, J. Pediatr. **82**:945, 1973.

Rhea, J. W., Ahmed, M. S., and Menge, M. S.: Nasojejunal (transpyloric) feeding, J. Pediatr. **86**:451, 1975.

Rhea, J. W., Ghazzawi, O., and Weidman, W.: Nasojejunal feeding: an improved device and intubation technique, J. Pediatr. **82**:951, 1973.

Shaw, J. C. L.: Parenteral nutrition in the management of sick low birth weight infants, Pediatr. Clin. North Am. **20**:333, May, 1973.

Sinclair, J. C., Driscoll, J. M., Jr., Heird, W. C., and Winters, R. W.: Supportive management of the sick neonate. Parenteral calories, water, and electrolytes, Pediatr. Clin. North Am. **17**:863, 1970.

Ziegler, E. E., and Fomon, S. J.: Fluid intake, renal solute load and water balance in infancy, J. Pediatr. **78**:561, 1971.

9

Infections of the perinate

Neonatal morbidity and mortality from acquired infection exceeds that from all other causes after the first few days of life. The inability of macroglobulin IgM* to be transmitted across the placenta, its lag in reaching optimum levels after birth, less efficient phagocytosis, undernutrition, and frequent immaturity render the small infant particularly susceptible to invasion by microorganisms. Special precautions for preventing infection, as well as prompt recognition when it occurs, are necessary for the optimal management of the infant of low birth weight. Any change in behavior suggesting infection is an indication for treatment with antibiotics after diagnostic procedures have been undertaken. Often overlooked is the important task of identifying noninfected infants and avoiding or discontinuing antibiotic therapy when warranted.

RECOGNIZING INFECTION IN THE PERINATE
Period of exposure

1. Infections acquired in utero
   a. Placentally transferred organisms, usually viruses (e.g., rubella), pass directly across the placenta to the fetus.
   b. In ascending infection, microorga-

nisms pass through the cervix, with entry into the amnion encouraged by long labor and premature and prolonged rupture of the membranes (Chapter 16). The route of fetal infection is through the respiratory or gastrointestinal tract.
2. Infections acquired during delivery
   a. Generalized infections in which the pathways again are principally the upper airway and gastrointestinal tract
      1. Flora of the maternal genital tract such as group B streptococci
      2. Pathogenic organisms occasionally harbored in the intestinal tract of the mother, for example, *Listeria monocytogenes, Salmonella* and *Shigella* organisms, *Escherichia coli,* and enteroviruses
      3. Herpesvirus from maternal genital tract lesions
   b. Local infections
      1. Conjunctiva
         a. Gonococcus infection (profuse purulent discharge by 2 to 4 days of age)
         b. Inclusion blenorrhea (serosanguineous to yellow-whitish discharge at approximately 1 week)
      2. Oral cavity
         a. Thrush caused by the yeast *Candida albicans*
3. Infections caused by bacteria, for ex-

---

*Although the newborn have a paucity of IgM and bacterial antibodies to gram-negative organisms, they have a surprising resistance to invasion by these organisms.

119

ample, staphylococci and *Diplococcus pneumoniae*, during resuscitation from contamination from the placement of indwelling catheters or endotracheal tubes or mouth insufflation
4. Infections from within the nursery by organisms frequently inhabiting the area, for example, *Proteus, Pseudomonas*, and *Klebsiella-Aerobacter* organisms

These infections may be transferred by the hands of personnel or spread from contaminated equipment or incubators. The umbilicus is a receptive site for cutaneous infection leading to sepsis.

Viral infection (fetal)*

1. Factors suggesting viral infection
   a. Small-for-dates infants
   b. Microcephalus and occasionally hydrocephalus
   c. Early jaundice with an increased "direct" component of bilirubin
   d. Petechiae, purpura, or vesicular rash
   e. Hepatosplenomegaly, often firm in character
   f. Chorioretinitis, keratitis, conjunctivitis, cataracts, retinopathies, and microphthalmia
   g. Congenital anomalies
   h. Anemia with evidence of hemolysis, thrombocytopenia, disseminated intravascular coagulation (DIC)
2. Diagnosis of viral infection
   a. Obtain history of illness in the gravida.
   b. Perform hematocrit, platelet, and reticulocyte counts and fractionation of bilirubin.
   c. Take direct cultures of the throat, urine, stool, cerebrospinal fluid, and vesicular fluid (herpesvirus).
   d. Obtain urine specimen for cytology in suspected cases of cytomegalovirus infection.
   e. Perform IgM determination—over 25

mg/100 ml suggests active viral disease.
   f. Test for neutralizing hemagglutinin inhibition and complement-fixing antibodies—to be repeated later.
   g. Take x-ray films of the long bones (rarefactions) and skull (intracranial calcifications).
   h. Perform an electrocardiogram for evidence of myocarditis (Coxsackie B enterovirus).
   i. Examine retinas for evidence of chorioretinitis or cataracts.

Bacterial infection

1. The common recognizable clues of bacterial infection are
   a. Skin changes such as sudden pallor, intensification of jaundice, or cyanotic periods
   b. Lethargy or irritability
   c. Lack of interest in food, regurgitation, delay in stomach emptying (residual before gavage), and particularly abdominal distention
   d. Tachypnea and/or respiratory distress; tachycardia
   e. Unexpected weight loss and thermal instability (a rise or fall in body temperature)
2. The infant should be particularly examined for
   a. Enlargement of liver and spleen
   b. Changes in fontanel pressure
   c. Discomfort on extremity manipulation
3. Other factors suggesting the likelihood of infection are
   a. Meconium aspiration
   b. Bloody secretions in the upper airway
   c. Prolonged rupture of the membrane; amnionitis (Chapter 16)

General infection

1. Sepsis
   a. Suggested by pallor, lethargy, petechiae, hepatosplenomegaly, or jaundice

---

*See p. 124 for specific diseases.

b. May involve the lungs, urinary tract, and meninges in one third of cases
2. Pneumonia, indicated by one or more of the following:
   a. Increase in rate of respiration
   b. Costal retraction and movement of alae nasi
   c. Simple hyperpnea
3. Meningitis (Chapter 22)
   a. Lethargy
   b. Irritability
   c. Apnea and cyanosis
   d. Grayish color
   e. Full fontanel
   f. Seizures and head retraction in advanced states
4. Epidemic diarrhea
   a. Pallor
   b. Dehydration (sunken eyes)
   c. Lethargy
   d. Distention
   e. Watery stools

Diagnosis of bacterial infection

1. Routine procedures
   a. White blood cell and differential count
      A shift to the left, a reduction in number (under 5,000 white blood cells/mm^3), or an increase (over 20,000 white blood cells/mm^3) in number suggests bacterial infection.
   b. Urinalyses
      A fresh and clean-catch or bladder-tap specimen with over two or three white blood cells per low-power field in a centrifuged specimen or with one or more bacteria per oil immersion field in a concentrated smear indicates the possibility of infection.*

---

*Failure to discover pyuria or bacteria on a microscopic examination does not eliminate the possibility of urinary tract infection; properly performed bacterial counts are necessary for precise diagnosis. Conversely, the presence of pus or bacteria may represent contamination.

c. Smear and culture
   Make a smear and culture of any inflamed cord stump, discharge, repeated diarrheal stool, etc.
2. Special procedures
   a. Examine the chest x-ray film when any change in respiratory action occurs.
   b. Perform a spinal tap for the presence of meningeal inflammation when any significant change in behavior is noted that is not readily explained.
   c. Obtain cultures of blood, urine from bladder tap, and spinal fluid (include examination of stained smear). A 1 to 2 ml quantity is sufficient.

TREATING INFECTION
Management of bacterial infection

The majority of viral diseases cannot be treated effectively; since bacteria are responsible for most infections, therapy is aimed at them.

1. Treatment for suspected infection
   a. Begin administering kanamycin and penicillin or ampicillin promptly—a few hours' delay can be fatal.
   b. For infections acquired in a nursery with a high percentage of resistant organisms, treatment with agents such as nafcillin and/or gentamicin is to be considered.
   c. Reduce or eliminate oral feedings and give parenteral infusion of fluids, calories, and electrolytes (Chapter 8).
   d. Support infant for shock or respiratory failure if needed.
2. Interpretation of cultures
   a. If cultures are negative, discontinue antibiotics unless signs of possible infection persist.
   b. If blood culture is positive, continue treatment for 7 to 10 days with proper antibiotic agent; treat urinary tract infection or meningitis for a minimum of 2 weeks.

Table 9-1. Antibiotic therapy

Drug	Dose	Indication	Hazards
Kanamycin sulfate Limit to 7-12 days Supplied as Kantrex (75 mg/2 ml)	15 mg/kg/day, divided into two doses (IM)	Gram-negative pathogens, coliform bacteria, *Proteus, Neisseria,* and *Mycobacterium*	Ototoxic if dose excessive or prolonged; renal damage, particularly if fluid intake low
Gentamicin	Less than 7 days: 5 mg/kg/24 hr (IM) divided into 2 doses; more than 7 days: 7.5 mg/kg/24 hr in 3 doses	*Klebsiella-Aerobacter, Pseudomonas, Proteus,* staphylococci, *Escherichia coli, Salmonella*	Toxic to vestibular system; nephrotoxic
Potassium penicillin G (aqueous)	50,000-100,000 units/ kg/24 hr, divided into 2 doses (IM or IV) for infants less than 7 days; for older infant, divide into 3 doses	Hemolytic streptococci, pneumococci, and some strains of staphylococci	Procaine products avoided when muscle mass reduced
Ampicillin	50 mg/kg/24 hr (IM or IV); divided in 2 doses for infants less than 7 days; preterm infants over 7 days, 100 mg/kg/ 24 hr in 3 doses; term infants over 7 days of age, 150 mg/ kg/24 hr in 3 doses	Most gram-positive organisms, most gram-negative organisms, *Salmonella, Haemophilus influenzae, Streptococcus faecalis, Proteus mirabilis,* and *Escherichia coli*	Dangers not delineated for newborn infant

Treatment of minor infections acquired after birth

1. Pustules, abscesses, and local infections
   a. Open any collection of pus. Make a culture, smear, and Gram stain of the fluid.
   b. Clean with alcohol and expose to air.
   c. Sponge area daily with pHisoHex.
   d. Segregate the infant and observe strict hand-washing care.
   e. Isolate babies with multiple infections.
2. Eye discharges
   Eye discharges occur in many healthy premature infants during their nursery course. Prompt and vigorous treatment is important because the eye may be destroyed or septicemia may occur.
   a. Make a smear and culture of the discharge.
   b. Cleanse the eye and instill broad-spectrum antibiotics every 2 hours, for example, Neosporin ophthalmic solution, 1 drop in each eye every 2 to 3 hours.
   c. Treat gonorrheal ophthalmia by parenteral penicillin unless it is penicillin-resistant.
   d. Administer tetracycline locally for inclusion blenorrhea (intracellular inclusions identified from conjunctival scrapings).
3. Thrush and other candidal infections
   a. Instill nystatin (Mycostatin) in the infant's mouth after feedings for oral mucous membrane involvement.

Table 9-1. Antibiotic therapy—cont'd

Drug	Dose	Indication	Hazards
Nafcillin, sodium methicillin (Staphcillin)	100 mg/kg/24 hr, divided into 2 doses (IM or IV) for infant under 7 days; 200-300 mg/kg/24 hr in 4 doses for infants over 7 days	Penicillinase-resistant staphylococci	Low order of toxicity
Carbenicillin	200-400 mg/kg/24 hr (IV), divided in 3 doses for infants under 7 days; 4 doses for older infants	*Pseudomonas, Proteus*	SGOT elevation
Colistimethate sodium (Colistin), 5-7 days	5-8 mg/kg/24 hr, divided into 2 doses (deep IM)	*Pseudomonas*	Nephrotoxicity; overgrowth of *Candida*
Polymyxin B sulfate, 5-7 days	3.5 to 5 mg/kg/24 hr, divided into 2 doses (IM)	*Pseudomonas*	May have cumulative nephrotoxicity with kanamycin
Neomycin	50-100 mg/kg/24 hr, in 4 doses (by mouth only)	Pathogenic *Escherichia coli* and gram-negative organisms producing diarrhea	No significant intolerance
Nystatin (Mycostatin)	200,000 units, divided into 4 doses daily (by mouth only)	Local candidal infections	No significant intolerance
Amphotericin B	0.25-1 mg/kg/24 hr (by slow IV infusion)	Systemic yeast and fungous infections	Gastroenteritis; nephrotoxicity; dangers not specified for immature infant

b. Apply 1% aqueous gentian violet twice daily when skin surfaces are involved. Gentian violet may also be applied to the buccal cavity.

Prophylactic antibiotics

1. Precautions

a. Antibiotics should not necessarily be given prophylactically to infants subjected to prolonged ruptured membranes (Chapter 16),* exchange

transfusion, or difficult resuscitation. There must be a reasonable likelihood or suspicion of infection to justify their use.

b. No drug is free from dangerous effects, particularly when administered to the premature infant.

c. Infections may develop that are resistant to antibacterial agents.

d. Intestinal bacterial flora required to activate essential vitamins, for example, vitamin K and thiamine, may be inhibited.

2. Antibiotic drug dosage (Table 9-1)

In premature infants, as well as in the term infant and, to a lesser extent, in infants past the neonatal stage, detoxifying enzymes are deficient, and renal

---

*When amnionitis is present (Chapter 16) and the infant is contaminated (over 5 polymorphonuclear leukocytes per high-power field seen on a smear of stomach aspirate), we believe the small or depressed infant should be treated, since about 10% of such babies are likely to be infected. Absence of the polymorphonuclear leukocytes on the smear is a reliable sign of no fetal infection (Oliver).

function is relatively inefficient. In the absence of good urinary excretion even very small doses of some drugs may cause serious reactions. Knowledge of the metabolic fate and principal route of excretion is important for estimation of an effective and safe dosage.

SPECIFIC INFECTIONS
Infection with group B streptococci

Group B streptococci, which can be cultured from the vagina in 5% to 25% of pregnant women, have become a major cause of neonatal sepsis. In fact, the frequency of group B streptococcal infections in the neonate has risen in some parts of the country to that of *Escherichia coli*.

Epidemiologic studies reveal an attack rate in neonates of approximately 2:1,000 live births and a mortality rate of 1:1,000 live births.

Infection of neonates with this organism can be divided into the following categories:

1. Early-onset sepsis, most likely acquired at birth by contact with an infected birth canal
2. Late-onset sepsis or meningitis (2 to 3 weeks of age), probably transmitted from personnel carrying the organism (mostly Type III)

1. Symptoms
   a. Early sepsis due to group B streptococcus
      1. Premature delivery
      2. Prolonged rupture of the membranes
      3. Onset of disease usually within 12 to 24 hours of age
      4. Respiratory distress with apnea or grunting respiration and cyanosis resembling hyaline membrane disease
      5. Rapid downhill course with respiratory failure and shock
      6. Occasional chest x-ray findings of pneumonia
   b. Late-onset sepsis

   1. Irritability
   2. Failure to feed
   3. Fever
2. Diagnostic aids
   Growth of the organism from cultures of blood or cerebrospinal fluid.
3. Management
   a. Prompt treatment with penicillin at suspicion of disease
   b. Vigorous supportive therapy for respiratory failure and shock if needed
   c. Generally supportive measures
4. Prognosis
   The early-onset septic form has a reported mortality of about 70% even with proper treatment given promptly. Sepsis due to Subtype I is followed by fatality of almost 100%, compared with approximately 17% for Subtypes II and III. The delayed-onset cases have a reported mortality approaching 45%.
5. Prevention
   The disastrous results produced by this organism on invasion of the neonate have stimulated investigation and discussion concerning the feasibility of preventive measures.
   Treatment of the maternal carrier appears to eradicate the organism, but there is insufficient documentation that identification and treatment of all carriers will reduce the incidence of group B streptococcal sepsis in the neonate. Potential risk factors and extent of such management may outweigh any advantages.

Rubella (German, or three-day, measles)

Approximately 30% to 50% of fetuses of women who contracted rubella during the first three months of pregnancy will be adversely affected by the virus. This degree of involvement may well be greater if early abortuses are studied adequately. Certainly perinatal mortality is increased, and a high proportion of the infants are born with low birth weight, whether obviously defective or not. Because about 10% of urban and 25% of rural women are not immune to this disease, a substantial number of defective or undersized infants can be expected to be born during rubella epidemics. No correlation apparently exists between the severity of maternal rubella and teratogenicity. Fetal damage can occur without obvious illness in the mother. The 1965 rubella epidemic involved many thousands of nonimmune pregnant women and resulted in damage to an extremely large proportion of their offspring during early fetal development.

The rubella virus readily invades the placenta and the fetus during gestation. Viremia during embryogenesis and perhaps later in pregnancy may produce signs and symptoms of persistent infection at birth. Appropriate cultures at this time for the rubella virus can prove fetal invasion with or without clinical evidence of disease. Excretion of the virus may persist through the first year in spite of measurable antibody titer. This continued excretion creates a danger to nonimmunized nursing personnel and babies (Fig. 9-1).

1. Diagnosis (after exposure 2 to 3 weeks previously)
   a. In the child or adult, *rubella* causes no specific lesion but, in order of possible occurrence, it can cause
      1. Low-grade fever and slight malaise that coincide with eruption
      2. Lymphadenopathy (postcervical, postauricular)
      3. Fleeting, fine, maculopapular rash (face to trunk to extremities)
      4. Leukopenia
      5. Occasionally arthropathy and/or encephalitis
   b. In the neonate the *rubella syndrome* is a congenital infection.
      1. Teratogenic effects
         a. Intrauterine growth retardation
         b. Congenital heart disease, hypoplasia of myocardium
         c. Sensorineural deafness (occasional anomalies of the cochlear duct, organ of Corti)
         d. Cataract and/or glaucoma
         e. Neonatal purpura ("blueberry muffin baby")

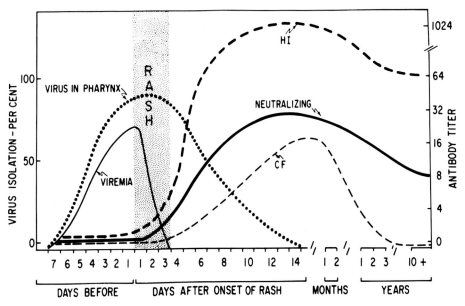

Fig. 9-1. Schematic illustration of the pattern of virus excretion and antibody response during rubella. (Modified from Cooper, L. Z., and Krugman, S.: Arch. Ophthalmol. **77:**434, 1967.)

f. Dermatoglyphic abnormalities (unusual fingerprints, palmar creases, skin folds)

2. Systemic involvement with or without malformation
   a. Adenitis, hepatitis, hepatosplenomegaly, jaundice
   b. Anemia, thrombocytopenia with petechial hemorrhages
   c. Areas of rarefaction in metaphyses of bones and irregularities of the epiphyseal lines of long bones shown by x-ray examination
   d. Encephalitis, meningitis
   e. Myocarditis (ECG changes)
   f. Eye lesions (iridocyclitis, retinopathy)
   g. Pneumonia (interstitial type)

3. Later effects
   a. Reduced growth, failure to thrive
   b. Multiple physical and behavioral handicaps

When the pregnant woman contracts rubella—confirmed by a rise in hemagglutinin-inhibition (HI) antibody over a 2-week period—in the first trimester, the incidence of malformation in the infant is about 35% in the first month, 25% in the second month, and 10% in the third month. After the fourth month, abnormalities are uncommon, except for hearing defects. (Congenital rubella has not been implicated as a cause of skeletal defects such as cleft palate, meningomyelocele, phocomelia.)

2. Laboratory tests
   a. A rapid rubella virus HI test and an IgM fluorescent antibody test are diagnostic.
   b. Culture of the rubella virus from nasopharyngeal washings is possible but difficult.
   c. Leukopenia that is present early may be followed by an increase of plasma cells.
   d. Delayed hypersensitivity reaction

with impaired cellular immunity is noted.

3. Treatment for the neonate with congenital rubella
   a. Strict isolation for as long as pharyngeal virus shedding or virus excretion in the urine persists
   b. Ophthalmologic consultation to avoid blindness due to glaucoma or cataracts
   c. Utilization of immunized nursery attendants who cannot or will not become pregnant
   d. Multidisciplinary care, since early recognition and treatment of handicaps will improve the child's chances of maximal development

4. Prevention
   a. Live attenuated rubella vaccine is highly effective and usually results in lasting immunity except for later gross exposure in an occasional individual. The vaccine should be given to all children before puberty. A pregnant woman in the immediate family is a contraindication to the use of the vaccine because of theoretical teratogenicity of the attenuated virus.
   b. Nonpregnant susceptible females (no HI antibody present) may be purposefully exposed or vaccinated provided it is certain they are not pregnant and will not conceive for at least 2 months after inoculation.
   c. Immune serum globulin (gamma globulin) will not prevent rubella. Although it may suppress outward evidence of the disease, the pregnant woman may develop a subclinical rubella, with its many congenital complications.
   d. First-trimester therapeutic abortion, when permissible, should be seriously considered in bona fide cases.

Herpes simplex virus infection

Herpesvirus infection in the neonate commonly is acquired by contact with the mother's infected birth canal. Though occasional case reports with intrauterine malformations and congenital infection of the infant have been published, transplacental passage of the virus appears to be infrequent.

The risk of acquisition of the virus by the neonate in a genitally infected mother may be as high as 10%. Approximately 90% of herpesvirus infection in infants is caused by herpesvirus 2, most likely because of the greater chance of contact, since this virus has a predilection for the genital area.

Incubation period for herpesvirus is apparently between 4 and 21 days.

1. Symptoms

   Typically in an infection acquired at birth, the infant will be asymptomatic for several days. Then the following may be observed:
   a. Lethargy
   b. Febrile episodes
   c. Mottled skin
   d. Hepatosplenomegaly
   e. Poor feeding
   f. Seizures
   g. Disseminated intravascular coagulation (DIC)
   h. Vesicular lesions on skin, including scalp

   In addition to these symptoms, a congenitally infected neonate at birth may demonstrate the following:
   a. Small for dates
   b. Microcephaly
   c. Intracranial calcifications
   d. Microphthalmia
   e. Chorioretinitis
   f. Inclusion bodies in urine
2. Laboratory results commonly observed in herpesvirus infections
   a. Elevated IgM
   b. Abnormal cerebrospinal fluid values
   c. Abnormal liver function studies
   d. Abnormal coagulation panel compatible with DIC (Chapter 23)
3. Diagnostic aids
   a. Isolation of virus from vesicle fluid, throat washing, urine, or cerebrospinal fluid
   b. Demonstration of neutralizing antibodies in serum
   c. Positive immunofluorescence (IgM)
   d. Identification of "owl-eye" inclusion bodies in vesicular fluid or urine (congenital infection)
4. Management
   Attempts to treat the disease with antiviral drugs that inhibit DNA synthesis such as idoxuridine and cytosine arabinoside have been discouraging. Infants with herpesvirus infection (or those who are suspect) should be
   a. Isolated
   b. Treated with general supportive measures
5. Prognosis
   The mortality of the disease, whether herpesvirus 1 or 2, is 50% to 70%. Infants with localized skin involvement have a better prognosis. The outcome for surviving infants is frequently complicated by abnormal neurologic development.
6. Prevention
   a. Identify mothers with genital lesions due to herpesvirus before delivery by culturing suspect cases.
   b. Deliver by cesarean section mothers with positive cultures from genital lesions to avoid inoculation. (Cesarean section more than 4 hours after rupture of membranes probably is not warranted.)
   c. Prevent contact of an infant with a mother having oral lesions due to herpesvirus.

Cytomegalovirus infection

The cytomegalovirus is by far the most common among other known infectious agents and has a propensity for producing various adverse effects on the brain. It can be isolated from the cervix in almost 20% of pregnant women. Approximately 6/1,000 infants have IgM antibody to cytomegalovirus in their cord sera. Of these 6, about one third have developmental abnormalities severe enough to predict school failure.

Although infection of a neonate is thought to occur only at the time of a primary infection in the mother, reports of a subsequently infected fetus have been documented. A positive correlation appears to exist between severity of neonatal infection and presumed duration of the disease in utero.

1. Symptoms (at or within 24 hours of birth)
   a. Jaundice
   b. Hemolytic anemia
   c. Thrombocytopenia with generalized petechiae
   d. Hepatosplenomegaly
   e. Central nervous system disease (including cerebral calcification)
   f. Chorioretinitis
   g. Retarded growth
2. Diagnostic aids
   a. Immunofluorescence (IgM)
   b. Specific intracellular inclusion bodies (An "owl-eye" halo appearance in the shed epithelial cells of a urine concentrate stained with hematoxylin-eosin may be seen. The saliva may also contain these cells. Pleocytosis is not uncommon in spinal fluid, in which similar inclusion bodies may be found.)
   c. Rising antibody titers
   d. Virus isolation from urine and/or throat
3. Treatment
   No effective prophylactic or therapeutic measures have been discovered.
   a. Give symptomatic, supportive treatment.
   b. Ensure parental support.
   c. Isolate infant while in nursery and avoid contact with pregnant women until virus excretion ceases.
4. Prognosis
   a. Early death is likely in the majority of symptomatic infants. Classic intracellular inclusion bodies will be present in the central nervous system and viscera in fatal cases.
   b. Mildly or even severely damaged offspring may live, but severe mental and motor retardation is likely in long-term survivors.
5. Prevention
   The development of a cytomegalovirus vaccine now under investigation offers hope for the prevention of congenital disease by this virus.

Syphilis

Untreated early syphilis complicating pregnancy is a major cause of midtrimester abortion, fetal death in utero, or premature labor and delivery the world over. Whether the neonate will or will not show stigmata of congenital syphilis depends on when the mother contracts the disease. If infection occurs less than 1 to 2 years prior to the gestation, the fetus probably will be affected seriously. When the onset of the disease coincides with conception or is very early in pregnancy, a deformed, congenitally afflicted, and premature infant probably will eventuate. Whether a woman who contracts syphilis during the second half of a pregnancy will deliver a diseased offspring or one that is spared by syphilis cannot be determined.

A serologic test for syphilis (STS) at the first obstetric visit is essential for the identification of a syphilitic mother. The symptomatology of syphilis may be unnoticed during pregnancy; even the secondary nonpruritic rash may be insignificant. Tertiary syphilis rarely complicates pregnancy.

The severity of syphilis is diminished by pregnancy in many gravid women. Gestation will not modify relapses after insufficient treatment, however, nor will it alter late syphilis.

1. Symptoms
   Congenital syphilis in the neonate can present a major diagnostic problem. Clinical findings frequently are absent

or unapparent. A primary stage is absent, since *Treponema pallidum* is directly introduced into the fetal circulation.
a. Early stage (under 2 years of age)
1. Vesicular bullous cutaneous lesions
2. Mucous membrane lesions (affected nose and pharynx produce "snuffles")
3. Osteochondritis
4. Hepatosplenomegaly
5. Hemolytic anemia
6. Abnormal cerebrospinal fluid findings (up to 50% of infants)
b. Late congenital syphilis (over 2 years of age)
In the majority of cases disease is latent except for a reactive serologic test for syphilis. The following signs may be present:
1. Interstitial keratitis
2. Hutchinson's teeth
3. Eighth nerve deafness
4. Neurosyphilis
5. Bone involvement with sclerotic gummatous lesions, as in saber shin, destruction of nasal septum, or rhagades
2. Diagnostic aids
a. Identify *Treponema pallidum* in serum from a chancre by dark-field examination.
b. IgM specific fluorescent treponemal antibody-absorption test (FTA-ABS test) is diagnostic, since IgM does not cross the placenta. The test will be positive usually before clinical symptoms occur; therefore it is very useful.
c. Since VDRL and regular FTA-ABS tests are usually for IgG antibodies, they are not as diagnostic unless repeated titers demonstrate a rise.
3. Treatment
a. Indications
1. Evidence of active disease in the mother for whom treatment

has been inadequate or omitted
2. A positive IgM-specific FTA-ABS test in the infant
3. A positive, quantitative STS in which the titer rises or fails to decrease in the first 6 weeks of life
4. A positive STS with clinical evidence of syphilis, for example, rhinitis, skin eruptions, x-ray evidence of osteochondritis or periostitis
b. Specific treatment likely to obviate sequelae
1. Isolate if open lesions are present.
2. Administer aqueous penicillin 100,000/kg/24 hr in two doses for 10 days, or administer 50,000 units/kg of benzathine penicillin G at one injection.

Toxoplasmosis

Placental transfer of the parasite *Toxoplasma gondii* to the fetus in the nonimmune gravida is increasingly common.

Although 5% to 20% of women have positive titers during pregnancy, the infection is likely to have antedated pregnancy, with the parasite in the encysted form and not dangerous to the fetus. As few as 1:1,000 women acquire the active disease in pregnancy, of whom 10% to 30% have infected infants. Identification of positive titers during pregnancy in women with previous negative titers suggests a proliferative disease dangerous to the fetus.
1. Symptoms and signs
a. Early
1. Hepatosplenomegaly with jaundice
2. Chorioretinitis and microphthalmia
3. Lethargy and/or convulsion
b. Later
1. Hydrocephalus or microcephalus
2. Mental retardation
3. Cerebral calcification
2. Diagnosis
a. IgM fluorescent antibody test may be positive.

b. A Sabin-Feldman dye test remains elevated for many months, in contrast to the passively transferred antibody from the mother.

c. Differentiate from erythroblastosis, sepsis, and cytomegalovirus inclusion disease.

3. Treatment

a. Once the infant shows the classic findings of toxoplasmosis, the prognosis is poor.

b. Active disease in the mother has been treated with pyrimethamine and sulfonamides, but teratogenic effects justify avoidance in first trimester.

Coxsackie virus disease

The Coxsackie virus, type A or B with many serotypes, causes an acute, influenza-like enteric or respiratory illness in adults. It also affects the fetus by (1) transplacental passage of the submicroscopic agent or (2) exposure of the neonate to diseased individuals. Occasionally the mother and attendants will have no clinical evidence of a viral disorder. Coxsackie virus may cause fetal malformations and is very serious for the premature infant. Several days after birth the newborn infant with the disease will have a cough, loose stools, fever, and tachycardia. Meningoencephalitis or myocarditis may develop. Neonatal death is often due to circulatory collapse or respiratory failure. Routine laboratory studies reveal no typical abnormalities. The virus may be isolated from throat washings or stools. Only symptomatic therapy is available. The prognosis depends on the extent of the disease.

Tuberculosis

Congenital tuberculosis is rare. Neonates born of mothers with tuberculosis have no specific affinity for the disease. It is essential to segregate the mother with pulmonary tuberculosis from her infant, however, to avoid neonatal acid-fast infection.

Patients undergoing treatment of tuberculosis should strictly avoid conception until the disorder has been inactive for 2 to 5 years, depending on severity. All obstetric patients should have chest x-ray examinations as soon as gestation is confirmed. Women who have arrested pulmonary tuberculosis should have chest films taken every 3 months during pregnancy and 6 months after delivery.

Isoniazid and para-amino salicylic acid probably are not teratogenic in the doses usually given for the chemotherapy of tuberculosis.

Listeriosis

Modern surveys have shown that up to 4% of pregnant women harbor *Listeria monocytogenes* in the cervix or vagina. Invasion of the placenta occasionally occurs, with influenza-like symptoms in the mother and the possibility of early delivery. A dirty brown amniotic fluid has been noted in instances of listeriosis.

Those infants infected either through direct invasion or from birth contamination may be seriously jeopardized. Mortality and morbidity are high, particularly from central nervous system complications.

1. Clinical findings

a. Fetal involvement with scattered foci or necrosis (granulomatosis infanticum).

b. Delayed infection of the newborn infant—vomiting, lethargy, and cardiorespiratory symptoms—often indicates listeriosis.

2. Diagnosis

a. Positive fluorescent antibody test is diagnostic.

b. Culture nasopharynx, stomach contents, and meconium (sometimes liquid) for gram-positive pleomorphic bacteria—*do not confuse with diphtheroids.*

c. Perform a spinal tap to identify listeriosis.

3. Treatment

a. Treat vigorously with penicillin or

tetracycline while awaiting results of specific drug sensitivity tests.

b. Maintain observation for sequelae of disease after dismissal from hospital.

SELECTED REFERENCES

Baker, C. J., and Barrett, F. F.: Transmission of group B streptococci from mother to neonate, J. Pediatr. **83**:919, 1973.

Dennis, S. M.: Comparative aspects of infectious abortion diseases common to animals and man (listeriosis, toxoplasmosis, vibriosus), Int. J. Fertil. **13**:191, 1968.

Desmonts, G., and Couvneur, J.: Toxoplasmosis, N. Engl. J. Med. **290**:1110, 1974.

Florman, A. L., Gershon, A. A., Blackett, P. R., and Nahmias, A. J.: Intrauterine infection with herpes simplex virus, J.A.M.A. **225**:129, 1973.

Franciosi, R. A., Knostman, J. D., and Zimmerman, R. A.: Group B streptococcal infections, J. Pediatr. **82**:707, 1973.

Gotoff, S. P., and Behrman, R. F.: Neonatal septicemia, J. Pediatr. **76**:142, 1970.

Hanshaw, J. B.: Herpes virus hominis infections in the fetus and newborn, Am. J. Dis. Child. **126**:546, 1973.

Hanshaw, J. B., Schultz, F. W., Melisch, M. M., et al.: Congenital cytomegalovirus infection in intrauterine infections, CIBA Foundation Symposium (New Series), Amsterdam, 1973, Association of Scientific Publishers, pp. 32-43.

Harner, R. E., Smith, J. L., and Israel, C. W.: The FTA-HBS test in late syphilis, J.A.M.A. **203**:545, 1968.

Katz, S. L.: The possible relationship of viruses, other than rubella and cytomegalovirus, to the etiology of birth defects, Birth Defects Orig. Art. Ser. **4**:57, 1968.

Mazzacuva, D., and Salvioli, G. P.: Incidence and pathologic features of congenital syphilis in the last 20 years, Clin. Pediatr. **49**:3, 1967.

McCracken, G. H.: Pharmacological basis for antimicrobial therapy in newborn infants, Am. J. Dis. Child. **128**:407, 1974.

Modlin, J. F., Brandling-Bennett, A. D., Witte, J. J., Campbell, C. C., and Meyers, J. D.: A review of five years' experience with rubella vaccine in the United States, Pediatrics **55**:20, 1975.

Monif, G. R. G., Egan, E. A., Held, B., and Eitzman, D. V.: The correlation of maternal cytomegalovirus infection during varying stages of gestation with neonatal involvement, J. Pediatr. **80**:17, 1972.

Nahmias, A. J.: Perinatal risk associated with maternal genital herpes simplex virus infection, Am. J. Obstet. Gynecol. **110**:823, 1971.

Nahmias, A. J.: The torch complex, Hosp. Pract. p. 65, May, 1974.

Overall, J. C., Jr.: Neonatal bacterial meningitis, J. Pediatr. **76**:499, 1970.

Overall, J. C., Jr., and Glasgow, L. A.: Virus infections of the fetus and newborn infant, J. Pediatr. **77**:315, 1970.

Rawls, W. E., Desmyter, J., and Melnick, J. L.: Serologic diagnosis and fetal involvement in maternal rubella, J.A.M.A. **203**:627, 1968.

Rowan, D. F., McCraw, M. F., and Edward, R. D.: Virus infections during pregnancy (ECHO, Coxsackie), Obstet. Gynecol. **32**:356, 1968.

Sever, J. L., editor: Conference on Immunological Responses to Perinatal Infections, J. Pediatr. **75**:111, 1969.

Sever, J. L., Fuccillo, D. A., and Gilkeson, M. R.: Changing susceptibility to rubella, Obstet. Gynecol. **32**:365, 1968.

Skinner, W. E.: Routine rubella antibody titer determinations in pregnancy, Obstet. Gynecol. **33**:301, 1969.

Stagno, S., Reynolds, D. W., Lakeman, A., Charamella, L. J., and Alford, C. A.: Congenital CMV infection: consecutive occurrence due to viruses with similar antigenic compositions, Pediatrics **52**:788, 1973.

10

Possible teratogens affecting the fetus and neonate

Care of the pregnant patient includes a concern for related medical problems. Regard for the welfare of the fetus imposes certain restrictions on the physician in performing diagnostic studies or instituting treatment of the mother. The list of drugs potentially hazardous to the fetus is immense and expanding. Knowledge of any drugs the mother may be taking on her own could help to obviate any harmful effects if the drug can be withdrawn. Diagnostic procedures should be held to a minimum. Nevertheless, life-threatening conditions that have to be treated with agents known to be teratogenic necessitate the consideration of an elective abortion. A pregnant woman addicted to heroin, alcohol, etc. should be entered in a treatment program to reduce, hopefully, the danger to her fetus. Methadone replacement for a heroin-addicted mother, on the other hand, creates similar problems for the fetus and neonate. Minimal doses that will avoid consequences for the offspring are not yet known.

Table 10-1 tabulates certain maternal medications that may be harmful to the perinate.

When the insult occurred is an important consideration in possible teratogenesis. The insult cannot influence the target structure if development is completed (but it may affect growth). For this reason Table 10-2

may be of assistance in counseling a patient concerning the possibility of malformation from teratogens. It may also be useful to refer to Fig. 3-1.

EFFECTS OF MATERNAL DRUG ADDICTION ON THE FETUS AND NEONATE

Occasional withdrawal reactions have been reported in infants of mothers who excessively use such drugs as barbiturates, alcohol, or amphetamines. Serious reactions are seen with an increasing frequency in neonates (approximately 85% of those exposed) whose mothers are addicted to heroin or treated with methadone. Almost 50% of pregnancies of women addicted to these narcotics result in low birth weight infants—not necessarily preterm.

1. Possible factors contributing to the greater incidence of low birth weight infants
   a. Acute infections in the mother, often resulting in premature onset of labor
   b. Poor maternal nutrition, leading to fetal undergrowth
   c. Direct influence of the drug on the fetus (based on animal experiments)
2. Withdrawal reaction
   Symptoms usually occur within 24 hours but can begin as late as 2 to 3 weeks, especially if methadone was taken by the mother. Symptomatology varies from

132

Table 10-1. Human fetotoxic medicaments

Maternal medication	Fetal or neonatal effect
Anesthetics	
Ether	Neonatal depression related to duration and depth
Halothane (Fluothane)	of anesthesia; ether has direct narcotic effect on
Trichloroethylene (Trilene)	infant
Antibiotics	
Chloramphenicol	Gray syndrome; neonatal death (not reported if
	gravida alone received the drug)
Chloroquine	Death; deafness; retinol hemorrhage
Erythromycin	Possible hepatic injury
Nitrofurantoin	Megaloblastic anemia; G6PD deficiency
Novobiocin	Hyperbilirubinemia
Quinine, quinidine	Possible ototoxicity; thrombocytopenia
Streptomycin	Nerve deafness
Sulfonamides	Kernicterus sulfonamides complete with bilirubin for
	albumin-binding sites
Tetracyclines	Inhibition of bone growth; discolored teeth
Anticoagulants	
Coumarins	Fetal death; hemorrhage; calcifications
Antidiabetics	
Chlorpropamide	Fetal death; prolonged neonatal hypoglycemia
Tolbutamide	Possible teratogenic effects (not proved)
Antiepileptics	
Diphenylhydantoin	Possible teratogenic effects
Phenobarbital	Neonatal depression; withdrawal reaction
Antithyroid agents	
Propylthiouracil	
Methimazole	Goiter; occasional hypothyroidism
Potassium iodide	
^{131}I	Congenital hypothyroidism
Cancer chemotherapeutic agents	
Aminopterin	
6-Mercaptopurine	Abortion; fetal malformation
Busulfan	
Cyclophosphamide	
Methotrexate	
Ethyl alcohol	Fetal growth retardation; congenital anomalies;
	withdrawal reactions in neonate
Heavy metals	Abortion; growth retardation
Lysergic acid	Chromosome breakage
Narcotics	
Heroin	Neonatal withdrawal reaction
Methadone	
Radiation	Fetal death; congenital anomalies
Reserpine	Neonatal nasal congestion
Smoking	Fetal growth retardation
	Reduction in O_2 transport to fetus

Continued.

Table 10-1. Human fetotoxic medicaments—cont'd

Maternal medication	Fetal or neonatal effect
Steroids	
Cortisone	Cleft palate (?)
Progestin	
Testosterone	Masculinization
Diethylstilbestrol	
Thalidomide	Fetal death; congenital anomalies
Thiazides	Thrombocytopenia
Vitamins	
Vitamins A and D	Congenital anomalies
Vitamin K	Hyperbilirubinemia
and analogues	Kernicterus

Table 10-2. Potential malformations related to the time of the insult*

Week since ovulation	Potential malformation	Week since ovulation	Potential malformation
Third	Ectopia cordis	Sixth	Microphthalmia
	Omphalocele		Carpal or pedal ablation
	Ectromelia		Hairlip, agnathia
	Sympodia		Lenticular cataract
			Congenital heart disease
Fourth	Omphalocele		Gross septal and aortic anomalies
	Ectromelia		
	Tracheoesophageal fistula	Seventh	Congenital heart disease
	Hemivertebra		Interventricular septal defects
			Pulmonary stenosis
Fifth	Tracheoesophageal fistula		Digital ablation
	Hemivertebra		Cleft palate, micrognathia
	Nuclear cataract		Epicanthus, brachycephaly
	Microphthalmia		
	Facial clefts	Eighth	Congenital heart disease
	Carpal or pedal ablation		Epicanthus, brachycephaly
			Persistent ostium primum
			Nasal bone ablation
			Digital stunting

*Modified from Kaiser, I. H.: Physiology and development of fetus and placenta. In Danforth, D. N., editor: Textbook of obstetrics and gynecology, ed. 2, New York, 1971, Harper & Row, Publishers.

mild to severe and may last for several weeks.

a. Symptoms commonly seen
  1. Hypertonicity
  2. Irritability
  3. Tremors
  4. Vomiting
  5. Diarrhea
b. Symptoms occasionally present
  1. Tachypnea
  2. Elevation of temperature
  3. Convulsions
  4. High-pitched cry
3. Treatment
  a. Drugs of choice
    1. Phenobarbital, 5 to 10 mg/kg/24 hr
    2. Paregoric, 3 to 10 drops/4 hr
    3. Chlorpromazine, 3 mg/kg/ 24 hr
  Drug dosage is reduced gradually after improvement of symptoms.
  b. Give close attention to feeding and to fluid requirements (parenteral fluids may be necessary).
  c. Monitor blood glucose levels by Dextrostix to avoid hypoglycemia.

ALCOHOLISM AND THE PERINATE

A rising incidence of alcoholism has been reported in the childbearing population. Only recently have its adverse effects on the perinate been documented. The following variants were noted in infants of alcoholic mothers compared to matched controls (Jones and colleagues):
1. Undergrowth
2. Mental subnormality
3. Congenital anomalies, with increase in
  a. Short palpebral fissure
  b. Ptosis
  c. Strabismus
  d. Joint anomalies
  e. Cardiac murmurs

No evidence has been marshalled against the children of mothers who are heavy social users of alcohol.

Recommendation: Severe alcoholism in the gravida justifies a consideration of abortion not only because of its apparent detrimental effect on the fetus but because it is a likely deterrent to reasonable parent-child interaction.

SELECTED REFERENCES

Apgar, V., and Gause, R. W.: Teratology, Med. World News **11**:59, 1970.

Cohlan, S. Q.: Fetal and neonatal hazards from drugs administered during pregnancy, N. Y. J. Med. **64**:493, 1964.

Connor, B. E.: Infections and pregnancy: a review, South. Med. J. **62**:275, 1969.

Heller, M. B., Terdiman, J. F., and Pasternack, B. S.: A procedure for calculating the gonadal x-ray dose in diagnostic radiography, Br. J. Radiol. **39**:686, 1966.

Hill, R. M., Verinand, W. M., Hornig, M. G., McCulley, L. B., and Morgan, N. F.: Infants exposed in utero to antiepileptic drugs, Am. J. Dis. Child. **127**:645, 1974.

Jones, K. L., Smith, D. W., Streissguth, A. P., and Myrianthopoulos, M. C.: Outcome in offspring of chronic alcoholic women, Lancet **1**:1076, 1974.

Kandall, S. R., and Garner, L. M.: Late presentation of drug withdrawal symptoms in newborns, Am. J. Dis. Child. **127**:58, 1974.

Nora, J. J., Nora, A. H., Sommerville, R. J., Hill, R. M., and McNamara, D. G.: Maternal exposure to potential teratogens, J.A.M.A. **202**:1065, 1967.

Reddy, A. M., Harpes, R. G., and Stern, G.: Observations on heroin and methadone withdrawal in the newborn, Pediatrics **48**:353, 1971.

Zelson, C., Lee, S. J., and Casalino, M.: Neonatal narcotic addiction, N. Engl. J. Med. **289**:1216, 1973.

11

Transport of the high-risk perinate

FETAL TRANSPORT

With proper evaluation of pregnant women and identification of the factors that significantly increase the risk of perinatal disaster, the development of special centers for the care of high-risk pregnancy is now at hand. Analyses of perinatal deaths in a Wisconsin study (Schneider, Sixty-Sixth Ross Conference) indicated that two-thirds of the neonatal deaths and half of fetal deaths at that time were preventable. Further observation in that state showed that 80% to 90% of perinatal care in the hospital was given by nurses who in general had had no special training.

Therefore it would seem appropriate that the 10% to 20% of women who contribute to the majority of perinatal mortality (Chapter 1) must be identified so that they can be referred for evaluation and perhaps delivery in a specialized 24-hour specialty team setting. This team care may include house staff, but it should be emphasized that such personnel are in the learning process and should not have the prime responsibility for critical decisions. Of more urgent nature is the fetus discovered to be at high risk when the pregnant mother demonstrates actual or threatened labor. Such complications are delineated in Chapter 2.

When these complications are identified in a community hospital, the physician in charge should consult with a perinatal center. The degree of progress toward birth

can be assessed and the time factor judged in relation to emergency transfer.

If transport is elected:
1. Arrange a means of conveyance appropriate for the distance and climatic conditions.
2. Send appropriate personnel.
3. Include adequate equipment and supplies to meet intertransport emergencies (Appendix F).

NEONATAL TRANSPORT

The development of intensive care units for the severely ill infant during the last 10 years has been followed by the development of specialized transport systems in many areas of the country. The modern neonatal transport has become a necessary community and regional medical resource. The transfer of sick and small preterm infants is not new, but the utilization of full intensive care during the trip, after any necessary stabilization—temperature, acid-base balance, and oxygen requirements—prior to the transport, has almost eliminated the hazards of travel. In fact, most jeopardized infants may arrive at a specialized center in better condition than they exhibit while they are in the referring hospital.

The time has come when all regions will have a coordinated program of intercommunication and specialized teams for transport of the neonate to a specialized center in keeping with the infant's level of risk and home locale. For the type of infant problems suggesting need for transport, see the discussion in Chapter 12 on regionalization.

High-risk infants
Modes of transport

1. Specially equipped ambulance or van suitable for transport up to 75 miles from center (depending on traffic density and type of highway)
2. Helicopter for transport 50 to 150 miles from center
3. Fixed-wing airplane with two-motor, all-weather capability for transport 100 to 500 miles from center

Transport team (in addition to driver, pilot, and auxiliary personnel between hospital and airport or helipad)

1. For infants in respiratory distress, in shock, or with an acute surgical emergency
   a. Team leader—a physician experienced in full neonatal support
   b. Supporting neonatal nurse
2. For infants at moderate risk
   a. Team leader—a neonatal nurse trained in specialized neonatal care, such as temperature control, suction, oxygen therapy, mask ventilation, and parenteral fluid infusion
   b. Supporting specialized nurse

Arrangements to be made by admitting or transport officer

1. Ensure availability of nursing coverage and transport equipment.
2. Obtain pertinent clinical information, for example, prolonged ruptured membranes, condition at birth (Appendix C).
3. Give referring physician specific information on temporary care, including
   a. Support of infant's temperature
   b. Administration of sufficient ambient oxygen to keep infant pink
   c. Request for x-ray films, hematocrit,

and pH and blood gas determinations
4. Coordinate specific travel requirements and flight plans.
5. Have referring hospitals photocopy chart forms, collect x-ray films, obtain maternal blood (clotted and unclotted), and obtain placenta if possible.
6. Notify members of other services who might be involved, for example, pediatric surgeon, cardiologist, or respiratory therapist.
7. Request usual permits and check on the signed discharge.
8. Notify hospital admission and neonatal center and provide appropriate information.

Transport team arrangements

1. Check transport incubator, heat-regulating sources, and oxygen supply.
2. Check transport equipment (Appendix G).
3. Check fuel supplies in relation to travel distance.

Equipment and supplies for transport

1. Transport open-view incubator with full temperature support—120-volt AC, 12-volt DC converter
2. Tanks—735 L* O_2 and compressed-air tanks with pressure-regulating valves and tank volume meter connected to an air-oxygen blender
   Following is a formula for estimating O_2 reserves:

$$t = k \frac{P}{V}$$

   t = Minutes
   P = Pressure (psi)
   V = Flow in L/min
   k = 0.28

3. Oxygen analyzer
4. Heart rate monitor with skin electrodes (Parks Electronics)

---

*80's cylinders that have three times as much volume are necessary for use of a respirator and on extended trips.

5. Holter pump with complete intravenous administration set
6. Telethermometer and skin probe (Yellow Springs)
7. Doppler blood pressure equipment, with sphygmomanometer (Parks Electronics)
8. Bulb syringe, DeLee suction trap
9. Small plastic hood for O_2 administration
10. Penlon bag with tail and appropriate masks
11. Apparatus for delivering continuous positive airway pressure (CPAP) or intermittent positive-pressure breathing (IPPB) with positive end-expiratory pressure (PEEP)
12. Miscellaneous—crescent wrench, stethoscope, flashlight, clipboard for forms
13. Equipment
    a. Additional resuscitation equipment, for example, endotracheal tubes with adapters; laryngoscope with spare bulb and battery; suture set for tube fixation
    b. Umbilical vessel catheterization tray with gloves, skin antiseptic, Argyle catheters, iris forceps
    c. Peripheral intravenous administration set, complete with razor and blades, scalp-vein needles, tubing, and intravenous fluid
    d. Emergency drugs such as sodium bicarbonate, epinephrine, digoxin, isoproterenol (Isuprel), Lasix, Plasmanate, antibiotics, phenobarbital
    e. Miscellaneous—tape, syringes, drapes, blood-collecting tubes, adhesive tape

Care and stabilization of high-risk infants, particularly those with respiratory distress

Before infants are transported between hospitals, sufficient stabilization and diagnostic procedures, for example, blood gas determinations, x-ray films for lung disease, and tube placements, are justified to avoid unnecessary emergencies en route and to ensure safe arrival.

1. Oxygenation/ventilation
   a. Determine patency of airway, color, respiratory efficiency, and need for assisted respiration and oxygen.
   b. Direct oxygen into plastic hood (Oxyhood), humidified with sterile H_2O (Medicone Co.).
   c. Intubate infants who need continuous respiratory assistance.
   d. If infant has respiratory distress syndrome, and an ambient O_2 of 60% or more is required to maintain color, attach CPAP apparatus.
   e. Be prepared to rule out and treat pneumothorax prior to transport.
2. Temperature control (Appendix D)
   a. Attach skin probe of battery-powered telethermometer, and note infant's temperature.
   b. If the infant is hypothermic (a temperature of less than 96° F, 35.5° C), increase environmental temperature by 1° to 2° F over infant's skin temperature.
3. Metabolic, fluid, and glucose support
   a. Place intravenous line for continuous infusion of 10% glucose by battery-powered infusion pump.
   b. Correct acidosis (Chapter 19).
   c. Be mindful of hypoglycemia and assess infant's blood glucose with Dextrostix.
   d. Add medications as indicated.
4. Monitoring of vital signs
   a. Attach battery-powered heart rate monitor.
   b. Measure blood pressure (Doppler method).
   c. Check respiratory rate every 15 to 30 minutes.
5. Consider shock and be prepared to give blood or Plasmanate if
   a. Blood pressure is below normal (Chapter 20)
   b. Hematocrit is under 45
   c. Infant has mottled or pallid skin
6. Take blood culture and begin antibiotic therapy if sepsis is a possibility.

7. Prepare the patient for a surgical procedure.
   a. Empty stomach and leave large-bore orogastric tube in place if gastrointestinal obstruction or diaphragmatic hernia is suspected, particularly when transportation is by air.
   b. Elevate thorax above abdomen and suction esophageal pouch continuously, or every 5 minutes in esophageal atresia.
   c. Cover gastroschisis or omphalocele with warm saline-soaked gauze pads.
8. Miscellaneous
   a. Explain to parents the need for special care.
   b. Show infant to mother before departing and encourage subsequent mother-infant contact when possible.
   c. Consider regulations and sensitivities of referring hospital and staff.

Care of infant during transport

1. Observe color, respirations, and heart rate.
2. Maintain skin temperature of 97° to 98° F. (An incubator temperature between 90° and 97° and a vehicle temperature between 75° and 85° may be required.)
3. Assist breathing, when necessary to maintain color and heart rate, by bag and mask or bagging by means of CPAP apparatus.
4. Note any abdominal distention and consider pneumothorax or displaced endotracheal tube with increasing cyanosis.
5. Meet special requirements.
   a. Diaphragmatic hernia
      1. Offer frequent gastric suction through indwelling orogastric tube.
      2. Try to maintain color with oxygen.
      3. Use no positive pressure unless there is increasing cyanosis, and then accomplish by endotracheal tube *only*, with pressures under 30 cm H_2O.
   b. Esophageal atresia
      1. Elevate head and shoulders.

   2. Offer gastric suction intermittently to keep esophagus empty.
   c. Choanal atresia
      1. Use oropharyngeal airway.
   d. Pneumothorax, or enclosed air space
      1. Recognize hazard on ascent to high elevations.
      2. Place chest tube (Fr 14) with Heimlich valve or underwater seal.
6. Notify parents (and hospital) of baby's arrival.
7. Note problems, if any, during transport. For care of infant on admission to the neonatal intensive care unit, see Chapter 7.

Summary

Neonatal transport for the infant in severe distress requires the prompt mobilization of a team not only trained in transport details but able to give emergency care aimed at the stabilization of the infant's physiologic state prior to transport. In most instances the infant will arrive at the neonatal center in better condition than he was found.

Infant at medium risk

Transport from a community or primary hospital to an intermediary hospital for infants at only moderate risk is a new concept in local regional neonatal care. Such transfers should be restricted to one geographic area, preferably within less than a 50-mile radius, and should include babies with hyperbilirubinemia, moderate prematurity (over 32 weeks and 1,500 gm), failure to thrive, and mild to moderate respiratory distress. Infants not responding can in turn be sent to a tertiary neonatal center.

Requirements

1. A carrying incubator that is heated by connecting it to an automobile cigarette lighter or an ambulance facility (12-volt DC)
2. A nurse experienced in temperature

control, suction, oxygen support, and emergency mask ventilation, with facility in maintaining parenteral infusion

Arrangements to be made are similar to those outlined on p. 137.

Summary

There are two services to be performed in medium-risk transport:

1. Removal of infants at medium risk from primary hospitals (usually delivering less than 1,000 babies per year) to a designated intermediary hospital able to give continuing specialized care
2. Transfer of infants from a tertiary center to the intermediate care center for the continued growth and recovery of an infant who no longer requires sophisticated intensive care

The parents will live closer to this unit, and thus better parent-infant relations can be established.

Problems of transport

The effectiveness of neonatal transport in lowering morbidity and mortality rates depends on the efficiency of team care before and during transport. The following unsatisfactory situations have been repeatedly documented before and during transport services:

1. Inadequate resuscitation at birth
2. Failure to give basic support before transport team arrives
3. Cooling of infant as a result of failure of equipment or inexperience of personnel
4. Hypoventilation with or without airway obstruction; failure to intubate and offer sufficient O_2
5. Missed pneumothorax or displacement of endotracheal tube
6. Failure to use essential monitoring equipment
7. Untrained personnel for transport responsibility
8. Inadequate physician communication between referring center and neonatal intensive care unit

SELECTED REFERENCES

Baker, G. L.: Design and operation of a van for the transport of sick infants, Am. J. Dis. Child. **118:**743, 1969.

Chance, G. W., O'Brien, M. J., and Swyer, P. B.: Transportation of sick neonates, 1972: an unsatisfactory aspect of medical care, Can. Med. Assoc. J. **109:**847, 1973.

Cunningham, M. D., and Smith, F. R.: Stabilization and transport of severely ill infants, Pediatr. Clin. North Am. **20:**359, 1973.

Segal, S., editor: Manual for the transport of high-risk newborn infants: principles, policies, equipment, techniques, Vancouver, 1972, Canadian Pediatric Society.

Shepard, K. S.: Air transportation of high-risk infants utilizing a flying intensive care nursery, J. Pediatr. **77:**148, 1970.

12

Regionalization and guidelines for perinatal care

The regionalization of perinatal care is now an established fact in many areas of North America. Organization of such care for the fetus and neonate at high risk is advocated by major medical groups, including the American Medical Association. Pregnant women whose fetuses have been identified at increased risk of death or damage are referred increasingly to perinatal centers for full perinatal team support. Approximately 5% to 10% of all deliveries will be at high risk, and another 10% to 25% will be at moderate risk. The criteria for selecting those at risk are given in Chapter 2.

Unfortunately, not all of those at risk are identifiable prior to labor or even delivery. Unsuspected complications or premature labor will continue to occur in primary hospitals, resulting in the delivery of a possibly jeopardized infant and the need for special care. Although some maternity units are of sufficient size and have the capability to offer 24-hour intensive neonatal coverage, most hospitals do not. Therefore an emergency plan should be formulated for transport of an infant in distress to a perinatal center when the infant's condition does not stabilize and improvement fails to occur. Perinates at high risk are best transferred by a specialized physician-nurse transport team capable of providing full intensive care in transit.

Infants in severe respiratory distress and those with major congenital defects require, in most instances, transport to a neonatal center that offers what has come to be called tertiary care. Infants in moderate distress born in a primary or smaller community hospital often require transfer to an intermediate or secondary hospital capable of giving continuing specialized care. Special care units must not be developed indiscriminately, since the staffing requirements are demanding in terms of numbers as well as skills.

The concept of regionalization for obstetrical and neonatal care, designed to reduce maternal and infant mortality and morbidity, represents an obstetric and newborn health care system composed of three distinct types of facilities.

The highest-level facility is the *regional perinatal center*, which is fully equipped to handle any type of obstetric or newborn problem. Serving patients having complications beyond the treatment capability of other facilities, the regional center would become the primary source for referral and consultation for those patients requiring specialized care not available at other hospitals.

A second level of care would be provided by the *intermediate or larger community hospital*, which presently serves the bulk of obstetric and newborn patients. It should be capable of offering continuing special care, with only a small number of unusual or complicated problems referred from it to the regional center.

The third and final type of facility, the *small community or rural hospital*, providing a sharply limited amount of care, is nonetheless necessary in locations where geographic conditions limit access to other facilities.

SMALL COMMUNITY OR RURAL HOSPITAL (PRIMARY CARE)

The continuing move to consolidation of smaller maternity units and development of perinatal centers allows for care of moderate-risk patients, as well as affording the unanticipated infant at risk (up to 40% of problem babies) a better chance for optimum care and intact survival. Most hospitals in the smaller communities will of necessity have an insufficient number of deliveries to give other than temporary specialized care. Approximately 75% of infants are fortunately born at the lowest risk—those born at term (40 ± 2 weeks' gestation) and between 3,000 and 4,000 gm in weight. Unless these babies show disability, they may be placed in the regular nursery after an observation period of 6 to 8 hours near the nurses' station.

Sufficient facilities and skilled personnel must be available so that the physician is able to give adequate resuscitation and initial intensive care for any unexpectedly sick or distressed infant until the infant is stabilized or has been placed in the care of a transport team. In addition, transitional care of babies who are recovering must be available to the 10% to 20% of infants who are at medium risk. (See Chapter 6.) These infants include the following:

1. Large- and small-for-dates infants
2. Transitional preterm infants (35 to 37 weeks' gestation)
3. Dysmature or wasted infants who demonstrate no asphyxia at birth and who can accept early feedings

4. Infants with depressed Apgar scores (4 to 6) who have improved on admission to the nursery

These infants are at increased risk until good health is demonstrated, and any hospital that has a maternity department should supply the basic care outlined. (See Chapter 6.)

Transfer of infants to regional center (see Chapter 11)

Three to six percent of infants born in the smaller community hospital require transfer to a hospital giving continuing specialized care. Approximately one third of these infants need the team support of a tertiary center, including those who are severely depressed at birth, demonstrate increasing respiratory distress, show significant congenital anomalies, are under 30 weeks' gestation, or weigh less than 1,500 gm. In addition, a small percentage will develop the following problems not evident at birth that often require transfer:

1. Delayed respiratory distress, for example, aspiration, pneumothorax
2. Apneic or cyanotic spells, for example, in congenital heart disease or sepsis
3. Disorders of behavior and activity, including regurgitation, distention, and hypotonia
4. Seizures and sepsis
5. Hemorrhage or pallor
6. Jaundice before 24 hours of age or over 15 mg/100 ml

Special care requirements and facilities

The nursery area can serve as an admission, recovery, observation, and special-procedure area for infants at increased risk. These babies preferably are placed near the nurses' station. At least 2 feet of space is needed between units.

1. Medical, nursing, and paramedical personnel at all times should include the following:
   a. Ability to resuscitate by positive-

pressure methods and intubate if necessary

b. Ability to infuse $NaHCO_3$, glucose, blood, Plasmanate, or other blood volume expanders through an umbilical vessel for temporary support

c. Ability to give known monitored concentration of oxygen sufficient to control central cyanosis and to record these levels

d. Ability to ensure an appropriate thermal environment for the infant from the time of birth (which infers a delay in bathing)

e. Knowledge in using simple monitoring equipment, phototherapy for otherwise well babies, and Dextrostix testing, particularly for the distressed or the inappropriately grown

f. Ability to identify significant variations from the usual during the first 4 to 6 hours of life (transitional care)

g. Access by phone to a regional center for consultation regarding problems

h. A prearranged plan with a transport center for the immediate transfer of sick newborn infants

2. Utilities

a. Oxygen, compressed air, and suction availability

b. Electrical equipment—sufficient 120-volt outlets to a common ground (half on hospital emergency power circuit)

c. Washbasins—one for each four to six patient stations; with foot or knee controls

3. Equipment

a. Incubators or radiant warming systems: at least one radiant warmer in the labor and delivery suite, four (at least two) incubators or warmers for each 100 infants born per month for transitional care

b. A warmed nebulized oxygen source and hood (not less than one per 50 infants born per month)

c. Oxygen analyzer

d. Heart rate or heart rate and apnea monitors (two per 100 deliveries per month)

e. Phototherapy units (two per 100 deliveries per month)

f. A means of blood pressure measurement

g. An accurate scale ideally calibrated in grams

h. Resuscitation and stabilization equipment and medications

    1. Bag and mask with oxygen adapter suitable for the small neonate

    2. Laryngoscope and endotracheal tubes

    3. Bicarbonate with H_2O for dilution

    4. Glucose solutions

    5. 10% calcium gluconate

    6. Plasmanate or volume expander

    7. Epinephrine

    8. Isoproterenol (Isuprel)

    9. Sodium phenobarbital

    10. Digitalis

    11. Lasix

The drugs listed are primarily for temporary support of the infant and not for continued use in a primary hospital. After resuscitation it is recommended that an infusion of 10% dextrose containing 3 ml of 10% calcium gluconate/100 ml of solution be given and oral feedings withheld.

Obstetric requirements are dependent on the capabilities of the medical and nursing staff and on the size of the maternity unit, which is often limited by its geographic location. Because women at high risk often will be referred to the nearest maternity center for delivery, emphasis is placed on the following:

1. Early identification of the pregnancy at high risk to allow the primary physician to share in its management with the center

2. An established communication arrangement, particularly in evaluation of impending labor and delivery

3. An emergency transport service with capability for management of women in labor
4. Availability of an electronic fetal monitor for those cases which may develop intrapartum distress

LARGER COMMUNITY HOSPITALS FOR CONTINUING SPECIAL CARE (INTERMEDIARY CARE)

Centers for special care should be planned to meet patient, medical, community, and regional needs. The intermediate hospitals would provide a standard of care sufficient for most of the contingencies encountered by an obstetric or newborn service. The care provided would be of high quality and in no way inferior to comparable services available at the regional center. Because of rising costs and falling birth rates, consolidation of maternity services is necessary for maximum efficiency in providing quality service. Ideally a minimum of 2,000 infants should be delivered each year to offer efficient continuing care to both fetus and neonate at high risk. However, a more limited number of deliveries is justified when the hospital, by its geographic character, supplies special services to adjacent rural hospitals. An organized system of communication and transport for an interchange of patients at risk is required.

Specific obstetric requirements

1. Obstetric personnel and staffing
   a. A staff physician-in-charge who is knowledgeable in perinatal technology
   b. In-house obstetric and anesthesia coverage, 24 hours a day
   c. A specially trained obstetric registered nurse on each shift, with an adequate number of circulating nurses trained in obstetric nursing
   d. Programs for special and ongoing training and staff meetings to ensure high standards of perinatal care

2. Facilities and services
   a. Sufficient space and equipment to permit
      1. Fetal heart rate monitoring (more than one unit)
      2. Rapid surfactant test
      3. A decision to perform a cesarean section within 20 minutes or less (emergency section room)
      4. Emergency transfusion of 0-negative blood, with the decision to transfuse made 20 minutes or less beforehand
      5. Closely monitored postdelivery or postoperative recovery room
      6. Resuscitation capability in delivery and section room
   b. Hospital services on a 24-hour basis, including
      1. Full laboratory support, with blood bank
      2. Inhalation therapy and radiologic services
      3. Social service

Specific neonatal requirements

A minimal unit of at least four intensive care "beds" is required to justify the specialized care program as outlined. The following basic recommendations are in addition to the emergency and observational care and are suggested for the primary hospital:

1. Pediatric personnel and staffing
   a. A physician-in-charge who has had special training or experience in neonatal care, on call 24 hours a day
   b. A registered nurse, trained in neonatal care, on each shift
   c. Paramedical personnel trained in respiratory therapy and in engineering and electronic supervision
   d. Nurse-patient ratio of 1:3 (may vary from 1:2 to 1:4)
   e. A committee responsible for planning and maintaining standards of care, policy, and regular review of the special care service, with particular attention paid to infection control

f. Programs for special and ongoing training of key personnel

g. Public health nurse and social worker consultation services

2. Utilities

   a. Two outlets each per patient for oxygen; one each for compressed air and suction

   b. Eight to ten 110-volt outlets per patient module—with half on hospital emergency power circuit

   c. 220-volt outlet per room for portable x-ray unit

   d. Adequate, convenient washbasins

3. Equipment

   a. Four intensive care beds of the isolette type or four open radiant warmers per 100 deliveries per month; additional modules if infants are admitted from regional hospitals

   b. Ward services

      1. Adequate resuscitation equipment

      2. Hematocrit centrifuge

      3. T-S (total solids) meter

      4. Glucose monitoring (urine and blood)

      5. Transillumination light (and darkroom)

      6. X-ray view box

4. Laboratory capabilities (24 hours)

   a. pH, P_{CO_2}, and P_{O_2} determinations

   b. Bilirubin measurement, direct and indirect

   c. Microelectrolyte determination

   d. Assessment of coagulation status, microhematologic service, typing, minor incompatibility

5. Special diagnostic and supportive service

   a. Immediately available x-ray services

   b. Blood bank

   c. Respiratory therapy (therapist on call, responsible for maintenance of equipment)

   d. Electroencephalograph and electrocardiograph recorders with newborn leads

   e. Rapid infant transport without heat loss (Chapter 11)

REGIONAL CARE CENTERS (TERTIARY CARE)

Regional care centers provide the ultimate in perinatal care for the very high–risk pregnancy and neonate.

Approximately 5% to 10% of women have sufficiently critical problems in pregnancy to be delivered with a full perinatal team in attendance. These conditions include eclampsia, severe diabetes, hydramnios, severe bleeding, premature rupture of membranes at less than 35 weeks' gestation, and heart disease.

Between 2,000 and 6,000 births in an area are necessary to justify 24-hour inhouse coverage by a skilled staff and to make a hospital economically viable. Fifteen-minute cesarean section time, emergency fetal scalp blood gas and pH capability, B-scan ultrasonography, and one-day estriol and rapid surfactant tests are among the requirements of such a center, in addition to those mentioned for the intermediary center.

Approximately 2% to 3% of newborns require the most critical care. This care covers infants requiring extended ventilatory assistance, cardiac catheterization, neonatal surgery, genetic and metabolic evaluation, and prolonged parenteral alimentation. This type of neonatal unit may need to draw from a population of approximately 10,000 annual births to justify its classification as a tertiary center that should be contiguous to the regional maternity center.

Those centers which intend to offer assisted ventilation for severe respiratory distress or insufficiency should recognize the effort and expertise such care requires. To justify the manpower and provide the experience in ventilatory support and related requirements, at least 3,000 to 5,000 annual births are desirable.

Personnel and staffing requirements

1. A neonatologist or pediatrician with special neonatal training on stand-by call

2. Twenty-four–hour in-house physicians capable of providing emergency life-support measures, including pediatric resident and anesthesiologist; perhaps also a neonatal nurse specialist
3. Registered nurses on each shift who have had at least 3 months' training in specialized neonatal care
4. Ability to offer one-to-one nurse-patient ratio for the extremely sick infant
5. Emergency consultative services (perinatal hotline) and a physician-nurse team for organized transport of infants between hospitals, involving ground and air travel—available 24 hours a day and 7 days a week
6. When neonatal care is offered in the subspecialties, e.g., cardiology or surgery, an appropriate team that has been organized in detail and that has diagnostic facilities, so that total care for these special problems can be integrated in the center
7. Clearly defined administrative responsibilities

Recommended facilities and services (in addition to the requirements of other specialized nurseries)

1. Incubators or open-air warmers with eight to ten electrical outlets, and two oxygen, compressed air, and suction outlets for each unit
2. An area of 60 to 100 square feet for each intensive care module
3. Cardiac-respiratory and central blood pressure monitoring
4. Capacity for delivering continuous positive airway pressure (CPAP) or continuous negative pressure (CNP) and intermittent positive-pressure breathing (IPPB) or intermittent negative-pressure breathing (INPB), with constant support by respiratory therapists
5. Complete 24-hour emergency radiologic services and laboratory support for blood gas and microelectrolyte determinations; the capability to perform blood coagulation studies and serum and urine osmolality tests
6. Ability to offer prolonged "parenteral alimentation" prepared under controlled conditions
7. Educational programs for center personnel as well as for physicians and nurses from referring hospitals
8. Full-time social service and public health nurse support
9. Follow-up studies of graduates to evaluate methods of care and mortality and morbidity rates

SELECTED REFERENCES

Blackman, L. R., and Brown, A. K.: Recommended standards for hospital nursery services, Augusta, 1973, Medical College of Georgia.

Carrier, C., Doray, B., Stern, L., and Usher, R.: Effect of neonatal intensive care on mortality rates in the province of Quebec (abstract), Pediatr. Res. 6:408, 1972.

Dinermon, B.: Obstetric services in the central area of Los Angeles County, 1973, Comprehensive Health Planning Council of Los Angeles County.

Hospital care of newborn infants, ed. 5, Evanston, Ill., 1971, American Academy of Pediatrics.

Lucey, J. F.: Why we should regionalize perinatal care, Pediatrics 52:488, 1973.

Sunshine, P., editor: Regionalization of perinatal care, Report of 66th Ross Conference, Columbus, Ohio, 1974, Ross Laboratories.

Swyer, P. R.: The regional organization of special care for the neonate, Pediatr. Clin. North Am. 17:761, 1970.

13

Malpresentation and cord accidents

BREECH

Breech is a longitudinal presentation in which the cephalic pole of the fetus occupies the fundal segment, and the caudal or podalic pole lies in the lower segment of the uterine cavity or within the birth canal. There are three major types of breech presentation:
1. *Frank breech:* hips flexed, knees extended, buttocks presenting
2. *Complete breech:* hips extended, knees partially flexed, buttocks and/or feet presenting
3. *Incomplete breech:* hips extended, knees extended, foot or feet presenting
    a. Single footling if one leg is completely extended and the other flexed
    b. Double footling if both legs are extended below the level of the buttocks

The incidence of term breeches is 3% to 4%, with approximately two thirds presenting as frank breeches. A previous breech or habitual breech is found in approximately 20% of cases. The incidence of breech is higher with decreasing gestational age.

Correlations predisposing to breech presentation

As the fetus grows, it occupies a greater volume in the uterine cavity and tends to accommodate to the shape of the corpus. The etiology of breech may be an aberra-

tion of this adaptation process or of the fetal attitude. In other cases the site of implantation of the placenta may encourage breech presentation. The following factors are known correlates of breech presentation:
1. Prematurity
2. Placenta previa
3. Fetal hydrocephalus
4. Multiparity
5. Multiple pregnancy
6. Hydramnios
7. Congenital uterine abnormality
8. Tumors of the uterus, cervix, vagina, or ovaries

Diagnosis

A wise dictum urges the assumption that all gestations are in the breech position until proved otherwise.
1. Examine the uterus by the four maneuvers of Leopold (Fig. 3-5).
2. Confirm by listening to the fetal heartbeat (which should be heard best over the back).
3. Order radiography or ultrasonography if in doubt.
4. Perform pelvic examination when the patient is in labor.

Management

1. External cephalic version
   External cephalic version is a method of treatment whereby the obstetrician at-

147

tempts to avert the breech presentation and its inherent dangers. This maneuver is usually performed prior to the thirty-fourth week of gestation and rarely after the thirty-eighth week. Although the procedure has been performed under anesthesia, we do not recommend it. The primary dangers to the fetus are separation of the placenta and cord entanglement.

2. Cesarean section

In view of the increased morbidity and mortality in breech presentation and the emphasis on smaller families of maximum quality, a more aggressive use of cesarean section is recommended in breech delivery. This procedure must at all times be performed at the most opportune time by a competent team in a properly equipped hospital. The morbidity from the procedure may be less than that from external cephalic version and is definitely less than that from breech extraction. Perform section immediately when there is

a. Any evidence of fetopelvic disproportion
b. A fetus weighing over 8 lb (3.5 kg)
c. A gestation of 42 weeks or more
d. Any prior history of dystocia or injury at previous breech birth
e. Any abnormality of the first stage of labor
f. Any need for oxytocin augmentation of labor
g. A prolonged second stage of labor
h. Any evidence of fetal distress
i. A primipara
j. A complete or incomplete breech
k. An undergrown fetus
l. A multiple gestation, with one or more infants in breech presentation
m. A prolapsed cord

3. Vaginal delivery

Assessing the possibility of vaginal delivery may be assisted by the breech scoring index, as proposed by Zatuchni and Andros (Table 13-1). Configuration and size of pelvis are not directly evaluated in this schema but are indirectly reflected by cervical dilatation, fetal descent, and previous pregnancy. In addition, the scoring index is not utilizable in patients who are considered for induction, because it is applicable only to patients admitted in labor. If the total score achieved is 3 or less, a cesarean section should be performed. A score of 4 demands a careful reevaluation, and a score of 5 or more may justify vaginal delivery.

Factors predisposing to fetal injury during labor and delivery are as follows:

1. Greater incidence of umbilical cord prolapse
2. Pressure on umbilical cord occurring in the first stage of labor

Table 13-1. Criteria for scoring*

	Points		
	0	*1*	*2*
Parity	Primigravida	Multipara	
Gestational age	39 weeks or more	38 weeks	37 weeks or less
Estimated fetal weight	More than 8 lb (3,630 gm)	7 lb to 7 lb 15 oz (3,176 to 3,629 gm)	Less than 7 lb (3,175 gm)
Previous breech†	None	1	2 or more
Dilatation‡	2 cm	3 cm	4 cm or more
Station‡	−3 or higher	−2	−1 or lower

*From Zatuchni, G. I., and Andros, G. J.: Prognostic index for vaginal delivery in breech presentation at term, Am. J. Obstet. Gynecol. **98:**855, 1967.
†Greater than 2,500 gm.
‡Determined by vaginal examination on admission.

3. Increased incidence of placental separation
4. Entrapment of the head by the cervix
5. Injury of the head and neck by more rapid descent through the birth canal
6. Injury of the head and neck by the mode of delivery
7. The arms are more likely to be swept over the head, which may increase the chance of nerve damage

Every effort should be made to decrease the possibility of any of these injurious factors occurring; therefore, if a vaginal delivery is to be anticipated for a breech, there are many critical factors in addition to the "breech index" that determine feasibility. Of paramount importance are the experience and ability of those in attendance.

Other keys to management of labor in the breech presentation must include the following:

1. Early detection of fetopelvic relations and aberrations, and prediction of whether they will permit vaginal delivery (x-ray pelvimetry and ultrasonography)
2. Determination of the exact position of the extremities
3. Observation for prolapse of the cord or for cord complications
4. Observation for fetal distress (electronic fetal monitoring)
5. Careful evaluation of labor's progress, in terms of both dilatation and descent of the presenting part
6. Immediate delivery by cesarean section if any augmentation of labor is necessary

In addition, ideal management would include the following:

1. Avoidance of early artificial rupture of the membranes
2. Examination of the patient vaginally at the time of rupture of the membranes and at the onset of labor to rule out prolapse of the cord
3. Delay in pudendal block anesthesia until breech is crowning, to maintain the patient's voluntary expulsive efforts
4. Interference during the second stage as little and as late as possible
5. Loosening and drawing down a short loop of cord when the umbilicus comes into view
6. A generous episiotomy
7. Allowing the fetus to be expelled to the level of the umbilicus before manipulation
8. Planning the delivery of a breech so that descent and rotation occur while the cervix is relaxed (Inhalation of the contents of a sodium nitrite pearl or injection of epinephrine, 0.2 ml, 1:1,000 solution intravenously, may relax the cervix temporarily if it has already begun to contract.)
9. Directing a second twin into the pelvis as a vertex rather than a breech presentation, if possible

Average analgesia (or less) should not harm even the small fetus. An experienced obstetrician and an assistant should be scrubbed for vaginal delivery of a breech. Vaginal examination at the time of rupture of the membranes is important in checking for possible prolapsed cord. The patient should avoid expulsive efforts until full dilatation of the cervix occurs. Pudendal block and a wide episiotomy are desirable.

However, the selection of the proper anesthetic for breech delivery is as varied as are the approaches to effecting that delivery. One popular method is local infiltration or nerve block for the episiotomy, with general anesthesia for the assisted breech portion of the delivery. However, some physicians urge the use of caudal and/or epidural anesthesia.

Following are three methods for delivery of the fetal body:

1. Total breech extraction, in which one and then both of the lower extremities are grasped and used literally to extract the

fetus from the uterus, is by far the most hazardous method of vaginal delivery.

2. Spontaneous expulsion allows for full delivery of the body without manipulative interference. It is the next most hazardous mode of delivery.

3. Assisted breech, in which the fetus is spontaneously expelled to the level of the umbilicus and the remainder extracted, is the least hazardous.

The mode of delivery for the aftercoming head remains in debate. Some believe that routine use of forceps may protect the head from trauma, but others disagree and recommend manual control of the head.

Complications in the perinate

Breech delivery is associated with a perinatal mortality of 18% (British Perinatal Study), and thus it is the leading factor in perinatal death. In the main, the hazard of the small breech-delivered infant is due to the following:

1. Complications of pregnancy (placenta previa, etc.)
2. Low birth weight related to complications of pregnancy
3. Injuries associated with low birth weight

In contrast, the large (term or postterm) breech-delivered infant generally is jeopardized by complications of labor, such as the following:

1. Prolapsed cord
2. Uterine dysfunction
3. Hypoxia and trauma during delivery—the consequences of relative feto-pelvic disproportion

The perinatal mortality of infants delivered in the breech position is 10 to 25 times greater than that of those delivered by vertex. This difference is largely due to premature birth. However, when mortality is compared, with correction for birth weight, the breech-delivered infant is still at a disadvantage in regard to higher mortality rates, increased neurologic damage, and subnormal intellectual levels.

Infant morbidity may reach 16%, with nearly half showing signs of permanent injury, primarily the result of asphyxia and intracranial hemorrhage. The breech infant of the multipara may suffer equally with that of the primipara because of the following:

1. Increasing size of subsequent fetuses
2. False sense of security in dealing with a "proved" pelvis
3. Repetition of breech presentation in approximately 20% of cases

Early identification of breech presentation and related problems is important to the outcome. Consultation and more liberal use of cesarean section in borderline cases are necessary to improve the salvage in breech presentation.

Neonatal care

Chapter 6 presents the birth-room attention given to infants who require special care. In addition to birth-room observations outlined, observe neonate for the following occasional injuries:

1. Fracture of clavicle or humerus; epiphyseal injury
2. Brachial plexus injury (unlikely if adequate Moro reflex)
3. Dislocation of hips
4. Paralyses of legs (cord injury)
5. Intracranial hemorrhage (Chapter 22)

OTHER MALPRESENTATIONS
Transverse lie

When the long axis of the fetus lies at right angles to the long axis of the mother, the presentation is described as a transverse lie. This complication occurs in less than 0.5% of all term gestations. It most frequently is associated with increasing multiparity because of relaxation of the abdominal wall and uterus. Other correlates are bony pelvis contraction and placenta previa.

The diagnosis is usually readily made by inspection and/or palpation. Should there be any difficulty in diagnosis by Leopold's maneuvers, confirmation by ultrasonographic or radiographic means should be undertaken. Since this presentation is not amenable to vaginal delivery and there is great hazard of prolapse of the umbilical cord if the patient presents in labor, cesarean section should be performed as soon as feasible. Perinatal mortality is markedly increased with transverse lie, about 140/1,000 live births.

Face presentation

When the face of the fetus is the presenting part, it is termed a face presentation. The point for designation of position is the mentum (chin). This condition occurs in only 0.2% of pregnancies. The diagnosis may be suspected by the abdominal examination; however, it is usually ascertained or confirmed by vaginal examination. In most cases, x-ray pelvimetry is necessary for adequate pelvic evaluation for vaginal delivery. Indeed, cesarean section will be necessary in nearly all primiparas and many multiparas. If, however, the pelvis is adequate in relation to the fetal size, spontaneous delivery or easy low forceps may be anticipated when the mentum is anterior or transverse. The mentum posterior precludes vaginal delivery, and all fetuses in this position except the very smallest will require cesarean section. For prevention of maternal morbidity (deep tears in the perineum), wide episiotomy should be performed. Exact clinical correlates have not been developed for this unusual presentation. Perinatal mortality is as high as 70 to 163/1,000 live births if the condition remains unidentified and untreated.

Brow presentation presents roughly the same set of risks as face presentation. However, it occurs less frequently (0.1% of cases).

PROLAPSE OF THE UMBILICAL CORD

Prolapse of the umbilical cord is a condition in which the funis lies alongside (occult) or lower than the presenting part (overt) in the birth canal. With the overt (or complete) variety, the cord may be contained entirely within the vagina or may protrude through the introitus. The greatest predisposition for cord prolapse occurs when the presenting part does not fill the lower uterine segment and impinges on the cervix. Thus the cord may enter this space and lie alongside or lower than the presenting part.

Overt prolapse occurs in 0.4% to 0.5% of all deliveries. The incidence of occult prolapse of the cord is difficult to ascertain because it is usually asymptomatic unless cord compression occurs. In the Collaborative Perinatal Study carried out by the National Institute of Neurological Diseases and Stroke (NINDS), occult prolapse of the cord was detected in 0.3% to 0.7% of all cases; however, electronic fetal monitoring reveals that approximately one fourth of high-risk patients will have cord compression patterns. Unfortunately, accurate data have not been accumulated concerning the percentage of variable decelerations (cord compression patterns) created by occult prolapse. Although infrequent, cord prolapse is important in perinatal wastage because of the great fetal hazard if it does occur. With occult cord prolapse, the normally expected perinatal mortality is doubled, and with overt prolapse it is increased approximately twelvefold.

Diagnosis
Clinical correlates

1. Abnormal presentation
   a. Breech
      Footling breech is at greatest risk of cord prolapse; however, all breeches are at some degree of risk. The overall incidence of this complication with breeches is fivefold greater than with vertex presentation.
   b. Shoulder (transverse lie)
   c. Face
   d. Brow

e. Transverse
f. Compound
2. Multiple pregnancy
3. Prematurity (45.5% of pregnancies complicated by this condition)
4. Artificial rupture of the membranes in the presence of a floating presenting part
5. Polyhydramnios and increasing gravidity, both of which have been correlated with umbilical cord prolapse, although to a lesser degree than with the factors noted above

Occult cord prolapse

Occult cord prolapse is detected most commonly by the presence of variable deceleration in electronic fetal monitoring patterns. Occasionally, sterile vaginal examination may reveal the presence of the umbilical cord along the presenting part.

Overt prolapse

With complete prolapse the patient may feel the cord slide through the vagina and over the vulva after rupture of the membranes. Usually compression of the cord causes violent fetal activity, obvious to both patient and observer. The cord may be seen or palpated by the patient, an attendant, or a physician during external or internal examination. Auscultation of the fetal heart with a head stethoscope or an electronic fetal monitoring device may reveal fetal distress. (See Chapter 4.)

Treatment

1. The patient should be placed immediately in the knee-chest or deep Trendelenburg position.
2. Using aseptic technique, upward pressure should be exerted on the presenting part to relieve cord compression.
3. Repositioning of the cord within the uterus may be attempted; however, it is rarely successful.
4. Careful palpation of the umbilical cord must be performed to ascertain fetal

viability. About 17% of pregnant women with this complication have a dead fetus on admission to labor and delivery, and it is possible to err by rushing to deliver the dead fetus.
5. The fetal heart tones should be monitored continuously until the time of delivery.
6. Delivery should be effected immediately and is most often accomplished by cesarean section with the mother under general anesthesia.
7. Consideration must also be given to other factors that may alter the above management.
   a. If the pregnancy is 27 weeks' duration or less, it may be ill advised to increase the maternal risk in an effort to salvage a very immature fetus.
   b. If the cervix is nearly completely dilated and the fetal presenting part is well within the pelvis, a vaginal delivery utilizing forceps or vacuum extractor may be accomplished.

Complications

As anticipated, fetal death rates are increased with prolapse of the cord. Occult prolapse of the cord in the Collaborative Perinatal Study of the NINDS was not associated with low birth weight infants, whereas overt prolapse of the cord occurred more commonly with low birth weight infants. The perinatal death rates (per 1,000 births) with occult prolapse of the cord varied between 57 and 185, and with overt prolapse, between 337 and 361. There was no consistent increase noted in the risk of neurologic abnormalities at 1 year of age among babies born after prolapse of the cord if they survived the original insult.

VELAMENTOUS INSERTION OF THE CORD (VASA PREVIA)

In velamentous insertion of the cord, its proximal end is attached to the membranes. Fetal vessels then extend across a membranous bridge to the placenta. The abnormality may be the result of growth of the placenta away from the implantation site, with concomitant atrophy of villous units in the bare zone about the point of cord insertion. When one or more fetal vessels actually cross the internal os, this variation is called *vasa previa*.

1. Occurrence
   a. One in 100 singleton placentas
   b. Five to ten out of every 100 twin placentas, with the velamentous insertion invariably attached to the smaller of the pair
2. Associations
   a. Late abortions
   b. Low birth weight infants
3. Complications
   a. Tear of a bridging vessel
      1. Fetal bleeding–fetal red blood cells or hemoglobin in vaginal blood
      2. Fetal distress, then fetal death
4. Therapy imperative to save the offspring
   a. Rapid delivery
   b. Transfusion

SELECTED REFERENCES

Alexopoulos, K. A.: Importance of breech delivery in the pathogenesis of brain damage: end results of long-term follow-up, Clin. Pediatr. **12:** 248, 1973.

Allen, J. P., Myers, G. G., and Condon, V. R.: Laceration of the spinal cord related to breech delivery, J.A.M.A. **208:**1019, 1969.

Barham, K. A.: The diagnosis of a vas praevium by amnioscopy, Med. J. Aust. **55:**398, 1968.

Benson, W. L., Boyce, D. C., and Vaughn, D. L.: Breech delivery in the primigravida, Obstet. Gynecol. **40:**417, 1972.

Bird, C. C., and McElin, T. W.: Five hundred consecutive term breech deliveries, Obstet. Gynecol. **35:**451, 1970.

Galloway, W. H., Bartholomew, R. A., Colvin, E. D., Grimes, W. H., Fish, J. S., and Lester, W. M.: Premature breech delivery, Am. J. Obstet. Gynecol. **99:**975, 1967.

Helfferich, M., and Favier, J.: Breech delivery, Am. J. Obstet. Gynecol. **110:**58, 1971.

Jurado, L., and Miller, G. L.: Breech presentation, Am. J. Obstet. Gynecol. **101:**183, 1968.

Mark, C., III, and Roberts, P. H. R.: Breech scoring index, Am. J. Obstet. Gynecol. **101:**572, 1968.

Medina, J. E., and Townsend, C. E.: Vasa praevia, report of a case and brief review of the clinical features, Med. Ann. DC **36:**748, 1967.

Niswander, K. R., and Gordon, M.: The women and their pregnancies (The Collaborative Perinatal Study of the National Institute of Neurological Diseases and Stroke), Philadelphia, 1972, W. B. Saunders Co., p. 416.

Rovinsky, J. J., Miller, J. A., and Kaplan, S.: Management of breech presentation at term, Am. J. Obstet. Gynecol. **115:**497, 1973.

Serreyn, R., et al.: Fetal hypoxia and breech delivery, Int. J. Gynaecol. Obstet. **11:**11, 1973.

Tank, E. S., Davis, R., Holt, J. F., and Morley, G. W.: Mechanisms of trauma during breech delivery, Obstet. Gynecol. **38:**761, 1971.

Woodward, R. W., and Callahan, W. E.: Breech labor and delivery in the primigravida, Obstet. Gynecol. **34:**260, 1969.

Zatuchni, G. I., and Andros, G. J.: Prognostic index for vaginal delivery in breech presentation at term, Am. J. Obstet. Gynecol. **98:**854, 1967.

14

Hypertensive states in pregnancy

The hypertensive disease states of pregnancy are certain vascular derangements (usually vasospastic) that either antedate pregnancy or arise during pregnancy or the early puerperium. The synonyms include toxemias of pregnancy, eclamptogenic toxemia, the edema-proteinuria-hypertension complex, and gestoses. These disorders are of unknown etiology and involve mutliple metabolic aberrations, often including low-protein intake. In addition to the vasospasm, sodium and water retention occurs, and there is depletion of serum albumin and globulin because of proteinuria. Primigravidas and women who have chronic hypertensive or renal disease are predisposed. The lower socioeconomic groups of all races are especially prone to eclamptogenic toxemia.

In this country, between 3% and 10% of pregnant women develop preeclampsia, but the incidence is as high as 20% in areas where poor medical care prevails. Eclampsia affects about 5% of toxemic patients in the United States.

Maternal mortality with preeclampsia is exceptional, but with eclampsia it may reach 15%. Perinatal mortality is two or three times the average in preeclampsia, whereas with eclampsia it is at least 20%, most of the infants being of low birth weight.

DIAGNOSIS

A vigorous screening program is necessary for the detection of the various degrees of the hypertensive states of pregnancy. There are certain *predispositions* that bear especially rigorous scrutiny:

1. Primigravida
2. Multiple gestation
3. Hydramnios or fetal hydrops
4. Hydatidiform mole
5. Obesity
6. Diabetes mellitus
7. Renal disease (especially chronic hypertension)
8. Positive family history
9. Pheochromocytoma
10. Lupus erythematosus

The diagnostic criteria for the various components of the hypertensive states of pregnancy are discussed in the following paragraphs.

Hypertension

Hypertension is a rise in the systolic pressure of 30 mm Hg or more; a rise in the diastolic pressure of 15 mm Hg or more; or the presence of a blood pressure reading of 140/90 or more. Hypertension may also be determined by a mean arterial pressure of 105 mm Hg or more or by a rise of 20 mm Hg or more. The level cited must be manifest on at least two occasions at least 6 hours apart and should be based on previously known blood pressure levels.

Gestational hypertension

Gestational hypertension is the development of hypertension during pregnancy or within the first 24 hours postpartum in a previously normotensive woman. No other evidence of preeclampsia or hypertensive vascular disease persists or develops. The blood pressure returns to normal levels within 10 days after parturition. Some patients with gestational hypertension may have preeclampsia or hypertensive vascular disease, but they do not satisfy the criteria for either of these diagnoses, for example, lack of proteinuria or generalized edema to substantiate preeclampsia.

Chronic hypertensive disease

Chronic hypertensive disease is the presence of persistent hypertension of whatever cause before pregnancy or before the twentieth week of gestation, or of persistent hypertension beyond the forty-second postpartum day.

Unclassified hypertensive disorders

Unclassified hypertensive disorders are those in which information is insufficient for classification. They should compose a minority of the hypertensive disorders in pregnancy.

Gestational edema

Gestational edema is a general accumulation of fluid in the tissues greater than 1+ pitting edema *after* 12 hours' rest in bed, or a weight gain of at least 5 lb in 1 week due to the influence of pregnancy.

Gestational proteinuria

Gestational proteinuria is the presence of proteinuria during (or under the influence of) pregnancy, in the absence of hypertension, edema, urinary tract infection, or known intrinsic renovascular disease. The protein must occur in concentrations greater than 0.3 gm/L in a 24-hour urine collection, or greater than 1 gm/L (1+ to 2+ by standard turbidimetric methods) in a random urine collection on two or more occasions at least 6 hours apart. The specimens must be clean voided, midstream, or obtained by catheterization.

Preeclampsia

Preeclampsia is the development of hypertension with proteinuria, edema, or both due to pregnancy or the influence of a recent pregnancy. It occurs after the twentieth week of gestation, but it may develop before this time in the presence of hydatidiform mole or choriocarcinoma. Preeclampsia is predominantly a disorder of primigravidas. For basis of treatment we divide preeclampsia into mild preeclampsia and severe preeclampsia.

1. Mild preeclampsia
   a. Hypertension: blood pressure greater than 140/90 or a 30/15 rise on two occasions 6 hours apart
   b. Weight gain: more than 5 lb/wk (2.3 kg)
   c. Edema: 15% to 50% of pregnant women have slight generalized edema, and about 4% have mildly elevated blood pressure and proteinuria
   d. Proteinuria: 0.3 gm/L or more on a random specimen on two occasions 6 hours apart
2. Severe preeclampsia (in addition to the above)
   a. Hypertension: blood pressure 160/110 or more on two separate occasions 6 hours apart with the patient at bed rest
   b. Proteinuria: 5 gm/24 hr or more
   c. Oliguria: 400 ml/24 hr or less
   d. Other symptoms (noted primarily if the condition is worsening):
      1. Headache: violent, persistent, and generalized
      2. Ocular abnormalities
         a. Symptoms: visual disturbances, blurred vision, or scintillating scotoma
         b. Sign: retinal arteriolar spasm on funduscopic examination
      3. Epigastric pain
      4. Nausea or vomiting
      5. Nervousness and irritability
      6. Pulmonary edema or cyanosis

3. Differential diagnosis
   a. Essential hypertension
   b. Adrenal hyperplasia
   c. Coarctation of the aorta
   d. Unilateral or bilateral renal arterial disease
   e. Hyperaldosteronism
   f. Glomerulonephritis
   g. Nephrotic syndrome
   h. Pyelonephritis
   i. Pheochromocytoma

Eclampsia

1. Diagnosis
   The diagnosis of eclampsia is based on the presence of the signs listed previously for severe preeclampsia, plus one or more of the following:
   a. Convulsions (tonic and clonic) or coma (often after an unobserved seizure) not attributable to other central nervous system disorders such as epilepsy or cerebral hemorrhage
   b. Hypertensive crisis or shock
2. Differential diagnosis
   a. Grand mal epilepsy
   b. Water intoxication
   c. Hysteria
   d. Cerebral tumor
   e. Hypoparathyroidism
   f. Acute porphyria
   g. Hypoglycemia
   h. Subarachnoid hemorrhage
   i. Alkalotic tetany
   j. Meningitis
   k. Systemic lupus erythematosus
   l. Strychnine poisoning
   m. Toxic reaction to local anesthetic agents

Superimposed preeclampsia or eclampsia

Superimposed preeclampsia or eclampsia is the development of preeclampsia or eclampsia in a patient with chronic hypertensive vascular or renal disease. When the hypertension antedates the pregnancy, as established by previous blood pressure recordings, a rise in the diastolic pressure of 15 mm Hg and the development of proteinuria, edema, or both is required during pregnancy to establish the diagnosis.

LABORATORY STUDIES

The following laboratory studies should be obtained on every patient who is affected by the hypertensive states of pregnancy seriously enough to require hospitalization:
1. Hematocrit, hemoglobin
2. White blood count
3. Urinalysis
4. Culture and sensitivity of urine
5. Serum protein with albumin/globulin ratio
6. Serum electrolytes
7. Blood urea nitrogen
8. Uric acid
9. Creatinine clearance
10. Twenty-four–hour urinary protein
11. Urinary vanillylmandelic acid (VMA)

Additionally, depending on the stage of gestation, it may be desirable to obtain the following:
1. Urinary estriol (24-hour specimen) or serum estriol
2. Amniotic fluid lecithin/sphingomyelin ratio and/or rapid surfactant test
3. A chest x-ray film for all patients who have had a seizure, to rule out aspiration

TREATMENT

The objectives of all treatment for the hypertensive diseases of pregnancy are (1) to prevent or control convulsions, (2) to ensure survival of the mother with minimal morbidity, and (3) to deliver a surviving infant with minimal trauma.
1. General measures
   a. Diet
      1. Calories, 1,500 to 2,500, depending on height and weight
      2. Protein, 1.5 to 2 gm/kg/24 hr
      3. Balanced sodium diet
   b. Diuretics
      Avoid diuretics for the patient with

mild disease who responds to bed rest in the lateral recumbent position (which increases renal blood flow and aids in the elimination of edema fluid).

c. Provide high-risk prenatal care as outlined in Chapter 2, with acute care for any complication that may develop.

2. Mild preeclampsia
   a. Hospitalize gravida.
   b. Give phenobarbital, 15 to 30 mg, three times a day, orally.
   c. Discharge to home on bed rest if the response is favorable, especially in control of the proteinuria. Persistence of proteinuria may contraindicate discharge from the hospital.
   d. Rehospitalize if any exacerbation occurs.
   e. Deliver when fetal maturity is sufficient to assure neonatal survival.

3. Severe preeclampsia (in addition to treatment for mild preeclampsia)
   a. Determine fetal maturity (lecithin/sphingomyelin ratio or rapid surfactant test) and follow at frequent intervals so that delivery can be effected as soon as the fetus is sufficiently mature for likely survival.
   b. Deliver fetus if the condition markedly worsens.
      1. Attempt induction if favorable.
      2. Perform cesarean section immediately if fetal distress develops or if induction is unsuccessful.
   c. Consider additional medication.
      1. Phenobarbital, 15 to 30 mg, four times a day intramuscularly, if delivery is not imminent.
      2. MgSO$_4$, to a blood level of 7 mg/100 ml for control of irritability and hyperreflexia.
      3. Antihypertensives may have to be added for control of hypertension. However, to guarantee uterine perfusion the blood pres-

sure should be lowered no more than 20% to 25%.
      4. Heparin* may be added if disseminated intravascular coagulation develops.
      5. With severe oliguria Lasix* may be helpful.
      6. Heart failure may be treated with digitalis* and oxygen.

4. Eclampsia
   Eclampsia is a medical emergency and requires the following:
   a. Airway maintenance (usually a plastic airway will suffice)
   b. Separate teeth with padded tongue blade or plastic airway to prevent maceration of the tongue
   c. Suction as necessary to remove regurgitated stomach contents and thus prevent aspiration
   d. Nasal oxygen at 6 L/min
   e. One of the following for control of the convulsion:
      1. Diazepam (Valium), 10 mg intravenously, by slow push
      2. MgSO$_4$, 4 gm intravenously over 5 to 10 minutes, then 1 gm/hr (1 gm/100 ml D$_{10}$W) by intravenous drip if urine output is satisfactory
      3. Amobarbital, 100 to 500 mg intravenously, slowly (only if delivery is not expected within 6 hours)
   f. Place bladder catheter for record of urine output per hour.
   g. Obtain a chest x-ray film to rule out aspiration.
   h. When the mother is stable, the maturity status of the fetus should be determined and delivery projected.

5. Chronic hypertension
   Mild hypertension may be followed

---

*Exact type and dosage are not given because therapy is best individualized for each of these critically ill patients. Interdisciplinary consultation is also a key feature of successful management.

closely and treated symptomatically; however, the following are key features in successful management of mild to severe chronic hypertension:

a. Consider abortion and sterilization.

b. Permit pregnancy to continue if the patient responds to hospitalization, as outlined under severe preeclampsia.

c. Obtain serial estriol levels from 26 weeks' gestation until delivery. If the blood pressure remains above 150/110, antihypertensives may be indicated.

d. Deliver immediately if
   1. Blood pressure rises above 200/120.
   2. Retinal exudates or hemorrhages occur.
   3. Congestive heart failure develops.
   4. Renal insufficiency ensues.

6. Decision for delivery
   The decision for delivery is based on the severity of the disease and the fetal maturation. The mode of delivery is dictated by a total assessment of both patients.

7. Analgesia and anesthesia (Chapter 5)
   Analgesia should be avoided in prematurity and used very cautiously in all pregnancies with this complication because of the already-compromised fetoplacental exchange.

   General anesthesia or epidural, caudal, or local blocks supplemented with nitrous oxide and oxygen may be effectively utilized for delivery or cesarean section. Regional anesthetic blocks (of the subarachnoid type) often have created severe hypotension that may be difficult to control.

8. General charting and laboratory studies for appropriate treatment of hospitalized patients

9. Laboratory studies
   a. Every 6 hours obtain
      1. Hematocrit (a rising hematocrit indicating a worsening of the disease process)
      2. Urinary protein (increasing urinary protein indicating a worsening of the process)
   b. Every 24 hours obtain
      1. Serum electrolytes
      2. Creatinine or BUN
      3. Uric acid
      4. Twenty-four–hour urine protein and creatinine
      5. Estriol (if undelivered)
   c. As needed, obtain
      1. Lecithin/sphingomyelin ratio and/or rapid surfactant test
      2. Serum proteins with albumin/globulin ratio

10. Vital signs
    a. Every 15 minutes to 1 hour, depending on the patient's condition, obtain
       1. Blood pressure, pulse, respiration
       2. Fetal heart tones
       3. Fluid intake and output
       4. Quality of deep tendon reflexes
    b. Daily
       1. Funduscopic examination for retinal arteriolar spasm
       2. Weight

COMPLICATIONS

1. Maternal complications
   a. Development of preeclampsia into eclampsia when the metabolic derangement cannot be controlled
   b. Blindness from retinal detachment or cerebral hemorrhage, resulting from hypertension and vascular fragility
   c. Premature separation of the placenta, with antepartum bleeding and postpartum hemorrhage (more common in hypertensive states)
   d. Coma, delirium, and confusion (manifestations of toxicity, central nervous system pathology, or oversedation, usually after convulsions of eclampsia)
   e. Injuries accompanying convulsions (vertebral fracture, laceration of the lips or tongue, aspiration pneumonia)

f. Protein depletion
g. Renal failure
h. Death
2. Factors apparently increasing chronic hypertension
   a. Age of the patient (older patients have a greater chance)
   b. High blood pressure in early pregnancy
   c. Higher blood pressure during the acute episode
   d. Duration of elevated blood pressure
   e. Extent and degree of proteinuria
   f. Persistence of hypertension in the puerperium
   g. Degree of obesity (more obese have a greater incidence)
3. Fetal complications
   a. Fetal distress
      1. Decreased uterine blood flow
      2. Abruptio placentae
   b. Premature labor
   c. Death
4. Complications of treatment
   a. Magnesium sulfate overdosage (the therapeutic range is 7 mg/100 ml, and the LD$_{50}$ is approximately 15 mg/100 ml) may create hyporeflexia, respiratory depression, and cardiac asystole. The antidote is calcium. It is our policy to have 10% of calcium gluconate in a syringe at the bedside whenever MgSO$_4$ is being administered, so that the toxic effects of magnesium sulfate overdosage will be vitiated by direct intravenous injection of the calcium.
   b. If diuretic therapy is utilized, one must be extremely careful not to deplete the intravascular space and thus develop an extravascular low-salt syndrome.

PROGNOSIS

Hippocrates accurately stated the prognosis in inadequately or poorly managed hypertensive states of pregnancy: "In pregnancy, drowsiness with headache accompanied by heaviness and convulsions is generally bad." This prognosis could well apply to both mother and fetus, for toxemia continues to be one of the three leading causes of maternal death each year in the United States (along with hemorrhage and infection) and remains a leading cause of perinatal mortality.

Mother

The outlook for the toxemia patient is good unless convulsions ensue, whereupon about one woman in fifteen will die of an intracranial accident, hemorrhage, shock, or renal failure from premature separation of the placenta, aspiration pneumonia, cardiac or renal cortical necrosis, or lower nephron nephrosis.

Perinate

Perinatal mortality in eclampsia can be reduced from at least 20% to about 10% by current, intensive therapy. The necessity for early delivery will diminish with improved maternal management.

PREVENTION

1. Toxemia of pregnancy is avoidable in most instances.
2. Early, adequate antenatal care and proper nutrition often will protect against toxemia.
3. Prompt, vigorous treatment of pre-eclampsia will limit the incidence of eclampsia drastically.
4. Definitive therapy of the convulsive state will reduce maternal and perinatal mortality considerably.

NEONATAL CARE

1. Major problems
   a. Prematurity
   b. Undergrowth
   c. A combination of prematurity and undergrowth
   d. Perinatal asphyxia
   e. Hypotonia resulting from hypermagnesemia (because of MgSO$_4$ therapy to mother)

2. Management
   a. Deliver in a maternity center equipped with neonatal intensive care unit
   b. Resuscitate immediately (Chapter 6)
   c. Assess infant for growth retardation and manage accordingly, for example, hypoglycemia (Chapter 17)
   d. Obtain magnesium level if indicated —over 5 mEq/L requires special care (Chapter 24)
3. Other problems of the neonate in toxemia of pregnancy
   a. Paralytic ileus—due to antepartum blocking agents to mother
   b. Nasal stuffiness with respiratory obstruction—due to antepartum therapy with reserpine
   c. Thrombocytopenia—antepartum administration of thiazides
   d. Neonatal depression—antepartum administration of tranquilizers and sedatives
   e. Methemoglobinemia—antepartum administration of nitrites

SELECTED REFERENCES

Craig, C. J. T.: Eclampsia and the anesthetist, S. Afr. Med. J. 46:248, 1972.

Del Greco, F., and Krumlovsky, F. H.: The renal pressor system in human pregnancy, J. Reprod. Med. 8:98, 1972.

Felding, D. F.: Pregnancy following renal disease, Clin. Obstet. Gynecol. 11:579, 1968.

Felding, D. F.: Obstetric aspects of women with histories of renal diseases, Acta Obstet. Gynecol. Scand. 48(supp.):43, 1969.

Heather, H. M., Humphries, D. M., Baker, R. S., and Chadd, M. A.: A controlled trial of hypotensive agents in hypertension in pregnancy, Lancet 2:488, 1968.

Heys, R. F., Scott, J. S., Oakey, R. E., and Stitch, S. R.: Estriol excretion in abnormal pregnancy, Obstet. Gynecol. 33:390, 1969.

McAllister, C. J., Stull, C. G., and Courey, N. G.: Amniotic fluid levels of uric acid and creatinine in toxemic patients—possible relation to diuretic use, Am. J. Obstet. Gynecol. 115:560, 1973.

McQueen, E. G.: Management of hypertension in pregnancy, Medicine Today 2:7, 1968.

Mengert, W. F.: Lifetime observations on the etiology of eclampsia, South. Med. J. 61:459, 1968.

Pahe, E. W.: On the pathogenesis of preeclampsia and eclampsia, J. Obstet. Gynaecol. Br. Commonw. 79:883, 1972.

Perel, I. D., and Forgan-Smith, W. R.: Thrombotic thrombocytopenic purpura presenting as eclampsia, Aust. N.Z. J. Obstet. Gynaecol. 12: 257, 1972.

Prachakvej, P.: Retinal changes in toxemia of pregnancy, J. Med. Assoc. Thai. 54:552, 1971.

Thompson, D., Patterson, W. G., Smart, G. E., MacDonald, M. K., and Robson, S. J.: Renal lesions of toxemia and abruptio placentae studied by light and electron microscopy, J. Obstet. Gynaecol. Br. Commonw. 79:311, 1972.

Wiser, W. L., et al.: Laboratory characteristics in toxemia, Obstet. Gynecol. 39:866, 1972.

Yogman, M. W., Speroff, L., Huttenlocher, P. R., and Kase, N. G.: Child development after pregnancies complicated by low urinary estriol excretion and pre-eclampsia, Am. J. Obstet. Gynecol. 114:1069, 1972.

15

Placental bleeding

Bleeding in late pregnancy occurs in 5% to 10% of all gravidas. The bleeding more commonly affects multiparas and may be classified according to its site of origin. Nonplacental bleeding is generally slight, and there are many causes, for example, cervical infection, vaginal infection, neoplasia of the lower genital tract, varicosities, and blood dyscrasias. The more serious hemorrhages, however, occur in 2% to 3% of all cases and are placental in origin. The two most common causes are abruptio placentae and placenta previa. They remain vexing problems even in modern obstetric practice and create a major portion of maternal morbidity and mortality. The full extent of fetal jeopardy with anoxia or even fetal hemorrhage is not known, but it must be considerable, since these conditions also contribute markedly to perinatal morbidity and mortality.

PREMATURE SEPARATION OF THE PLACENTA (ABRUPTIO PLACENTAE, ABLATIO PLACENTAE, SOLUTIO PLACENTAE, ACCIDENTAL HEMORRHAGE)

Premature separation of the normally implanted placenta is ablation of the afterbirth prior to the third stage of labor. Bleeding, either concealed or apparent, invariably accompanies this mishap. Abruptio placentae is extensive separation, often with concealed hemorrhage. Intrinsic placental vascular deficiency, sudden or marked vasodilatation, venous stasis, toxemia of pregnancy, and trauma to the pelvic organs are important causes of accidental hemorrhage. Although race is not a factor, older gravidas and women who have borne numerous children are more prone to premature separation of the placenta. The incidence of placental ablation is one in 175 to 200 pregnancies. Detachment of the placenta occurs in half the cases before the onset of labor, although it may occur as late as the second stage of labor. About 10% of patients with premature separation have abruptio placentae.

Slight premature placental separation

Even minimal uterine bleeding during the last half of pregnancy causes anxiety and the fear of hemorrhage and premature delivery. Minor degrees of premature separation of the normally implanted placenta often are responsible for such blood loss. Other causes are cervicitis, bleeding from the decidua, or unknown reasons. Pain, fetal distress, and early labor are unlikely unless the area of separation is large or retroplacental. Even so, strict bed rest and mild sedation for several days usually will arrest the bleeding temporarily, and the pregnancy may continue. Initial visualization of the vagina and cervix to rule out nonplacental bleeding is necessary. In addition, gentle palpation about the cervix, with ballottement of the presenting part, may help to rule out placenta previa. Un-

161

less the patient has excessive or persistent bleeding, however, palpation through the cervical canal is unwise. When a complete appraisal is necessary, a "double setup" will be required. Reassurance, increased bed rest, and close observation are necessary.

1. Pathogenesis
   a. Predisposition to early separation of the placenta occurs with
      1. Advanced age and multiparity (highly significant)
      2. Uterine distension (in multiple pregnancy or hydramnios)
      3. Previous abruptio placentae
      4. Hypertensive states of pregnancy
      5. Defective folate metabolism
   b. Precipitating causes of premature separation of the placenta
      1. Circumvallate placenta
      2. Abrupt or extreme vascular congestion, shock, and supine hypertensive syndrome (vena caval syndrome)
      3. Sudden reduction in the volume of the uterus—rapid loss of amniotic fluid or delivery of first twin
      4. A direct or indirect blow to the uterus
      5. Abnormally short cord
      6. Uterine anomaly or tumor
      7. Vascular deficiency, deterioration —eclamptogenic toxemia, diabetes mellitus, or chronic renal disease complicating pregnancy
      8. Possible predisposition occurring in mothers with type O blood
2. Pathology
   Two types of premature separation of the placenta are recognized:
   a. Marginal separation of the placenta, with leakage of blood behind the membranes through the cervix (This so-called external bleeding generally is painless.)
   b. Central separation of the placenta, with blood trapped behind the placenta and no external evidence of bleeding (This is painful, concealed bleeding—abruptio placentae. Failure of blood coagulation occurs in about 5% to 8% of serious cases of concealed hemorrhage.)
      1. Bleeding, with disruption of the vascular bed behind the placenta, results in extensive localized clotting and necrosis of the decidua basalis.
      2. Depletion of fibrinogen from the general circulation follows "fixation" of fibrinogen in retroplacental clotting.
      3. If peripheral blood fibrinogin falls to less than 100 mg/100 ml, generalized ecchymosis, free bleeding from all mucosal surfaces, and extravasation into the myometrium (Couvelaire uterus) often ensue.
         a. Couvelaire uterus is tetanic, ligneous, agonizingly painful, and tender.
         b. Dysrhythmic or arrested labor occurs.
         c. Maternal shock out of proportion to the estimated blood loss is the rule.
         d. Fetal death is nearly certain.
3. Clinical findings
   a. Symptomatology
      1. Painless vaginal hemorrhage may indicate unrestricted bleeding from the margin or a segment of the placenta.
      2. Suspect concealed hemorrhage and perhaps premature separation of most of the afterbirth when severe pain, backache, marked and unremittent uterine tenderness, an increased uterine tonus, enlargement of the uterus, or fetal distress develop prior to or during labor. Shock, bleeding from the nose, mouth, and needle puncture site, etc. and loss of fetal heart tones indicate severe abruptio placentae and hypofibrinogenemia (consumption coagulopathy).

b. Laboratory studies
 1. Hemoconcentration is usual; anemia, especially in concealed hemorrhage, may be noted later.
 2. Hypofibrinogenemia in association with abruptio placentae is confirmed by the following tests:
  a. Failure of clotting or fragile clot after 1 hour in Lee-White tube at 37° to 38° C
  b. Poor coagulation or no clot with Fibrindex test after 1 minute (reconstituted human thrombin added to one drop of the patient's plasma)
  c. Fibrinogen determination (gravimetric test) less than 100 mg/ 100 ml
  d. Disseminated intravascular coagulation is indicated if the plasma protamine coagulation test is positive.
 c. X-ray studies will not diagnose premature separation of the placenta but may identify placenta previa.
 d. Ultrasonography may reveal the retroplacental blood clot and assist in determination of placental location.
4. Differential diagnosis
 a. Nonplacental causes of bleeding—consider hemorrhagic lesions of the cervix or vagina, "show" of cervical dilatation and effacement, and rupture of the uterus.
 b. Placental bleeding may reveal placenta previa by "double setup" sterile vaginal examination in the operating room readied for cesarean section. vasa previa can be diagnosed before delivery only by amnioscopy.
5. Complications
 a. Mother—hemorrhage, shock, hypovolemia, hypofibrinogenemia, small pulmonary emboli, renal cortical and lower nephron nephrosis, and fibrinolysis may occur, especially with abruptio placentae.
 b. Fetus—hypoxia with resultant fetal

distress may cause damage to the fetal central nervous system with later cerebral palsy, mental retardation, or actual death of the fetus. Premature birth is also frequently seen with abruptio placentae.
6. Treatment
 a. Emergency measures
 1. Institute antishock measures.
 2. *Rupture the membranes*—without regard to the likely method of delivery—to permit drainage, reduce the risk of consumption coagulopathy, and speed labor.
 3. Obtain appropriate laboratory studies—complete blood count, type and cross match (3 to 6 units), fibrinogen, clot for observation, and appropriate studies as indicated by hematologic consultation.
 4. *Restore blood clotting mechanism,* if deficient before attempting any type of delivery.
 5. Mark the upper limit of the fundus to monitor uterine expansion from intrauterine bleeding.
 6. Institute direct electronic fetal monitoring.
 7. Institute central venous pressure monitoring.
 8. Measure urinary output hourly.
 9. Administer mannitol, 12.5 gm intravenously (supplied as 25% solution in 50 ml ampules), to protect against lower nephron nephrosis after shock, if severely oliguric or anuric.
 b. Specific measures
 1. Premature separation of the placenta accompanied by external bleeding probably will require no operative intervention, unless hemorrhage or prolonged labor develops. Type, match, and hold blood for possible transfusion or cesarean section.
 2. Treat the lesser degrees of abrup-

tio placentae in the same manner. In severe abruptio placentae, if vaginal delivery is likely to occur within a reasonable time (less than 6 hours), plan on delivery from below; if a longer labor is likely, do a cesarean section on a strictly maternal indication. Cesarean section is also indicated for any fetal distress.

c. General measures
  1. Give oxygen by face mask for fetal distress.
  2. Transfuse the gravida if she is in shock or anemic.
  3. If rapid labor or hasty delivery transpires, deny excessive analgesia, despite severe pain, to minimize fetal central nervous system depression.
  4. Monitor fetal heart tone and record maternal pulse and blood pressure every 5 minutes.

d. Surgical measures
  1. Utilize low forceps assistance to expedite delivery (Dührssen incisions are rarely, if ever, justified, even for fetal distress in a multipara, because of the danger of further hemorrhage and shock.)
  2. Employ cesarean section when
    a. Desultory labor does not respond to amniotomy and cautious oxytocic stimulation.
    b. Fetopelvic dystocia is recognized.
    c. Hemorrhage cannot be checked by amniotomy or restoration of the coagulation mechanism.
    d. Fetal distress occurs.
  3. Hysterectomy rarely will be necessary in abruptio placentae if normal blood coagulation has been achieved.

e. Treatment of complications
  1. Hypofibrinogenemia—treat with intravenous fibrinogen. If fibrinogen is unavailable, use quadruple-strength plasma (1 pint contains approximately 4.4 gm of fibrinogen). Do not rely on whole blood for replacement of fibrinogen, or hyperbulemia will result.
  2. Renal cortical necrosis—administer hydralazine hydrochloride, 25 to 40 mg diluted, by slow intravenous drip to possibly increase renal blood flow and thereby prevent or reverse renal ischemia; obtain nephrology consultation for possible dialysis.
  3. Cor pulmonale—give oxygen by mask or tent. Limit intravenous fluids. Administer digitalis.
  4. Lower nephron nephrosis—balance fluid intake and output. Deny potassium-containing materials. Dialyze the patient or begin peritoneal lavage when serum potassium approaches 7 mg/100 ml.
  5. Serum hepatitis in 10% to 20% of patients is a calculated risk with fibrinogen therapy. Gamma globulin, 20 ml administered intramuscularly, may prevent homologous serum jaundice. Order a low-protein, high-carbohydrate diet. Segregate the patient if jaundice develops.

7. Prevention
  a. Avoid trauma and toxemia.
  b. Diagnose and treat promptly, especially by artificial rupture of the membranes.

8. Prognosis
  a. Maternal mortality after premature separation of the placenta is 0.5% to 5% throughout the world. Hemorrhage and renal failure are major causes of maternal death.
  b. Perinatal mortality is 50% to 80%, of which almost half involves a shortened gestation. In approximately a fifth of the cases, the fetus is dead at the time of the parturient's entry into the hospital. Hypoxia, birth

trauma, and prematurity are the principal causes of perinatal death.
9. Care of neonate (Chapter 6)

Pathophysiology of concealed hemorrhage

In abruptio placentae, gross clotting occurs behind the placenta, and considerable decidua and endometrium are destroyed. With this tissue decomposition, clotting then occurs in small vessels in the uterus and elsewhere. Plasminogen is converted to plasmin, and secondary fibrinolysis starts. This process may be so extensive and rapid that many clotting factors may be expended in a very short time. Additionally, the secondary fibrinolysis digests fibrinogen to smaller molecules that exert a heparin-like anticoagulant action. In such instances the patient will begin to bleed from the uterus, the sites of needle puncture, mucous membranes, etc. The bleeding time will be prolonged secondary to thrombocytopenia, and although a small, fragile clot may form, it soon disintegrates by lysis. This coagulation disorder is termed consumption coagulopathy, or defibrination syndrome.

Shock often develops, and although the patient may remain normotensive for a time before becoming hypotensive from hypovolemia, the microcirculation particularly becomes constricted. Erythrocytes become damaged by being forced through a contracted vasculature partially blocked by clots. As a result, many broken, misshapen red blood cells ("helmet cells," schistocytes) appear in the peripheral blood smear as evidence of the microangiopathic hemolytic anemia.

Laboratory indices of consumption coagulopathy

1. Thrombocytopenia (notable even in smear of peripheral blood)
2. Coagulation consumption of factors I, II, V, and VIII (prothrombin and partial thromboplastin)
3. Demonstration of fibrin monomer, fibrinogen degradation products (FDP) complexes, in the plasma by the prothrombin (3P) test. (This is due to an increase of FDP and can be proved by specific assay.)
4. Prolonged thrombin time

Treatment of abruptio placentae with consumption coagulopathy

1. Do not attempt a vaginal delivery or cesarean section until the coagulation problem is corrected.
2. Treat for shock with a *fresh* blood transfusion. If serious bleeding persists:
   a. Give cryoprecipitate in amounts sufficient to restore coagulation mechanisms. Cryoprecipitate contains both fibrinogen and factor VIII and is therefore more effective in restoration of normal coagulation than the previously used lyophilized fibrinogen. Additionally, it has the advantage of minimizing transmission of serum hepatitis (between 10% and 30% of patients undergoing fibrinogen therapy acquire homologous serum jaundice).
   b. In some cases, fresh frozen plasma and/or platelet administration will be necessary.
   c. Rarely, when the uterus cannot be emptied or when there is continued disseminated intervascular coagulation, heparin will be necessary. It should be administered only after appropriate investigative studies and usually in consultation with a hematologist. If used, it is proper to administer heparin, 75 to 150 units/kg of body weight every 6 hours intravenously, to maintain coagulation time at about 20 minutes. If the uterus remains well contracted postpartum, persistent or delayed bleeding is unlikely. (Protamine sulfate will counteract heparin if unusual bleeding ensues.) Heparin has an antithrombin effect and blocks intrinsic activation of prothrombinase as

well. Because the consumption of coagulation factors is secondary to the proteolytic effect on thrombin, which increases the induction of a release phenomenon of platelet components, heparin corrects the problem.

3. When bleeding is checked and the coagulation defect is corrected, empty the uterus in the easiest, most expeditious way.

PLACENTA PREVIA

Placenta previa is the implantation of the placenta in the lower uterine segment. In this abnormality the afterbirth covers all or a portion of the internal os and precedes the fetus in vaginal delivery. Reduced vascularity in the fundus probably is of etiologic significance, but the cause in most cases cannot be determined. Older age of the mother and multiparity increase the likelihood of placenta previa, but race is unrelated to the occurrence of this disorder. The incidence of placenta previa during the third trimester is approximately 1:200 pregnancies. In 10% of cases the placenta completely covers the cervical os.

1. Pathogenesis, pathology, pathologic physiology
   a. Tumors and scarring in fundus encourage placentation low in uterus.
   b. Afterbirth covers a one-third greater area to obtain adequate circulation.
   c. Antepartum or intrapartum bleeding occurs with the following:
      1. Spontaneous dilatation, effacement of cervix
      2. Rectal or vaginal examination
   d. Low situation of placenta causes delay in, failure of, engagement of presenting part. Breech and transverse presentations frequently occur.
   e. If more than a small portion of pla-

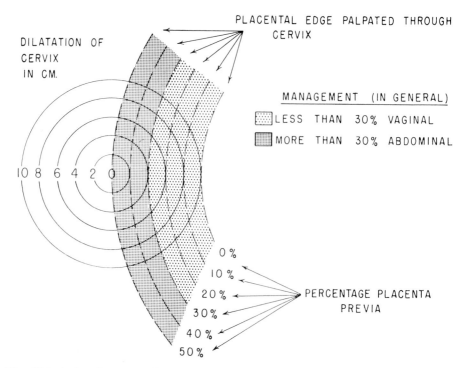

Fig. 15-1. A classification of placenta previa. (Redrawn from Tatum, H. J., and Mulé, J. G.: Am. J. Obstet. Gynecol. 93:767, 1965.)

centa is over the os, even after rupture of the membranes and full dilatation of the cervix, vaginal delivery may not occur without
1. Disruption of a portion of placenta and hemorrhage
2. Operative assistance
  f. Laceration of the edge of the afterbirth may result in fetal, as well as maternal, blood loss. Fetal hemorrhage may be severe when placenta previa is greater than 20% coverage of the internal os. Maternal hemorrhage may be extreme when placenta previa is greater than 30%.
2. Degree of previa
  a. Older designation as marginal, partial, or complete placenta previa is not recommended because such nomenclature does not aid in prognosis or therapy.
  b. Estimate the extent of coverage of the internal os by the placenta, assuming full dilatation of the cervix (Fig. 15-1).
3. Clinical findings
  a. Symptomatology
    1. Uterine bleeding with placenta previa is painless unless the patient is in labor or has other complications (infection, tumor, etc.).
    2. Bleeding may be continuous or intermittent.
  b. Laboratory findings are not diagnostic of placenta previa, but blood from the placenta
    1. Clots
    2. May contain fetal red blood cells
  c. X-ray studies
    1. *Sonography.* This method will usually delineate the abnormal placental location.
    2. *Radioisotope placentography.* Radioisotope placentography using technetium or radioactive iodinated human serum albumin (RISA) is a simple and generally reliable method for the antepartum

localization of the placenta by delineating the maternal vascular pool within the placenta. A single injection of the radioactive material into an arm vein is accomplished. A scintillation-scan over the abdomen minutes after injection usually reveals the placenta as the greatest concentration of radioactivity.

The posterior or low-lying placenta is the most difficult to predict and represents the main source of error because lateral scans are not helpful.

A lower radiation dose is given to mother and fetus during radioisotope placentography than during roentgenographic placental localization. Oral administration of 10 ml of Lugol's solution to the mother several hours prior to RISA injection and the same amount three times a day until delivery will saturate the fetal thyroid and minimize the uptake of radioactive iodine.

3. *Vesicouterine contrast.* If vertex is presenting at term, instill 200 ml of 10% sodium iodide solution into bladder. Obtain an anteroposterior x-ray film. If the distance from the bladder to the skull is greater than 4 cm on film, suspect placenta previa (this approach is not diagnostic with breech or transverse presentation).
4. *Soft tissue roentgenography.* If placenta is not in the fundus, assume placenta is in the lower portion of the uterus—perhaps placenta previa.
5. *Amniography* (Chapter 3).
6. *Percutaneous transfemoral aortography.* Anteroposterior and lateral films (supine) usually will reveal a forelying placenta, but not the degree of previa.

d. Special management procedures
1. Hospitalize the patient for definite bleeding.
   a. Treat anemia, infection.
   b. Visualize the cervix and vagina with a speculum (bleeding will cease in 24 hours in more than 90% of patients, with bed rest alone, irrespective of the cause of antepartum bleeding).
   c. Attempt to carry the patient to at least 36 weeks' gestation or until surfactant test is mature.
2. To determine degree of previa, especially if the patient is in labor or hemorrhaging, do "double set-up" sterile vaginal examination in the readied operating room.
   a. Type and match blood. Have more than 2 units available for transfusion.
   b. Prepare for vaginal delivery or cesarean section in the same operating room (depending on findings).
   c. Using sterile technique, inspect the vagina and cervix for ulcerative, bleeding lesions.
   d. Palpate around the cervix; ballot presenting part; attempt to identify placenta between the cervix and presenting part.
   e. Insert finger through the cervix; feel for placenta; estimate percentage of coverage, assuming full dilatation required for vaginal delivery of the fetus at or near term.
   f. Anticipate a vaginal delivery after trial of labor if placenta previa is less than 30%. *Rupture membranes as soon as labor ensues to aid engagement and tamponade of bleeding portion of placenta.*
   g. If placenta previa is more than 30% and the fetus is alive, do immediate cesarean section,

preferably low cervical type under regional anesthesia.
4. Differential diagnosis
   a. Rule out nonplacental causes for vaginal bleeding: carcinoma, tuberculosis of the cervix or vagina, polyps, ruptured vaginal varices, lower genital tract infections, blood dyscrasias.
   b. Rule out the other major placental cause for bleeding: premature separation of the normally implanted placenta (often with painful uterine bleeding).
5. Complications
   a. Fetus
      1. Delivery of a premature neonate occurs in one third to one half of cases.
      2. Early delivery accounts for 60% of perinatal deaths in placenta previa.
      3. Prolapse of the cord may occur when membranes rupture and presenting part is unengaged.
      4. Hypoxia, birth injury, and transplacental hemorrhage exact an incalculable morbidity.
      5. When placenta is torn at cesarean section, the fetus may bleed.
   b. Mother
      1. Hemorrhage and hypovolemic shock may develop.
      2. Operative trauma, especially cervical laceration and uterine rupture, may occur.
      3. Vascular thrombosis and embolism often develop postpartum.
      4. Placenta previa accreta may account for lack of separation of forelying placenta.
6. Treatment
   a. Emergency measures
      1. Hospitalize at once; treat for hemorrhage and shock.
      2. Postpone delivery until 36 weeks' gestation, if possible.
   b. Specific and supportive measures

1. Type and match blood and have it available for transfusion.
2. Avoid oxytocics and enemas for stimulation of labor (to minimize bleeding) unless contractions are desultory and vaginal delivery is chosen.
3. *Rupture membranes if possible,* with the patient in a high Fowler's position, to bring down presenting part. (The cord is more likely to prolapse when the patient is in supine position.)
4. Deliver the patient in the manner least hazardous to the gravida and offspring.
   a. Vaginal delivery usually is best if previa is 20% to 30%, particularly when the patient is a multipara.
   b. The use of a vacuum extractor or of Willett sclap forceps and traction (0.25 kg) is inadvisable for delivery of the premature infant.
   c. Monitor the fetal heart rate, checking it at least every 15 minutes in the first stage and every 5 minutes during the second stage of labor, or more often with fetal distress.
   d. Apply low forceps for assisted delivery, if feasible. Avoid internal version or difficult vaginal manipulation.
   e. Do a cesarean section, preferably low cervical under block anesthesia, unless placenta is anterior—when a classic entry may avoid placenta and serious hemorrhage. Suture bleeding sinuses within the uterus for control of placental site.
   f. Placenta previa accreta will require cesarean total hysterectomy.
7. Prevention: none
8. Prognosis
   a. Maternal mortality is now less than 0.8% in major medical centers.
   b. Perinatal mortality is still more than 20%, even in large hospitals, despite improved methods.
   c. Approximately ten times as many offspring die if the mother has placenta previa, as compared with normal obstetric patients.
   d. Perinatal mortality can be reduced to less than 10% with optimal treatment, including avoidance of reckless intervention at delivery of the undersized fetus.
   e. Cesarean section increases the likelihood of placenta previa in a subsequent pregnancy by about 5%.
   f. Multiparity and infection raise the incidence of placenta previa.
9. Care of the neonate
   The high perinatal mortality in placental bleeding suggests that the labor and delivery should occur in a maternity center in which an experienced team can be present for both mother and infant. A neonatal intensive care unit should be part of the center.
   a. Special problems to be anticipated at birth
      1. Prematurity (labor usually is established before term is reached)
      2. Asphyxia (result of disruption of fetal-placental circulation)
      3. Hypovolemia (loss of blood* from fetal side of placenta)
      4. Hyaline membrane disease (intensified by asphyxia, which reduces surfactant production in the preterm infant)
   b. Management
      1. Resuscitate immediately.
      2. Offer plasmanate for shock unless

---

*Check vaginal blood in advance of delivery for fetal bleeding by the Kleihauer technique (resistance to acid elution). Fixed blood smear is immersed in a citrate-phospate buffer of acid pH (3.3 to 3.4). Hemoglobin A is eluted from the erythrocytes, but hemoglobin F (fetal) is not.

forewarned by knowledge of fetal blood loss with appropriate blood available.

3. Perform serial hematocrits three times per hour—a falling hematocrit indicates acute blood loss.
4. Transfuse if hematocrit is less than 45.
5. Support respiratory failure (Chapter 19).

CIRCUMVALLATE OR CIRCUMMARGINATE PLACENTA (EXTRACHORIAL PLACENTA)

Extrachorial placenta (circumvallate or circummarginate) is associated with increased rates of slight or moderate antepartum bleeding, early delivery (which is a major cause of second-trimester losses), and perinatal death. Older multigravidas often have a much greater predisposition. Nevertheless, circumvallate placenta and circummarginate placenta together represent only about 6% of the total deliveries. Despite well-documented obstetric-pediatric complications, extrachorial placenta is an uncommon, rarely serious clinical obstetric problem. Nevertheless, our experience demonstrates a high incidence of low birth weight infants of white mothers who had extrachorial placentas.

SELECTED REFERENCES

Beischer, N. A., Brown, J. B., MacLeod, S. C., and Smith, M. A.: Value of urinary estriol determinations in patients with antepartum vaginal bleeding, J. Obstet. Gynaecol. Br. Commonw. **74**:51, 1967.

Benson, R. C., and Fujikura, T.: Circumvallate and circummarginate placenta, Obstet. Gynecol. **34**:799, 1970.

Cohen, W. N., Chaudhuri, T. K., and Christie, J. H.: Correlation of ultrasound and radioisotope placentography, Am. J. Roentgenol. **116**:843, 1972.

DeValern, E.: Abruptio placentae, Am. J. Obstet. Gynecol. **100**:599, 1968.

Gruenwald, P., Levin, H., and Yousan, H.: Abruption and premature separation of the placenta: the clinical and pathologic entity, Am. J. Obstet. Gynecol. **102**:604, 1968.

Lunan, C. B.: The management of abruptio placentae, J. Obstet. Gynaecol. Br. Commonw.

McHattie, T. J.: Placenta previa accreta, Obstet. Gynecol. **40**:795, 1972.

Naftolin, F., Khudr, G., Benirschke, K., and Hutchinson, D. L.: The syndrome of chronic abruptio placentae, hydrorrhea, and circumvallate placenta, Am. J. Obstet. Gynecol. **116**:347, 1973.

Niswander, K. R., Friedman, E. A., Hoover, D. B., Pietrowski, H., and Westphal, M. C.: Fetal morbidity following potentially anoxigenic obstetric conditions. I. Abruptio placentae, Am. J. Obstet. Gynecol. **95**:838, 1966.

Ramzin, M.: The condition of the newborn after placenta praevia with premature detachment of the placenta, Gynaecologia **166**:221, 1968.

Schlesinger, E. R., Mazundar, S. M., and Logrillo, V. M.: The impact of placenta previa on survivorship of offspring to four years of age, Am. J. Obstet. Gynecol. **116**:657, 1973.

Semmens, J. P.: A second look at expectant management of placenta previa, Postgrad. Med. **44**:207, Oct., 1968.

Varma, T. R.: Fetal growth and placental function in patients with placenta previa, J. Obstet. Gynaec. Br. Commonw. **80**:311, 1973.

Wentworth, P.: Circumvallate and circummarginate placenta, their incidence and clinical significance, Am. J. Obstet. Gynecol. **102**:44, 1968.

Whalley, P. J., Scott, D. E., and Pritchard, J. A.: Maternal folate deficiency and pregnancy wastage. I. Placental abruption, Am. J. Obstet. Gynecol. **105**:670, 1969.

Wiesenhaan, P. F.: Fetography (and placentography), Am. J. Obstet. Gynecol. **113**:819, 1972.

16

Untimely termination of pregnancy

PREMATURE LABOR

Labor is the process by which the products of conception are expelled. It is subject to a variety of complications, but one of the more frequent is premature termination of pregnancy. Labor is defined as premature when it results in a live infant of under 38 weeks' gestation; nearly half of such infants weigh more than 2,500 gm at birth. Premature labor occurs in over 10% of all pregnancies* and accounts for nearly two thirds of infant deaths (approximately 40,000 infants annually in the United States). The exact etiology of premature labor may be difficult to determine. There are certain strong clinical correlates that will allow identification of many of the pregnancies at risk before the complication develops; however, if we could prevent premature labor, much perinatal mortality and morbidity would be avoided. Many direct approaches to the extension of gestation have been attempted, with limited success. On the other hand, indirect, supportive measures have been beneficial.

Numerous obstetric entities commonly associated with early birth are recognized. Although it is unlikely that the supportive methods employed by the physician can carry the patient to term in each instance, a surprising degree of fetal growth and maturity may be possible.

Chapter 27 attempts to focus on the social, economic, and educational factors that so often relate to early birth as well as to low birth weight. No doubt these influences have much to do with the fact that Sweden has one third the incidence of live born infants weighing less than 1,500 gm that the United States does (Table 25-2). Specific causes of early birth that are important contributors to perinatal mortality (e.g., multiple births) are discussed elsewhere.

Iatrogenic prematurity

Prevention of prematurity can be accomplished in the 7% to 10% of those infants who are premature because the physician misjudged fetal maturity and performed an untimely elective cesarean section or induction of labor. This continuing tragedy can be sharply curtailed or entirely eliminated if all elective deliveries are screened for maturity by the simple rapid surfactant ("bubble") test (p. 36) or lecithin/sphingomyelin ratio performed on the amniotic fluid. Although size of fetal head is not precisely related to gestational age, a biparietal diameter of 9.5 cm or more, measured by ultrasound, is an assurance that the fetus is of adequate size for delivery, if amniocentesis is not desirable.

Diagnosis of premature labor

The diagnosis of premature labor requires uterine contractions at least every

---

*Another 3% of pregnancies result in mature low birth weight infants (less than 2,500 gm).

171

10 minutes, and they must be associated with progressive dilatation and/or effacement of the cervix, often with descent of the fetal presenting part.

1. Clinical correlates of premature labor
   a. Previous obstetric history
      1. Premature or low birth weight babies
      2. Complications listed in **b** to **e**
   b. General medical complications
      1. Hypertension (primarily chronic hypertensive vascular disease)
      2. Renal disease
      3. Heart disease
      4. Pyelonephritis
      5. Acute systemic infections
      6. Heavy cigarette smoking
      7. Alcoholism and/or drug addiction
      8. Severe anemia
   c. Obstetric complication
      1. Severe hypertensive states of pregnancy
      2. Abruptio placentae
      3. Placenta previa
      4. Circumvallate placenta
      5. Placental insufficiency
      6. Premature rupture of the membranes (occurs in approximately 20% of all premature deliveries)
      7. Multiple gestation
      8. Polyhydramnios
      9. Malnutrition (excessive or inadequate nutrition) and inadequate or excessive weight gain with pregnancy
      10. Pregnancy occurring less than 3 months after the previous pregnancy's termination
   d. Genital tract anomalies
      1. Uterine
         a. Bicornuate
         b. Subseptate
         c. Unicornuate
      2. Cervical incompetence
         a. Congenital
         b. Acquired
            (1) Surgical (conization, abortion)
            (2) Obstetric (lacerations)
      3. Uterine leiomyomas
   e. Miscellaneous
      1. Trauma
      2. Surgical operation
      3. Low socioeconomic status
      4. Infections—genital mycoplasma, cytomegalovirus, herpes simplex (type II), toxoplasmosis, listeriosis

2. Presenting symptoms and signs
   a. Labor contractions
      In the majority of cases, strong premature contractions initiate labor.
   b. Premature rupture of the membranes occurs in approximately 20% to 25% of all premature deliveries and may be the first abnormal sign. The etiology of premature rupture of the membranes is unknown. Nevertheless, it has been shown that the membranes that rupture prematurely have a lower bursting tension than do membranes that do not rupture prematurely.
   c. Vaginal bleeding
      Second-trimester vaginal bleeding may be due to a circumvallate placenta, abruptio placentae, or placenta previa. Each of these creates relative placental insufficiency and gestational instability. They are discussed elsewhere (Chapter 15).
   d. Increased vaginal discharge and vaginal pressure
      Incompetent cervix is usually seen with discharge and pressure.

3. Examination in premature labor
   a. Fetal size
      Special care should be taken to determine fetal size (B-scan ultrasonography) and well-being (electronic fetal monitoring).
   b. Presenting part
      The presenting part should be noted (an increased incidence of breech presentation occurs early in gestation).
   c. Contractions and cervix

The duration and intensity of contractions, cervical dilatation, cervical effacement, and fetal station all are important in the evaluation of the labor.

Exclusions to treatment of labor

It would seem at first glance that one should attempt to suppress every instance of premature labor because of the devastatingly high perinatal mortality and morbidity with prematurity. This is illogical, however, because many cases of premature delivery and perinatal death are related to a serious disorder that cannot be diagnosed antepartum. Moreover, it may be best to actually encourage early birth in some conditions to spare the mother or her fetus. Nonetheless, one must identify instances in which the only threat to the offspring would appear to be premature labor. Thus we must exclude the following and permit labor to continue in these instances:

1. Maternal conditions that jeopardize the intrauterine environment or make birth the lesser risk (e.g., eclampsia or extensive placenta previa)
2. Fetal disorders that either tend to precipitate early delivery (e.g., polyhydramnios) or to make attempts to stop premature labor profitless (e.g., severe erythroblastosis fetalis)
3. Clinical conditions in which it should be obvious that attempts to check premature labor will be futile, (e.g., ruptured membranes or cervical dilatation of more than 3 to 4 cm)

If one excludes all patients in whom attempts at arrest of labor are either contraindicated or likely to be unsuccessful, only about 20% of the total "low birth weight" fetuses will remain as candidates for labor-suppression drug therapy. Also, the excellent prognosis for neonates who have mature lecithin/sphingomyelin ratios or mature rapid surfactant tests obviates any reasonable attempt to delay their delivery.

Pharmacologic control

1. **Sedation contraindicated**

   Many have confused sedation with analgesia. Thus, morphine or meperidine hydrochloride (Demerol) has mistakenly been given to sedate patients in prodromal labor in the hope that untimely birth could be averted. These narcotics are contraindicated. They may accelerate premature labor, and they may severely narcotize the neonate should prompt delivery ensue. Barbiturates are even more hazardous and are also contraindicated.

   Many other drugs potentially dangerous to the fetus, including opiates, anesthetics, progesterone, epinephrine, chlordiazepoxide (Librium), and diazepam (Valium), have been abandoned as effective agents against premature labor.

2. **Currently useful medications**

   The following drugs currently available may be effective for the suppression of uterine contractility in threatened premature labor:

   a. Ethyl alcohol, administered intravenously
   b. Isoxsuprine hydrochloride (Vasodilan), administered intravenously
   c. Ritodrine, *p*-hydroxyphenylethyl-*p*-hydroxy-norepinephrine, administered intravenously

   Isoxsuprine and ritodrine must still be considered experimental tokolytic drugs in advanced pregnancy. They are contraindicated in women with coronary insufficiency or hemorrhagic disorders because of the vasodilating effects of the drug. With these exceptions, they appear to be safe when used with caution. No undesirable fetal effects have been demonstrated.

3. **Determine before therapy**

   a. Fetal weight under 2,500 gm; less than 37 weeks' gestational age
   b. Membranes intact; cervix dilated less than 4 cm
   c. Healthy fetus

d. No obstetric and/or medical conditions that contraindicate continued pregnancy
4. Pharmacologic inhibition contraindicated
   a. Fetal death or fetal distress
   b. Critical fetal problems, e.g., polyhydramnios, gross anomalies, or severe isoimmunization
   c. Intrauterine infection
   d. Therapy likely to affect fetus adversely
   e. Ruptured membranes
   f. Cervix dilated over 4 cm
   g. Serious bleeding problems
   h. Severe preeclampsia, eclampsia
   i. Marked hypertensive cardiovascular or renal disease
5. General measures
   a. Bed rest
   b. Initial pelvic examination only
6. Tokolytic regimens
   a. Ethanol, administered intravenously
      1. Infusion fluid: 100 ml 95% (v/v) ethanol + 900 ml 5% dextrose water = 1,000 ml 9.5% (v/v) ethanol (75.4 gm/L)
      2. Loading dose: 15 ml/kg body weight/given over 2 hours
      3. Maintenance dose: 1.5 ml/kg body weight/hr
      4. Reloading dose: If treatment has been discontinued 10 hr earlier or less, the dose to reload the patient is calculated as follows (Fuchs and colleagues):

$$\text{Loading dose} \times \frac{\text{No. of hours}}{10}$$

   b. Isoxsuprine, administered intravenously
      1. Infusion fluid: Isoxsuprine, 60 to 120 mg (40 to 80 mg in 1 L of 5% dextrose in water, run at 5 ml/min). Continue for 6 to 12 hours; increase dosage if adequate uterine response is not obtained.
      2. Loading dose: Isoxsuprine, 20 mg in 1 L of 5% dextrose in water administered intravenously within 2 hours, followed by infusion fluid (above).
      3. Oral dose: If good uterine response is achieved by intravenous drug (above), isoxsuprine, 10 mg orally three times a day for 1 or 2 days, may be given (Krapohl and associates).
   c. Ritodrine hydrochloride, administered intravenously
      1. Infusion fluid: One ampule of ritodrine, 25 mg, is diluted in 250 ml of 5% glucose and water. This solution contains 100 μg of ritodrine/ml.
      2. Maintenance dose: 400 μg/min Maximum dose is limited by maternal tachycardia. Ritodrine is continued until at least 2 hours after uterine contractions have ceased.

Management of preterm delivery

See Chapter 5.

PREMATURE RUPTURE OF THE MEMBRANES

Spontaneous rupture of the membranes may ensue at any time during pregnancy. When it occurs prior to the onset of labor, the condition is termed premature rupture of the membranes; when more than 24 hours elapse after rupture of the membranes until the onset of labor, the problem is one of prolonged premature rupture of the membranes. Amniotic fluid may gush through the cervix, denoting a wide rent in the membranes; in other cases a persistent trickle suggests a small tear or perforation. With considerable loss of fluid, the onset of labor usually occurs within a few days. Periodic discharge of amniotic fluid may occur, but occasionally the presenting part will prevent marked loss, or the perforation may seal off. In these instances the mother and fetus usually are unaffected, and the pregnancy will continue. Regrettably, a preterm fetus often is involved. In most instances the etiology of premature rupture of the membranes is speculative. This complication involves up to 15% of all gravidas, many of whom have medical-social problems.

1. Pathogenesis and pathology
   a. The following have recognized relationships to premature rupture of the membranes:
      1. Lower genital tract infection
      2. Cervical incompetence
      3. Multiple pregnancy
      4. Hydramnios
      5. Fetal malpresentation
   b. Pathology generally is undetermined but may prove to be due to an inherent defect in the membranes, the duration of the pregnancy, or the age and/or parity of the patient.
2. Pathologic physiology
   a. Premature rupture of the membranes is an important cause of premature labor, prolapse of the cord, and intrauterine infection.
   b. So-called "dry labor," which eventually follows gross loss of amniotic fluid, may be desultory or prolonged if
      1. Patient is not at term.
      2. Uterus is not "sensitized" to labor.
      3. Malpresentation exists.
3. Clinical findings
   a. Symptomatology
      1. Persistent or recurrent loss of fluid, often including flecks of vernix
      2. Reduction in the size of the uterus
      3. Increased prominence of the fetus to palpation
   b. Laboratory findings
      The following tests are useful in the identification of rupture of the membranes:
      1. *Amniotic fluid test*
         Amniotic fluid is clear or milky, slightly alkaline (pH = more than 7; nitrazine test paper is deep blue), and has a seminiferous odor.

2. *Histochemical test*
   a. Spread vaginal fluid on a clean slide and allow to dry.
   b. Stain with a 0.5% aqueous Nile blue sulfate, a fatty acid stain.
   c. Identify exfoliated fetal sebaceous epithelial cells that stain yellow-orange to red-orange.
   The presence of orange anuclear cells may not be found prior to the thirty-third week of gestation, leading to false-negative reports before this period.
3. *Arborization test* (when fluid is uncontaminated with gross blood or meconium)
   a. Obtain fluid from the vagina approximately 3 cm from introitus.
   b. Spread fluid on a clean glass slide and allow to dry.
   c. Observe for a distinct pattern of crystallization resembling a palm or fern design, which indicates amniotic fluid.
4. Dye test
   a. Aspirate 5 ml of amniotic fluid transabdominally.
   b. Inject 5 ml of dilute Evans blue solution.
   c. Insert a vaginal speculum after 15 to 20 minutes.
   d. Blue-colored fluid in the vagina indicates ruptured membranes.
   In summary, the use of any three of the tests just mentioned, including a careful history within 2 hours of the presumed rupture of the membranes, will allow an accuracy of diagnosis of between 90% to 95% (Friedman and McElin).
4. Differential diagnosis
   a. Vaginal fluid is mucoid and acid and will not crystallize, nor does it contain exfoliated fetal cells, as noted in the histochemical test.
   b. The incontinent patient may have vaginal fluid that has the odor of

urine and contains urate crystals but does not reveal fetal elements and does not dry to form fernlike crystal patterns.

c. Hydrorrhea gravidarum fluid is periodic, profuse, often yellowish, and pus laden. It occurs most often during the second trimester. Presumably, the liquid represents discharge from deciduitis or seepage from the decidua behind the membranes. Reduction in the size of the uterus does not occur, nor are the laboratory characteristics of amniotic fluid met.

5. Prevention
   a. Treat vaginitis and cervicitis before and during pregnancy.
   b. Repair incompetent cervix when indicated.
   c. Provide prolonged bed rest for patients with a multiple pregnancy or hydramnios.
   d. Deny prophylactic antibiotics, but treat the specific infection.

6. Treatment
   a. Prepare the patient for impending labor.
   b. Check for evidence of a multiple pregnancy, malpresentation, fetal anomaly, or prolapsed cord.
   c. Avoid frequent vaginal or rectal examinations to minimize the chance of introducing intrauterine infection.
   d. Manage preterm delivery as discussed in Chapter 5.
   e. Offer care in prolonged rupture of membranes as on p. 177.

7. Prognosis
   a. Mother—good unless virulent infection develops; the incidence of operative delivery increased.
   b. Fetus—guarded; depends on the maturity of the fetus, the occurrence of intrauterine sepsis, and the trauma of delivery.

Amnionitis

Intrauterine infection after rupture of the membranes shows an almost linear progression beginning after a lag period of 12 to 18 hours for pregnancies under 36 weeks and a period of 6 hours for pregnancies over 36 weeks. As time passes after rupture of the membranes from any cause, the exposure of the fetus to infected fluid leads to intrauterine pneumonia; omphalitis and septicemia usually are secondary to placentitis but may follow amnionitis.

1. Fetal risk is much greater for the premature than for the term fetus because
   a. Resistance to infection is much less than that of a mature offspring and is directly related to the degree of maturity.
   b. The lag period prior to spontaneous or even induced labor is longer for the woman who is not at term than for one who is close to the expected date of confinement.
   c. Many a premature infant presents in the breech position, and trauma during vaginal delivery may cause injury.

2. Antibiotics of the broad-spectrum type, even in large doses, do little to protect the fetus from intrauterine infection.

3. Presence of amnionitis is indicated by the following signs:
   a. Fetid odor of amniotic fluid
   b. Fever in mother (often accompanied by a tender uterus)
   c. Placental membranes and cord showing "smoky" or "steamy" translucence (A frozen section of these structures will show abnormal collections of neutrophils with infection.)
   d. Polymorphonuclear leukocytes found on a smear of the chorionic surface of the amnion.
   e. Polymorphonuclear leukocytes found on a smear of a gastric aspirate from the infant.

4. Treat mother
   a. Administer appropriate broad-spectrum antibiotics.
   b. Delivery should be effected rapidly.

Prolonged rupture of membranes (PROM)

Leakage of amniotic fluid for over 24 hours is designated as prolonged rupture. Of great interest are recent reports suggesting that in the preterm infant, after leakage has continued for 16 hours prior to delivery, maturation of the fetal lung may be enhanced, as measured by the lecithin/sphingomyelin (L/S) ratio. The neonate in such an event may be at less risk for the respiratory distress syndrome. Therefore it would be advantageous to delay the onset of labor and delivery in such pregnancies, except for the increased hazard of amnionitis and its threat of pneumonitis and sepsis, particularly in the immature infant.

The increase in cortisol levels reported in PROM has encouraged clinicians to offer a course of cortisone therapy on an empiric basis to women with threatened premature labor. Although such therapy may be proved to render an advantage in the preterm infant as prophylactic therapy against hyaline membrane disease, the potential benefit must be weighed against possible risk.

1. Management of pregnancy under 37 weeks' gestation with PROM
   a. Delay delivery 48 to 72 hours when
      1. An immature rapid surfactant ("bubble") test or L/S ratio is observed on the amniotic fluid.
      2. No sign of amnionitis is present.
   b. Deliver infant promptly when
      1. Amniotic fluid study shows an intermediate or mature surfactant test (attempt induction followed by cesarean section if not delivered in 24 hours).
      2. Amnionitis is present.
2. Management of neonate

   Every infant born after prolonged rupture of the membranes or obvious signs of amnionitis in the mother (fever, tender uterus, foul-smelling amniotic fluid) should have a gastric aspiration (a swab from the external ear canal also can be used). Gram stain should be used to examine the material microscopically. More than five polymorphonuclear neutrophils (PMN) per high-power field indicates exposure to infection but not necessarily active infection (approximately 10% to 15% of such infants develop sepsis); thus treatment is not mandatory. For infants with a "positive" gastric aspirate, obtain a blood culture (not from an umbilical vessel) and consider antibiotic treatment with kanamycin and penicillin or ampicillin when

   a. Streptococci are observed on the smear (especially when the presence of group B streptococci are confirmed by immunofluorescence)
   b. The infant is delivered with a low Apgar score (under 7)
   c. The infant is preterm
   d. Evidence of respiratory distress, especially with an x-ray film demonstrating pneumonia, is observed
   e. There is abnormal behavior or change in behavior of the infant compatible with infection

   Duration of antibiotic treatment must be individualized depending on results of cultures, infant's clinical behavior, etc. We generally discontinue antibiotic treatment if blood culture remains negative for over 48 hours and the infant does not appear to be ill. For infants with obvious infection, treat as in Chapter 9.

INCOMPETENT CERVIX

Cervical incompetence, premature painless dilatation-effacement of the cervix, is caused in most cases by damage sustained during previous cervicouterine surgery or delivery. Repeated second trimester abortion or premature birth may be caused by cervical incompetence, which is found approximately once in every 500 to 600 pregnancies. Two percent of prematurity is ascribed to the incompetent cervix. No particular age or race is prone to this disorder.

Undoubtedly it is more common in communities where the practice of obstetrics and gynecology is inexpert.

1. Pathogenesis
   a. Forcible dilatation of the cervix in the nongravid patient and traumatic labor, delivery, or induced abortion lead to cervical damage. Lacerations may or may not be apparent, but as pregnancy progresses, containment of the products of conception becomes more and more difficult.
   b. A congenital shortness or weakness or abnormal function (perhaps psychogenic) is assumed in the occasional primigravida with cervical incompetence.
2. Pathology
   a. Note lacerations, even a site of rupture of the cervix into the lower uterine segment.
   b. Concealed damage—perhaps multiple tears—may be present.
3. Pathologic physiology
   a. The cervix (and perhaps the lower uterine segment) cannot "hold" the gestation within the uterus.
   b. With painless thinning and widening of the cervix, the membranes usually rupture; this will be followed by untimely delivery.
4. Clinical findings
   a. Progressive insensitive dilatation and effacement of the cervix after the first trimester, premature rupture of the membranes, and premature labor and delivery are typical of cervical incompetency.
   b. Neither laboratory findings nor x-ray studies are diagnostic during pregnancy.
   c. Repeated, gentle sterile-glove vaginal examinations may disclose an abnormal progressive opening of the cervix.
5. Differential diagnosis of midtrimester abortion
   a. Consider lower genital tract infection, severe isoimmunization, active maternal syphilis, premature separation of the placenta, placenta previa, extrachorial placenta.
   b. Congenital uterine deformity reduces uterine capacity, resulting in midtrimester abortion and premature labor and delivery.
6. Complications and sequelae
   a. Repeated midpregnancy pregnancy termination
   b. The offspring usually is considerably undersized; the prematurity rate is increased eight or nine times over the average in cervical incompetence.
7. Treatment
   a. Emergency measures
      Cervical cerclage may be successful if the os is not more than 2 to 3 cm dilated or 50% effaced, assuming an otherwise normal, viable pregnancy.
   b. Specific measures
      1. Bed rest and avoidance of stress
      2. Vaginal antiseptics such as nitrofurazone (Furacin) cream or suppositories
      3. Laxatives when needed
      4. Avoid hormone therapy
      5. Only mild sedation for the mother to avoid narcotizing the immature fetus if early delivery follows despite therapy.
   c. Surgical measures
      1. Cervical cerclage may be
         a. Temporary, in which two mattress sutures of heavy nonabsorbable type are placed through the cervix at right angles to each other (Würm procedure).
         b. Semipermanent, in which a ribbon of inert material (Mersilene) is passed around the cervix just over the fascia with tightening and securing of the strand followed by closure of the mucosa with additional absorbable sutures (Fig. 16-1). This procedure may also be accomplished in the nonpregnant state.
      2. When labor ensues

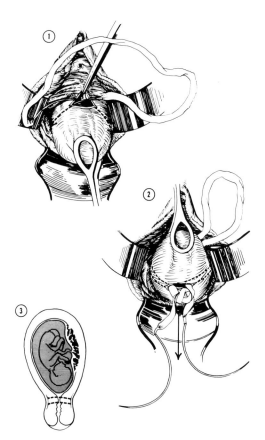

Fig. 16-1. Cerclage of the cervix (Shirodkar) with incompetent os in pregnant patient. (From Benson, R. C.: Handbook of obstetrics and gynecology, ed. 5, Los Altos, Calif., 1974, Lange Medical Publications.)

    a. The Würm sutures must be cut for vaginal delivery.

    b. If a buried cerclage is inserted, it may be severed for delivery from below, or a transverse lower-segment cesarean section may be elected.

    c. Cervicouterine infection, fetal death, or severe bleeding will require removal of the cerclage and emptying of the uterus.

8. Prevention

    a. Avoid trauma to the cervix in obstetric or gynecologic operations.

    b. Correct cervical lacerations or close

an abnormally patulous cervix before pregnancy.

9. Prognosis

    a. Repeated late abortions or premature deliveries will occur if the cervix is incompetent. Most fetuses are lost before the thirty-second week. A 25% to 75% perinatal mortality was usual prior to the use of cerclage.

    b. Currently, in otherwise uncomplicated cases, two thirds to three fourths of the offspring will go well beyond viability (28 weeks), with a perinatal mortality of 10% to 15%.

PROLONGED PREGNANCY

The majority of fetuses whose gestation is prolonged or who have reached 42 weeks of completed gestation from the last menstrual period will show the effects of impairment of nutritional supply—perhaps from an aging process of the placenta. Many of these infants will have suffered an actual loss of weight in utero, with evidence of reduced subcutaneous tissue, scaling, and parchmentlike skin—a condition usually referred to as dysmaturity. This common event in the postterm has led to the use of the term "postmaturity" to imply "placental insufficiency" even in infants who are not at term. Since many postterm babies do not suffer placental inadequacy but continue to grow and gain (Fig. 16-2), the term "postmaturity" should be abandoned as a term for fetal wasting. In contrast, see Fig. 16-3 for a postmature infant who has suffered chronic fetal distress (dysmaturity).

Incidence

At least 3% of infants are born after 42 completed weeks of gestation.

Management

    1. Recalculate expected date of delivery.

    2. Perform amniocentesis for maturity test by rapid surfactant and any evidence of meconium staining.

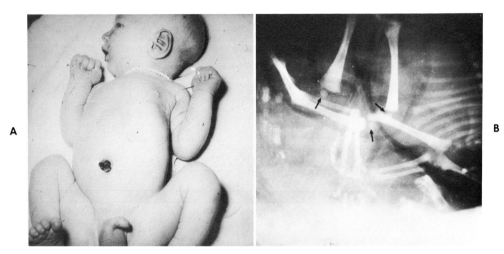

Fig. 16-2. A, An oversized (4,400 gm) postmature (44 weeks' gestation) newborn. **B,** Fetogram of infant in **A,** with large distal femoral and proximal tibial epiphyses.

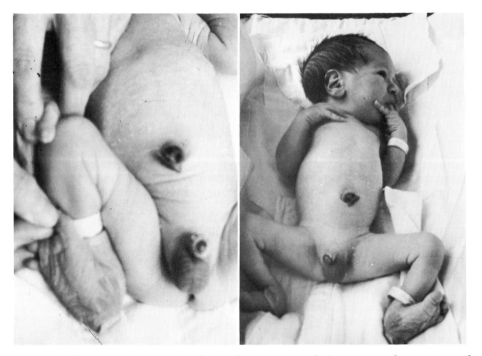

Fig. 16-3. This 2,600 gm infant was delivered after term and shows severe dysmaturity with scaling of the skin and loss of subcutaneous tissue. The open eye, hunger, wrinkled soles of the feet, and excessive fingernail length support a diagnosis of postmaturity.

3. Identify oversized fetus or fetopelvic disproportion (p. 32).
4. Identify fetal distress (serial estriol levels, oxytocin challenge test).
5. If there is no evidence of fetopelvic disproportion or fetal distress, induce labor with continuous fetal monitoring.
6. Perform cesarean section if fetus is in abnormal position, if there is evidence of fetopelvic disproportion, or if fetal distress is present.

Complications

1. A sharp rise in both fetal and neonatal mortality after 42 weeks' gestation (Fig. 16-4)
2. Fetal injury from fetopelvic disproportion
3. Asphyxial damage from fetal distress, which is particularly hazardous in the primigravida

These complications in the survivors increase the chance of mental subnormality and neurologic sequelae.

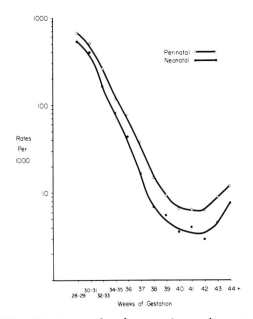

Fig. 16-4. Perinatal and neonatal mortality rates by weeks of gestation from over 40,000 births. (From Behrman, R. E., Babson, S. G., and Lessel, R.: Am. J. Dis. Child. **121:**486, 1971.)

SELECTED REFERENCES

Barden, T. P., Bieniarz, J., Cibils, L. A., Fuchs, F., Landesman, R., Mercer, J. P., Moawad, A. H., Pauerstein, C. V., and Zuspan, F. P.: Premature labor: its management and therapy, J. Reprod. Med. 9:93, 1972.

Bauer, C. R., Stern, L., and Colle, E.: Prolonged rupture of membranes associated with a decreased incidence of respiratory distress syndrome, Pediatrics 53:7, 1974.

Bieniarz, J., Motew, M., and Scommegna, A.: Uterine and cardiovascular effects of ritodrine in premature labor, Obstet. Gynecol. 40:65, 1972.

Bolognese, R. J.: Ampicillin: transfer into fetus and amnionic fluid, Rocky Mt. Med. J. 65:72, 1968.

Clark, D. M., and Anderson, G. V.: Perinatal mortality and amnionitis in a general hospital population, Obstet. Gynecol. 31:714, 1968.

Contifaris, B.: Habitual abortion and premature labor due to incompetence of the internal os of the cervix: cause—diagnosis—surgical treatment, Int. Surg. 51:156, 1969.

Friedman, M. L., and McElin, T. W.: Diagnosis of ruptured fetal membranes, Am. J. Obstet. Gynecol. 104:544, 1969.

Fuchs, F., Ruchs, A. R., Poblete, V. F., Jr., and Risk, A.: Effect of alcohol in threatened premature labor, Am. J. Obstet. Gynecol. 99:627, 1967.

Howmer, M. E., and Sprunt, K.: Screening method for identification of infected infant following premature rupture of maternal membranes, Pediatrics 49:283, 1972.

Hummer, W. K., and Sheldon, R. S.: Prolonged gestation, Minn. Med. 52:333, 1969.

Krapohl, A. J., Anderson, J. M., and Evans, T. N.: Isoxsuprine suppression of uterine activity, Obstet. Gynecol. 32:178, 1968.

Lanersen, W. H., and Fuchs, F.: Experience with Shirodkar's operation and postoperative alcohol treatment, Acta Obstet. Gynecol. Scand. 52:77, 1973.

Liggins, G. C., and Howie, R. N.: Prevention of respiratory distress with corticoids, Pediatrics 50:515, 1972.

Naeve, R. L.: Infants of prolonged gestation: a necropsy study, Arch. Pathol. 84:37, 1967.

Naver, E.: The incompetent cervix and its treatment in habitual abortion and premature labour, Acta Obstet. Gynecol. Scand. 47:314, 1968.

Richardson, C. J., Pomerance, J. J., Cunningham,

M. D., and Gluck, L.: Acceleration of fetal lung maturation following prolonged rupture of the membranes, Am. J. Obstet. Gynecol. **118:**1115, 1974.

Rovinski, J. J., and Shapiro, W. J.: Management of premature rupture of membranes, Obstet. Gynecol. **32:**855, 1968.

Scanlon, J.: The early detection of neonatal sepsis by examination of liquid obtained from the external ear canal, J. Pediatr. **79:**247, 1971.

Weingold, A. B., Palmer, J., and Stone, M. L.: Cervical incompetency: a therapeutic enigma, Fertil. Steril. **19:**244, 1968.

Yosowitz, E. E., Haufrect, F., Kaufman, R. H., and Gayette, R. E.: Silicone-plastic cuff for the treatment of the incompetent cervix in pregnancy, Am. J. Obstet. Gynecol. **113:**233, 1972.

Zlatnik, F. J., and Fuchs, F.: Controlled study of ethanol in threatened premature labor, Am. J. Obstet. Gynecol. **112:**610, 1972.

Zwerdling, M. A.: Factors pertaining to prolonged pregnancy and its outcome, Pediatrics **40:**202, 1967.

17

Disproportionate fetouterine growth

GROWTH-RETARDED FETUS

Moderate growth retardation indicates a perinate below the 10th percentile (Fig. 3-2). Severe growth retardation indicates one below 2 standard deviations from the mean (approximately 3rd percentile). Thus the incidence depends on the criteria used. Fig. 17-1 illustrates the linearity of normal growth and demonstrates the more common variations from it.

Growth impairment in the first half of pregnancy is most likely due to embryonic injury, genetic defect, or viral invasion of the fetus. Such fetuses often die in utero, whereas slowing of growth in the last half of pregnancy is usually related to a reduction in the flow of nutrients and/or oxygen supply to the fetus. Severe impairment of maternal-fetal transfer may cause arrest in cell division or even hypoxic damage to the brain. Moreover, there is decreased uterine blood flow with uterine contractions. Therefore the added asphyxial effects of labor further jeopardize the fetus. Early identification of the slowly growing fetus and intensive team management is imperative to assure intact survival.

1. Maternal-placental associations of fetal undernutrition (Fig. 3-2)
   Pathophysiologic changes that interfere with the nutritional supply line of the fetus are limitation of uterine blood flow, reduction in area of placental exchange, lowered maternal arterial con-

centration of essential nutrients, and impairment of diffusion across placental membranes. Factors to be considered are as follows:

a. Insufficiency of growth substrate due to
   1. Maternal undernutrition

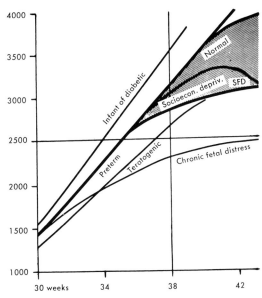

Fig. 17-1. Birth-weight curves of population (shaded range) and several abnormal groups. Subacute fetal distress (SFD) refers to the only curve representing a weight loss. The heavy line continuing straight above the normal range is the extrapolated curve. (From Gruenwald, P., and Babson, S. G. In Davis' gynecology and obstetrics, Hagerstown, Md., 1972, Harper & Row, Inc.)

2. Close spacing of pregnancies, and infants born after four pregnancies
3. Limited maternal weight gain or weight loss in the last trimester
   b. Maternal and placental disease or abnormality, such as
   1. Toxemia, hypertension, and renal and heart disease
   2. Bicornuate uterus and uterine surgery
   c. Placental variations, which include
   1. Multiple pregnancies with sharing of the placenta, twin-to-twin transfusion
   2. Circumvallate placenta, two-vessel cord, and velamentous insertion
   d. "Placental insufficiency," which may include
   1. Aging placenta in postmaturity
   2. Placental separation or infarction
   e. Later placental infection such as syphilis, toxoplasmosis, cytomegalovirus inclusion disease, and malaria
   f. Miscellaneous: tobacco smoking, high-altitude exposure, and drug addiction
   g. Idiopathic—constraint of infant size may be
   1. A family trait
   2. The result of growth impairment in the mother's childhood
2. Identification factors (clinical)
   a. A previous undergrown infant in a multipara
   b. Slowing in fundal measurements (under 1 cm/wk)
   c. Slowing of maternal weight gain or girth
   d. Presence of maternal disease or addictive habits
3. Diagnosis by ultrasonographic measurements of growth in biparietal diameter
   a. Under 2 mm/wk from the thirtieth to thirty-fourth week
   b. Under 1 mm/wk from the thirty-fifth week to term
4. Management
   a. Rule out fetal distress.

1. Serial 24-hour urinary estriol determinations (A falling of 40% from the previous value or under 10 mg/24 hr indicates grave fetal distress.)
2. Amnioscopy to determine amniotic fluid meconium staining
3. Oxytocin challenge test (Chapter 3)
   b. To determine the readiness for delivery, perform amniocentesis for rapid surfactant test or lecithin/sphingomyelin ratio (Chapter 3).
   c. Correct any maternal nutritive, habituative, or additive defects.
   d. Treat any disease process amenable to modern therapy.
   e. Place at bed rest in the lateral recumbent position in an attempt to increase uterine blood flow.
   f. Offer full team care during labor and delivery, with continuous monitoring (Chapters 4 and 5) for atraumatic delivery.

SMALL-FOR-DATES NEONATES

Infants whose birth weight is below the 10th percentile of the Denver weight grid (Fig. 3-3) are suspect for fetal undergrowth. Some of these infants are small because of family patterns but can be differentiated from undergrown infants by the presence of adequate subcutaneous tissue and proportionate body measurements. A substantial number of infants are adequate in size for gestational age but show signs of late fetal wasting and should be managed similarly to those with chronic fetal deprivation.

Undersized infants are classified into two groups: (1) those who are hypoplastic because of an intrinsic impairment of fetal cell division through injury or genetic influence and (2) those who suffered fetal undergrowth or weight loss imposed by limitation in the nutritional supply line. This may be chronic, subacute, or acute.

Hypoplastic infant

Hypoplastic infants usually, but not always, exhibit malformation.

1. Etiologic factors
   a. Genetic defects and chromosomal disarrangements, for example, trisomy syndromes, Down's syndrome
   b. Placental transfer of infection, for example, rubella
   c. Teratogenic drugs, such as thalidomide
   d. Ionizing radiation, such as from x-ray studies or therapy
2. Identification
   a. Careful inspection of the placenta and cord and knowledge of the volume of amniotic fluid may reveal placental abnormalities, hydramnios, oligohydramnios, amnion nodosum, or a single artery in the cord. Such findings vastly increase the chance of malformation.
   b. Examination of the infant for signs of anomaly (Chapter 6) should be carried out.

Nutritional impairment

Surprisingly the perinate tolerates well the anoxia and nutritional deprivation that accompany chronic placental impairment.

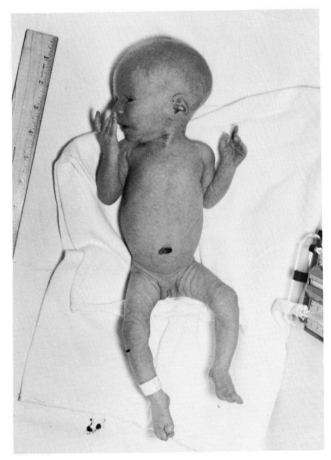

Fig. 17-2. Proportionately undergrown infant, 1,600 gm, who is 40 weeks of gestational age. Note the observation of the hand. She apparently contracted rubella in the second trimester without evidence of teratogenic effect.

Table 17-1. Comparison of clinical features of growth retarded term infants with those of large premature babies—both approximately 2,250 gm (5 lb)

	Growth retarded (38+ weeks)	Large premature (34 weeks)
Body size	Reduced body size for gestation; weight in general reduced more than length or head circumference; head circumference usually reduced least	Body measurements proportional and appropriate for gestational age
Weight loss	Minimal weight loss, if any, after birth, usually under 5%	5% to 10% of birth weight
External appearance		
Skin	Minimal subcutaneous tissue, often loose and wrinkled; scaly and cracked in dysmaturity	May be edematous and shiny
	Milia often present	Milia not seen
Color	Whiter from thicker epidermis in spite of higher hematocrit	Pink
Vernix	Minimal to absent	Abundant
Lanugo	None	Moderate
Hair	Sparse, straight, and silky	Fine and fuzzy
Sole creases	Extend over whole sole	Anterior third only
Skull bones	Firm on palpation to edges—often suture separation without increase in spinal fluid pressure	Soft and pliable—skull bones overlap at sutures
Ear cartilage	Erect, with sharp ridges	Soft and pliable
Scrotum	Testes pendulous with well-developed rugae	Not completely descended, few rugae
Labia	Labia minora tend to be covered	Labia minora more prominent
Breast tissue	Nodule with or without gland swelling, depending on degree of fetal malnutrition	Nodule absent
Cord stump	Thin and often discolored; dries early	White and thickened
Behavior		
Activity	Active—eyes open with anxious appearance	Inactive, torpid, eyes closed
Feeding	Takes nipple eagerly, sucks fingers; gains rapidly	Takes nipple poorly; slow to regain birth weight
Neurologic signs		
Tone	Increased tone—holds head well on traction; raises head from mattress	Head lag on traction; cannot raise head
Moro reflex	Brisk, complete, but often restricted	Incomplete
Eye response	Fixes and follows with eye	No recognition
Transillumination	Under 2 cm of reflected light	2 to 4 cm
Electroencephalo-gram	Mature cerebral waves, short response to photic stimulation (157.4 ± 2 msec)	Mean peak latency of photic response (212.5 ± 20 msec)
Physiologic signs		
Oxygen consumption	Increased per kilogram of body weight over preterm infant	Slightly decreased compared to term infants
Temperature control	Better able to defend against heat loss (muscular activity, brown fat presence); however, heat conservation limited by reduced subcutaneous fat	Supplemental heat required to maintain body temperature
	Perspires and shivers	Neither perspires nor shivers

Table 17-1. Comparison of clinical features of growth retarded term infants with those of large premature babies—both approximately 2,250 gm (5 lb)—cont'd

	Growth retarded (38+ weeks)	*Large premature (34 weeks)*
Organ systems	Regular respiration unless airway obstruction	Periodic breathing
	Concentrates urine well; minimal delay in bilirubin conjugation; decreased glycogen stores	Urine dilute; delay in conjugation of bilirubin; glycogen stores reduced, but usually adequate
Ossification centers		
Knee	Presence of both proximal tibial and distal femoral epiphyses—delay influenced by degree of fetal malnutrition	Absent

An acceptable theory indicates that to conserve limited oxygen supplies for the most vital organs (heart and brain), much of the circulation to the viscera and limbs is reduced. This reduction of oxygenation to skin may account for the parchmentlike scaling (less noticeable on the face) and absence of vernix in the moderately dysmature infant. Release of meconium and its staining of the skin represents the more severe effect of fetal distress.

Chronic fetal deprivation (chronic fetal distress) (Fig. 17-2)

Chronically decreased fetal exchange usually occurs after midpregnancy. A gradual restriction in growth results in a proportionately small infant in all growth parameters (under the 3rd percentile). Brain weight is least affected, but if nutritional restriction is sufficiently severe, brain cell division may cease.

Subacute fetal deprivation of dysmaturity (Fig. 16-3)

This common condition affects the fetus near the end of pregnancy and is identified at birth by loss in body weight and generalized wasting, with reduction in fat and muscle. These tissues have been consumed to support the metabolism necessary for survival. The skin is often cracked and dry, and there is a loss of vernix. The length and head size may be in the normal range but are proportionately greater than weight. The ponderal index—a weight/length ratio—may be under 2 SD, or under 2.20 (weight in grams $\times$ 100 $\div$ cm^3); yet the weight for gestation may be appropriate and over the 10th percentile. In other words, the infant is light for length but not necessarily small for dates. Nonetheless, metabolic jeopardy is often serious.

Acute fetal distress

Acute fetal distress indicates relatively sudden and uncompensated hypoxic insult, which is an added hazard for the fetus with growth retardation. The combination of growth retardation and asphyxia, the latter intensified by labor, is a leading cause of perinatal morbidity and death. In this case rescue by immediate delivery is justified.

Recognition of undergrown mature infant

The special problems and requirements of undergrown mature infants are such that they be differentiated from preterm infants. Table 17-1 compares their clinical characteristics.

Management of infants with nutritional impairment

1. Infants in good condition but undersized and undernourished or dysmature

a. Administer orally a 10% glucose solution to active infants as soon after birth as possible.
b. Offer full-strength and later 24 to 30 calories/30 ml formula if feedings are well tolerated.
c. Perform Dextrostix test every 4 to 6 hours for the first 48 to 72 hours of life as a screening test. A faint blue color or no color indicates the possibility of a low blood glucose level (under 30 mg/100 ml) and the necessity for quantitative measurement.
d. Give parenteral $D_{10}W$ if intake is not satisfactory or the blood glucose level is under 40 mg/100 ml.
e. Be prepared to lavage stomach several times if mucus vomiting occurs (common in dysmature).
2. Growth-retarded infants who have severe asphyxia and meconium aspiration
   a. Clear the airway thoroughly by tracheal aspiration.
   b. Insufflate lungs with oxygen.
   c. Correct metabolic acidosis.
   d. Maintain skin temperature at 97° ± 1° F (36° C).
   e. Administer 10% glucose in water intravenously, at the rate of 80 to 100 ml/kg of body weight; continue the infusion until oral feedings are established. (See feeding, Chapter 8.)
   f. Treat with aqueous penicillin, 50 to 100,000 units, and kanamycin, 15 mg/kg of body weight/24 hr in divided doses every 12 hours for 5 to 7 days in respiratory distress.
   g. Give ultrasonic mist vapor.
   h. Examine chest x-ray film for aspiration syndrome (Chapter 19), pneumothorax (increase in cyanosis and respiratory effort), and cardiomegaly (hypoglycemia or cardiac failure).
   i. Check pH and blood gases as necessary and the blood glucose level (Dextrostix) every 4 hours and 3 hours after glucose infusion is stopped.

Complications

The following complications are sufficiently common and serious that they are discussed in other sections of this book. Term gestations under 2 SD have eight times the perinatal mortality rate of infants of similar gestational age but who are appropriate in size.
1. Asphyxia neonatorum, often with meconium aspiration
2. Hypoglycemia (Chapter 24)
3. Pulmonary hemorrhage (Chapter 19)
4. Congenital anomalies (incidence approximately ten to twenty times that found in large mature infants)
5. Asphyxial convulsions (Chapter 22)

Late development

1. Neurologic deficit
   The neurologic damage of symptomatic hypoglycemia and perinatal asphyxia is well known. Brain weight and size is less affected than are other organs in fetal undernutrition; yet this potential handicap to future development must be faced in view of the possible limitation in cell division and number. Although animal studies indicate a clear relationship between fetal growth retardation and the suppression of brain development and the learning process, evidence of slowing of neurologic maturation and intellectual development in the human from intrauterine nutritional deprivation remains circumstantial.

   In studies of monozygotic twins severely discrepant in size by 25% or more at birth, the larger twin maintained a relatively small advantage over his smaller twin in IQ.

   Minkowski and associates have been impressed by the degree to which brain development during fetal life progresses independently of unfavorable gestational circumstances that may affect physical growth. Even if neurologic maturation of small-for-dates infants is appropriate for gestational age, cell multiplication may be suppressed. Drillien has shown that children who were "small for dates" did equally as well in their IQ scores at 10 to 12 years of age as did those of the same maturity who were much larger at birth when reared in better-than-average homes, but not if they were reared in poorer homes. We have reported that if the severely undergrown infant is free of disease and unhampered by significant asphyxia, normal school progress can be expected.

2. Growth retardation

Physical growth in undersized term new-borns continues at a reduced level during the early part of the growth period. Fig. 17-3 shows the longitudinal growth measurements of twelve severely undergrown term infants through the first year of life. The growth curves in weight and length are parallel at a much reduced level in comparison with those of normal infants. Head circumference less reduced at birth usually increases at a faster rate in that the curve approaches that seen in infants of normal size at 1 year of age. Twin studies demonstrate that the smaller twin of monozygotic pairs seldom attains the physical size of his twin even after growth is completed. Head circumfer-

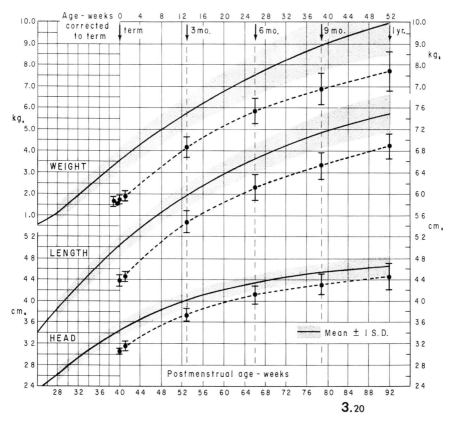

Fig. 17-3. Mean longitudinal growth of twelve severely undergrown term infants. Proportional reduction in body size is shown at the time of birth. (From Babson, S. G.: J. Pediatr. 77:11, 1970.)

ence is the least affected, although significant difference in this measurement still remains.

OVERSIZED, OR "LARGE," FETUS

During the past decade, especially, an increase in the weight of newborn infants has been recorded. Almost 2% of the neonates at our institution have a birth weight of 4,500 gm (9 lb 15 oz) or more, and 10% are over 4,000 gm in weight. The body length and other measurements have increased concomitantly with weight. Although racial differences and better nutrition are major reasons for heavier babies, women's pelvic dimensions have not increased proportionately. The vast majority of excessive-sized babies are born of multiparous mothers, a number of whom have "prediabetes," diabetes mellitus, or obesity.

The large infant is often exposed to serious birth trauma, which is most critical in breech presentation. Currently, the cesarean section rate for the excessive-sized fetus is about twice that for those of average weight. In addition, the baby of the diabetic mother is metabolically stressed.

It is well known that successive progeny are heavier and that excessive weight gain (over 24 lb) during pregnancy is associated with larger offspring. Moreover, if a woman produces a large baby, there is a very good chance that a later baby will be large, or even larger. About 35% of large babies are delivered after 293 days and are postmature.

Estimation of fetal size in utero is difficult. Nonetheless, the physician should think in terms of say, "small babies"—2,500 gm or less, "average babies"—2,500 to 4,000 gm, and "large babies"—4,000 gm or more.

Excessive development of the fetus is far more common (and more important) than a larger-than-normal (justo major) pelvis.

Prolonged, "difficult" labor is usual with the oversized fetus. Instrumental delivery is the rule. Shoulder dystocia is a common problem because of greater circumference, and posterior or transverse arrest is frequent. The mother suffers accordingly.

1. Associations (Fig. 3-2)
   a. Infants delivered of women who are more than 25% overweight or who had a prepregnant weight/length ratio of over 2.4
   b. Infants of women who gain more than 35 lb in weight during pregnancy
   c. Infants of diabetic or gestational diabetic mothers
   d. Infants with transposition of great vessels
2. Clues to excessive fetal development
   a. Past maternal history of large babies
   b. Large stature, multiparity, diabetes, or obesity
   c. Weight gain of over 35 lb in pregnancy
   d. Postmature pregnancy (294 days or more)
   e. Prolonged, dystotic labor
3. Diagnosis
   a. Biparietal head diameter (ultrasound) over 10 cm
   b. Fundal measurement over 42 cm
   c. Fetal cephalometry combined with x-ray pelvimetry
4. Management
   a. Consider fetal overgrowth in relation to the size and architecture of the mother's pelvis.
   b. Be prepared for a cesarean section for malposition and dystocia.
   c. Reevaluate all pregnancies that approach 42 weeks of gestational age.
   d. Monitor electronically in any trial of labor.
   e. Prepare for shoulder-girdle dystocia.
5. Clinical features of the infant
   a. Weight, head, and length are all proportionately large.
   b. Initial activity and hunger are usually reduced.

c. Weight loss is nearly double that of normal-sized infants.

d. Hyperbilirubinemia, hypocalcemia, and hypoglycemia are not uncommon in infants born before term.

6. Complications (when delivered vaginally)

a. Fetal asphyxia or trauma with dystocia or malpresentation

b. Observe for
   1. Broken clavicle
   2. Brachial plexus injury

c. Mental subnormality
   The increase in the incidence of mental subnormality reported may reflect excessive fetal stress. This potential tragedy should be prevented by the liberal use of cesarean section.

The large-for-dates perinate is defined as being over the 90th percentile in weight for gestational age. At term this percentile for middle-class, white infants peaks at approximately 4,250 gm (Fig. 6-3). This may be an excessive size for successful delivery. In a study of 70 infants who weighed over the 95th percentile at birth, we found that at least 50% of the mothers were obese and had gained over 35 lb in pregnancy. Only about one third of these babies were born after 42 weeks of gestation. Additionally the improved nutrition of many areas of the world has apparently resulted in increasingly larger fetuses, whereas pelvic capacities have not

increased proportionately. This discrepancy in size (fetopelvic disproportion) also places many fetuses of lesser size at increased jeopardy. North European parents produce the largest infants (nearly 2% are over 4,500 gm at birth). Contrary to the multitude of factors that slow fetal growth, maternal diabetes or its tendency is the only known pathophysiologic correlate to accelerated fetal growth (Fig. 17-1).

MULTIPLE PREGNANCY

Multiple pregnancy (usually twinning) is the result of either the abnormal segmentation of a single fertilized ovum (monozygotic, monovular, or identical twins) or the fertilization of multiple ova (dizygotic, binovular, or fraternal twins). Monozygotic twinning is a chance occurrence, the incidence being the same in all races and peoples; dizygotic twinning is determined by a female recessive trait. Blacks have a higher rate of twinning than whites, but Orientals have a lower rate. Younger primigravidas and older multiparas have a greater frequency of twinning than other gravidas.

The frequency of twins is about 1:90; triplets $1:90^2$; quadruplets $1:90^3$, etc. More males than females are born in plural births.

Twins account for nearly 2% of all neonates. They contribute over 15% of all infants weighing less than 2,500 gm; over

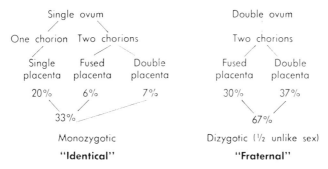

Fig. 17-4. Twin zygosity and placental form. (Based on data from Potter, E. L.: Am. J. Obstet. Gynecol. **87:**566, 1963.)

half are preterm. The mean weight of twins in North America is approximately 5 lb (2,300 gm). Thus multiple pregnancies account for more undergrown neonates than any other known cause. The perinatal mortality and morbidity for multiple gestation far exceeds that for singletons of similar gestational age. Early diagnosis of multiple pregnancy, elimination of obstetric complications, extension of gestation, avoidance of delivery problems, and optimal neonatal care are very special needs in multiple pregnancy.

1. Anatomy of twins (Fig. 17-4)

   Examination of the placenta and membranes is of help only in zygosity determinations in twins with monochorionic placentas because these twins are always monozygotic. Other placental forms, for example, single, fused, or double, do not aid in determining zygosity in individual twin pairs, since any of these forms may be associated with monozygotic or dizygotic twins. The differentiation of single-ovum twins can be accomplished in about two thirds of monozygotic pregnancies (20% of all twin pairs) or in those with a single chorion and one placenta.

2. Clinical findings

   Most cases of twinning should be diagnosed by the twenty-fourth to twenty-sixth week of gestation. Consider the following signs:

   a. Symptomatology
      1. Large uterus for dates
      2. Considerable fetal activity
      3. Marked maternal weight gain, unexplained by obesity or toxemia
      4. Identification of more than one fetus (before or after delivery of one)
      5. Auscultation of more than one fetal heart, each varying at least 8 beats/min from the other and from the mother's pulse

   b. Laboratory results showing significantly reduced maternal iron and abnormally low hematocrit

   c. X-ray films (oblique or lateral) that usually reveal the presence of more than one fetal skeleton by 14 to 16 weeks

   d. Sonography allowing a diagnosis of twins during the third or fourth month of pregnancy

   e. Fetal electrocardiogram identifying a multiple pregnancy (one major complex and more than one minor QRS complex)

3. Differential diagnosis

   a. Single fetus—larger than expected because of discrepancy of dates

   b. Hydramnios—expected with multiple pregnancy but occurring more often in singletons with anomalous development

   c. Pelvic tumor plus single fetus—suggestive of multiple pregnancy (However, paucity of small parts, sounds of the one fetal heart, and single ballotable presenting pole are contradictory.)

   d. Abnormal twin pregnancy—bony union of conjoined twins revealed by radiography

   e. Early intrauterine death of one fetus (fetus papyraceous, or compressus)

4. Complications and sequelae

   a. Mother
      1. Preeclampsia-eclampsia is three times more frequent in women with twins than in women with singletons.
      2. Premature labor, often after spontaneous rupture of the membranes, and delivery are seven times more likely in multiple pregnancy than in singleton pregnancy.
      3. Premature separation of the placenta is common, especially after delivery of the first twin.
      4. Postpartum hemorrhage occurs often after delivery of more than one fetus.

   b. Fetus
      1. Fetal death occurs three times as

often with twins as with a solitary fetus because of

    a. Abnormal fetal or placental development

    b. Circulatory competition

    c. Cord compression or other accidents

2. Central nervous system injury and other trauma may follow intervention and operative delivery. Asphyxia relates to prolapse of the cord or premature separation of the placenta. Thus cerebral palsy and mental retardation are increased.

3. Monozygotic twins have tripled the perinatal mortality of dizygotic twins and a greater chance of congenital malformations in one of the pair.

4. Twin-to-twin transfusion (monozygotic) is not infrequent because of circulatory communication; polycythemia in one and anemia in the other require prompt treatment.

5. Single umbilical artery occurs three times more often in twins.

6. Velamentous insertion of the cord occurs seven times more frequently with multiple pregnancy.

5. Treatment

  a. Optimal antepartum care

    1. Supervise weight control; allow a gain in weight approximately 50% greater than in single pregnancy—as much as 40 lb above nonpregnant weight if the latter was in the normal range.

    2. The patient must have a prenatal visit no less than every 2 weeks in the second trimester and weekly in the third trimester. In addition to the routine prenatal care, vaginal examinations for cervical effacement or dilatation must be performed.

    3. Monitor hematocrit and supply sufficient iron.

  b. Hospitalization

The value of bed rest for a week at the time of diagnosis (if under 30 weeks) and again at 32 weeks is undeniable. The patient should be encouraged to maintain the lateral recumbent position to maximize uterine blood flow. Offer bed rest when

    1. Toxemia, spontaneous labor, cervical dilatation, or other serious problems threaten

    2. Proper daily rest is impossible at home

  c. Delivery (Chapter 5)

    1. Multiple pregnancy is in a very high-risk category, and ideally the gravida should be delivered in a maternity center with a physician-nurse team for each infant in the delivery room.

    2. Cesarean section should be performed primarily in the monoamniotic twins (determined by amniography). Cesarean section should also be liberally used for malposition and fetal distress even if one twin has already been delivered vaginally.

    3. Electronic fetal monitoring must be employed.

    4. Neonates usually require intensive care.

6. Prognosis

  a. Mother

    1. Maternal morbidity is eight times that reported for singleton vaginal delivery because of hemorrhage, trauma, etc.

    2. Anemia is common.

  b. Fetus

    1. The smaller the fetuses, the poorer is the prognosis, especially for the second or smaller twin.

    2. Double-ovum twins fare better than single-ovum twins.

    3. Sets of triplets or quadruplets often do not live. Twice as many triplets die in the perinatal period as twins.

4. The prognosis for the second twin is best when prompt delivery and prophylactic (outlet) forceps are used or when delivery is spontaneous. Internal podalic version-extraction may be seriously traumatic.

HYDRAMNIOS AND OLIGOHYDRAMNIOS

Both excessive accumulation and a paucity of amniotic fluid are associated with great hazard to the perinate. Hydramnios (polyhydramnios) is an increase over the normally expected 800 to 1,200 ml of amniotic fluid near term gestation and usually is not detectable until 2,000 to 3,000 ml are present. It may occur either acutely (2%) or chronically (98%), and although the exact causes are unknown, there are certain clinical correlates:

1. Diabetes, 25% of cases
2. Congenital malformation, 20% of cases
3. Erythroblastosis fetalis, 12% of cases
4. Multiple gestation, 8% of cases

Despite these correlates, the largest group (33%) is still idiopathic. It complicates 0.4% of all pregnancies, and nearly 40% of the pregnancies so complicated have a perinatal demise. It is therefore imperative that any pregnancy with this complication be investigated by glucose tolerance test, repeat antibody screening, and B-scan ultrasonography, and be considered for amniography. Many modes of treatment have been attempted, and bed rest with diuretics may assist slightly. Ultimately, in the severe case, multiple amniocentesis may be necessary. It should be borne in mind, however, that this aggressive management is indicated only for maternal indications (relief of dyspnea).

Oligohydramnios is the rare condition in which there is a significant paucity of amniotic fluid (usually under 500 ml at term). It is difficult to make the diagnosis because of the decreasing amount of amniotic fluid with the lengthening gestation; however, the diagnosis is suggested when the uterus is tightly apposed about the fetus and any form of ballottement is impossible. There appear to be a multiplicity of causes; however, an exact etiology is undetermined. The clinical correlates are fetal renal agenesis and obstruction to the urinary tract.

1. Possible causes of hydramnios
   a. Increased production of amniotic fluid
   b. Decreased clearance of amniotic fluid
   c. Fetal urine excess or reduced swallowing of amniotic fluid
   d. Gross transudate
2. Marked congenital abnormalities associated with hydramnios (approximately 50% of cases)
   a. Central nervous system anomalies such as anencephaly or spina bifida
   b. Gastrointestinal anomalies—esophageal atresia
3. Maternal problems related to hydramnios
   a. Eclamptogenic toxemia
   b. Multiple pregnancy
   c. Cardiac and/or renal diseases with edema; diabetes mellitus
   d. Syphilis (tertiary) of the viscera
   e. Erythroblastosis
   f. Umbilical cord obstruction
4. Conditions associated with oligohydramnios
   a. A pregnancy with placental insufficiency
   b. A fetus with serious urinary tract abnormality—little or no urine excreted
   c. Fetal death and absorption of amniotic fluid
   d. Persistent, slight loss of fluid via a small membrane defect

Maternal diagnostic studies and observations in hydramnios and oligohydramnios

1. Obtain radiographs and/or ultrasound for
   a. Skeletal defects, for example, anencephaly or hydrocephaly
   b. Twinning and hydrops fetalis

c. Signs of fetal death, for example, cranial bone overlap and fetal gas

d. Skeletal age; observation of the presence and size of the distal femoral epiphyses

2. Identify fetal inactivity, for example, neuromuscular disease or cerebral defect

3. Note signs of toxemia and isoimmunization

4. Record appearance of abnormal amniotic fluid, for example, meconium or bile contamination (Pigment is increased in hemolytic disease.)

Treatment

1. Hydramnios
   a. Treat maternal disease appropriately: digitalize for cardiac failure; give diuretics for stasis edema.
   b. Accomplish amniocentesis when
      1. No gross fetal anomaly can be identified, and maternal distention is extreme and refractory to other therapy.
      2. Serious fetal or maternal disease is diagnosed, and premature termination of the pregnancy is necessary.

2. Oligohydramnios
   a. Recalculate and reestimate the duration of the pregnancy. A smaller uterus may indicate a later expected date of confinement, not placental dysfunction.
      1. Avoid intervention if fetal or maternal jeopardy is uncertain.
      2. Terminate the pregnancy if fetal anomaly is recognized or fetal death has occurred or when placental insufficiency is likely.
   b. Measure fetal growth by sonography.

SELECTED REFERENCES

Adamson, A. R., and Benster, B.: Renal agenesis, oligohydramnios, and diabetes mellitus, Postgrad. Med. J. **45**:189, 1969.

Allen, M. S., Jr., and Turner, U. G., III.: Twin birth—identical or fraternal twins? Obstet. Gynecol. **37**:538, 1971.

Arts, N. F. T., and Lohman, A. G. M.: The vascular anatomy of monochorionic diagnostic twin placentas and the transfusion syndrome, Eur. J. Obstet. Gynecol. **1**:85, 1971.

Babson, S. G., and Henderson, N. B.: Fetal undergrowth: relation of head growth to later intellectual performance, Pediatrics **53**:890, 1974.

Babson, S. G., Henderson, N., and Clark, W. M.: The preschool intelligence of oversized newborns, Pediatrics **44**:536, 1969.

Babson, S. G., and Kangas, J.: Preschool intelligence of undersized term infants, Am. J. Dis. Child. **117**:553, 1969.

Babson, S. G., and Phillips, D. S.: Growth and development of twins dissimilar in size at birth, N. Engl. J. Med. **289**:937, 1973.

Bolton, R. N.: Some considerations of excessive fetal development, Am. J. Obstet. Gynecol. **77**:118, 1959.

Chantler, C., and Baum, J. D.: Dextrostix in the diagnosis of neonatal hypoglycemia, Lancet **2**:1395, 1967.

Coer, R. W., and Sutherland, J. M.: Placental vascular communications between twin fetuses: a simplified technique for demonstration, Am. J. Dis. Child. **120**:332, 1970.

Corney, G., Robson, E. B., and Strong, S. J.: Twin zygosity and placentation, Ann. Hum. Genet. **32**:89, 1968.

DeGeorge, F. V.: Maternal and fetal disorders in pregnancies of mothers of twins, Am. J. Obstet. Gynecol. **108**:975, 1970.

Drillien, C. M.: The small-for-dates: etiology and prognosis, Pediatr. Clin. North Am. **17**:9, 1970.

Eriksson, A. W., and Fellman, J.: Acta Genet. **17**:385, 1967.

Fitzhardinge, P. M., and Stevens, E. M.: The small-for-date infant. II. Neurologic and intellectual sequelae, Pediatrics **50**:50, 1972.

Griffiths, M.: Cerebral palsy in multiple pregnancy, Dev. Med. Child Neurol. **9**:713, 1967.

Jonas, E. G.: The value of prenatal bed rest in multiple pregnancy, J. Obstet. Gynecol. Br. Commonw. **70**:461, 1963.

Lee, K. H.: Hydramnios in the Chinese: a clinical study of 256 cases, J. Obstet. Gynaecol. Br. Commonw. **74**:868, 1967.

McDonald, A.: Retarded foetal growth. In Dawkins, M., and MacGregor, W. G., editors: Gestational age, size and maturity, London, 1965, Spastics Society/Heinemann.

Miller, H. C., and Hassanein, K.: Fetal malnutrition in white newborn infants: maternal factors, Pediatrics **52**:504, 1973.

Minkowski, A., Larroche, J., Vignaud, J., Dreyfus-Brisac, C., and Saint-Anne Dargassies, S.: Development of the nervous system in early life. In Falkner, F. F., editor: Human development, Philadelphia, 1966, W. B. Saunders Co.

Naeye, R. L., Blanc, W., and Cheryl, P.: Maternal nutrition and the fetus, Pediatrics **52:** 494, 1973.

Nanda, U., and Patnaik, D. R.: A ten-year review of multiple pregnancy. J. Indian Med. Assoc. **51:**286, 1968.

Nelson, L. W., Horne, M. K., and Bradford, W. D.: Polyhydramnios: an infrequent etiology, South. Med. J. **65:**188, 1972.

Ounsted, M.: The regulation of foetal growth. In Jonxis, J. H. P., Visser, H. K. A., and Troelstra, J. A., editors: Aspects of prematurity and dysmaturity, Springfield, Ill., 1967, Charles C Thomas, Publisher.

Ounsted, M., and Taylor, M. E.: The postnatal growth of children who were small-for-dates or large-for-dates at birth, Dev. Med. Child. Neurol. **13:**421, 1971.

Pernoll, M. L., and Carnes, R. W.: Electronic fetal monitoring of twin gestations, Am. J. Obstet. Gynecol. **116:**583, 1973.

Queenan, J. T., and Gadaw, E. C.: Polyhydramnios: chronic versus acute, Am. J. Obstet. Gynecol. **108:**349, 1970.

Sack, R. A.: The large infant, Am. J. Obstet. Gynecol. **104:**195, 1969.

Scott, K. E., and Usher, R.: Fetal malnutrition: its incidence, causes, and effects, Am. J. Obstet. Gynecol. **94:**951, 1966.

Shorlaad, J.: Management of the twin transfusion syndrome, Clin. Pediatr. **10:**160, 1971.

Singer, J. E., Westphal, M., and Niswander, K.: Relationship of weight gain during pregnancy to birth weight and infant growth and development in the first year of life: a report from the Collaborative Study of Cerebral Palsy, Obstet. Gynecol. **31:**417, 1968.

Talukdar, P. K.: Placental transfusion syndrome, Indian Pediatr. **4:**302, 1967.

Usher, R. H.: Clinical and therapeutic aspects of fetal malnutrition, Pediatr. Clin. North Am. **17:** 9, 1970.

Van den Berg, B. J., and Yerushalmy, J.: The relationship of the rate of intrauterine growth of infants of low birth weight to mortality, morbidity, and congenital anomalies, J. Pediatr. **69:** 531, 1966.

Whitfield, C. R.: Effect of amniotic fluid volume on prediction, Clin. Obstet. Gynecol. **14:**537, 1971.

Wynter, H. H., and Hew, L. R.: Fetal mortality and morbidity in twin pregnancy, West Indian Med. J. **17:**204, 1968.

18

Other pregnancy complications

URINARY TRACT INFECTION

Urinary tract infection during pregnancy is a major cause of premature delivery, fetal death, and maternal morbidity. In most cases of urinary sepsis, gram-negative bacteria of the coliform *Aerobacter aerogenes* group are identified. A single organism *(Escherichia coli)* may be expected in four fifths of the cases of initial uncomplicated pyelonephritis, but a variety of organisms are found in the majority of recurrent cases and in women with even minor degrees of urinary tract obstruction and retention. Previous bladder or kidney sepsis—often in childhood, adolescence, or a prior pregnancy—predisposes to gestational or puerperal exacerbations. About 15% of obstetric patients suffer from symptomatic urinary tract infection; multiparas outnumber primigravidas with this complication. From 5% to 10% of all pregnant women have asymptomatic bacteriuria. Chronic and recurrent acute urinary tract infection during pregnancy is the rule unless long-term therapy is prescribed. Early delivery may be required in acute, persistent pyelonephritis to avoid fetal death.

1. Pathogenesis
   a. Vaginitis, cervicitis, contamination of the urethral meatus by leukorrhea, and urethral irritation by coitus or gynecologic or urologic instrumentation may initiate lower tract infection.
   b. Congenital or acquired obstruction reduces the free flow of urine.
   c. Bacteria usually reach the ureter and kidney pelvis by ascending lymphatics or by urinary reflux.
   d. Hematogenous nontuberculous infection of the urinary tract probably is exceptional.
   e. Urinary stasis during pregnancy occurs because of dilatation, displacement, elongation, and flaccidity of both ureters, usually more marked on the right as a consequence of high steroid sex hormone levels and compression of the ureters by the gravid uterus.
2. Pathology and pathologic physiology
   a. Fibrosis with long-standing or recurrent infection prevents the usual reversal of the physiologic pregnancy dilatation—elongation of the ureters postpartum.
   b. Scarring reduces elasticity, and periureteral inflammation causes matting and kinking of the ureters.
   c. Obstruction (hydroureter and hydronephrosis) often follows: pyelonephritis and renal abscess formation, permanent renal damage, reduced function, or, rarely, death may ensue.
   d. Urinary tract stricture, polyp, diverticulum, stone, and reduced resistance aggravate infection.
   e. Urethritis and cystitis are often progressive to upper tract involvement.
3. Clinical findings—symptomatology
   a. Acute signs

1. Rapidly progressive dysuria, urgency, anorexia, chills, fever, and occasionally hematuria are noted in acute lower and upper urinary tract infection.
2. Flank pain and costovertebral angle tenderness identify pyelonephritis.
3. Anemia, septicemia, and jaundice may develop in subacute cases.
4. Shock is a rare, acute complication of severe pyelonephritis.
5. Uterine irritability, premature labor, or fetal death may accompany urinary tract sepsis.

   b. Chronic signs
   1. Anorexia, urinary distress, flank pain, low backache, chills, fever, and anemia are recorded.
   2. Premature labor is a common sequel.

4. Laboratory findings
   a. Urinalysis
   1. A "clear-catch" (midstream) or catheterized urine specimen will reveal more than two white blood cells and/or red blood cells per low-power field in urinary tract infection. Often myriads of white blood cells, many clumped, are seen.
   2. Stained urinary sediment revealing even scattered bacteria indicates bacteriuria (infection).
   3. Gram-positive bacilli are probably *Staphylococcus aureus;* gram-negative may be *Escherichia coli.*
   4. Bacterial counts, usually by spread-plate technique, of more than 100,000 bacteria/mm³ are diagnostic of bacteriuria.
   5. Bacterial sensitivity tests will identify the best antibiotic for therapy.
   6. If urine is apyuric, without stained bacteria in the sediment, suspect tuberculosis and do a guinea pig inoculation or culture for tuberculosis bacilli.

   b. Blood studies
   Leukocytosis (to approximately 25,000 white blood cells/mm³), with many immature forms and an elevated sedimentation rate, characterizes acute urinary tract sepsis.
   c. X-ray studies are an important diagnostic aid in chronic urinary tract infections.

5. Treatment
   a. General measures
   1. Order bed rest and mild sedation (avoid salicylates—sulfa is inactivated).
   2. Eliminate foci of infection, especially vaginitis or cervicitis.
   3. Force fluids to 3 to 4 L/24 hr.
   4. Alkalinize urine with citrocarbonate, 1 gm orally every 2 hours, or similar preparations.

   b. Specific measures—prescribe intensive chemotherapy initially.
   1. If gram-negative bacilli are stained in the urinary sediment, assume *Escherichia coli;* treat with sulfisoxazole, 0.5 to 1 gm orally four times a day, or nitrofurantoin (Furadantin), 100 to 200 mg orally four times a day, or equivalent, for at least 7 days in a first attack. Sulfisoxazole, 0.5 gm orally four times daily, is effective and safe during pregnancy. Avoid all delayed-excretion sulfa preparations. They may cause neonatal hyperbilirubinemia.
   2. If gram-positive organisms are identified, consider the infection to be of the noncoliform type. Give ampicillin, 250 mg orally, four times a day for 1 week.
   3. If the patient is unimproved in 2 days with this therapy, substitute the best drug from the culture-sensitivity study; consider cystoscopy, ureteral catheterization, and retrograde pyelography.
   4. Continued bacteriuria or recur-

rence of infection requires supressive therapy with sulfisoxazole, 0.5 gm orally, four times a day, or nitrofurantoin (Furadantin), 100 mg orally daily, etc. throughout the antepartum period and the puerperium.

    5. Induce labor after viability is well established to save the fetus if the gravida continues to be seriously ill and unresponsive to therapy.

6. Differential diagnosis—consider appendicitis, cholecystitis, ureterolithiasis, and false labor.

7. Prevention

    a. Avoid trauma, catheterization, or other instrumentation during pregnancy, delivery, and the postpartum state.

    b. Provide prolonged and uninterrupted prophylactic chemotherapy of asymptomatic or recurrent symptomatic bacteriuria.

8. Prognosis

    a. Mother

        1. Approximately one third of obstetric patients with bacteriuria develop acute pyelonephritis during pregnancy or immediately thereafter if bacteriuria persists.

        2. The outlook is good if the antibiotic completely eliminates infective organisms and is continued postpartum. Recurrence will follow if there is a stone, obstruction, or maternal birth trauma present or if poorly chosen short-term therapy is given.

        3. Cure is established by three successively negative cultures or negative slides of urinary sediment stained for bacteria during a 10-day period.

    b. Fetus

        1. Prognosis is good with cure of bacteriuria.

        2. The likelihood of fetal death or premature labor and delivery is three times the usual expectancy

if urinary tract infection, especially the symptomatic type, persists.

DIABETES COMPLICATING PREGNANCY

Diabetes mellitus, the inability to metabolize glucose properly, is a disease of uncertain etiology. No race is prone, but heriditary predisposition (mendelian recessive trait) to the disorder is recognized. Obese and older individuals are more commonly afflicted than are slender or younger persons. At least 4% of women and about half as many men in the United States have latent or overt diabetes.

Diabetes mellitus complicates at least one in every 325 pregnancies, and latent or gestational diabetes may have an equal incidence. Maternal mortality is only slightly increased, but morbidity is considerably worsened by this abnormality; perinatal mortality is still 10% to 30%, and the incidence of anomalies in the offspring of diabetic parents is three to five times the average. Prematurity is a problem not only because of spontaneous premature labor but also as a result of the current medical policy to deliver many diabetic gravidas prior to term to avoid fetal death in utero.

1. Pathologic physiology

    a. Mother

        1. Gravida with diabetes mellitus is

          a. Prone to infection

          b. Subject to acidosis, diabetic coma, or insulin shock

          c. Likely to develop toxemia and hemorrhage

          d. Able to have a normal glucose tolerance test after 72 hours postpartum in the gestational type of the disease

        2. Adverse effects of pregnancy on diabetes

          a. Subclinical diabetes may be temporarily converted to clinical (gestational) diabetes.

          b. The renal glucose threshold is increased—the glucose tolerance test, including the 2-hour postprandial level, is elevated.

c. Insulin requirements usually are raised.

d. Metabolic complications (hyperemesis, food cravings) may be difficult to treat.

e. The "work" of labor depletes glycogen stores, and ketosis may result.

f. Anabolism becomes catabolism postpartum—a reversal that may severely confuse the regulation of diabetes.

3. Adverse effects of diabetes on pregnancy
   a. Infertility and spontaneous abortion are increased in the decompensated patient.
   b. The incidence of congenital anomalies is at least tripled.
   c. Edema is more difficult to control.
   d. Hydramnios is increased ten times.
   e. Preeclampsia-eclampsia complicates one third to one half of the cases.
   f. Premature labor and delivery are more frequent.
   g. Fetal death after 36 weeks is more likely to occur, often because of acidosis or placental dysfunction.
   h. The larger perinate (over 4,000 gm) is more prone to birth injury.

b. Newborn infant
   1. Overgrown in the majority of instances from intrauterine metabolic acceleration
   2. Development of function related to gestational age rather than size
   3. Subject to hypoglycemia, acidosis, hypocalcemia, and hyperbilirubinemia
   4. Increase in respiratory distress syndrome (hyaline membrane dis-

ease), perhaps related more to prematurity and frequency of delivery by cesarean section

2. Clinical findings
   a. Symptomatology
      1. Polydipsia, polyuria, pruritus, asthenia, somnolence, and paresthesias may occur.
      2. Mycotic vaginitis is common.
      3. Xanthomas and carotenemia may develop.
      4. Cataracts, retinopathy, atherosclerosis, nephrosclerosis, and neurosensory loss may afflict diabetic persons.
   b. Laboratory findings
      1. Seek glycosuria, hyperglycemia, and reduced glucose tolerance in suspected diabetes.
      2. Obtain a fasting blood glucose determination and a 2-hour postprandial glucose determination early in pregnancy in patients suspected of having diabetes.
         a. If the patient's fasting blood glucose determination exceeds 200 mg/100 ml, a glucose tolerance test will be unnecessary and may be harmful (threat of diabetic coma).
         b. A 2-hour postprandial glucose level less than 110 mg/100 ml is normal in pregnancy, a level of 110 to 120 mg suggests diabetes, one of 140 to 180 mg is indicative of gestational diabetes, and a level of greater than 180 mg designates clinical diabetes.
      3. Placenta—nonspecific lesions, but degenerative changes are common. Examine placenta for
         a. Defective investment of terminal villi
         b. Sclerosis of fetal vasculature
         c. Intervillous fibrin deposition
   c. X-ray examination
      1. Seek calcification of vessels of the

lower extremities. Such blood vessel changes, especially in the pelvis, are serious findings.

2. Obtain roentgenographic pelvimetry-fetometry near term to determine disproportion or fetal bony anomalies.

d. Special examinations, including those of the ophthalmologic, cardiovascular, and renal systems

3. Differential diagnosis

Abnormal carbohydrate metabolism may also occur during lactation and with ACTH or cortisone administration in Cushing's syndrome, hepatitis, pheochromocytoma, and acromegaly.

4. Complications and sequelae

a. Diabetic acidosis or coma, insulin shock, eclamptogenic toxemia, hydramnios, premature labor and delivery, and genital tract or other infection may afflict the gravida.

b. The fetus may die in utero or during the postnatal period.

c. Babies of mothers with gestational diabetes generally have the same fate as those born of mothers with clinical diabetes.

5. Treatment

a. Mother

1. Treat diabetic coma or insulin shock promptly and adequately.

2. Study diabetic suspects (based on history, physical findings), using appropriate laboratory tests. Do not rely on urinalysis; secure blood glucose determinations and perhaps carbon dioxide, serum sodium, and potassium determinations in specific instances.

3. Insist on obstetric and medical consultation; admit diabetic patients to the hospital for study and regulation early in pregnancy.

a. Supervise diet carefully.

b. Permit slight glycosuria while the patient is receiving insulin.

c. Restrict salt to 1 gm per day; forbid the patient excessive weight gain.

d. Deny steroid sex hormone therapy (valueless).

4. Readmit the gravida to the hospital for regulation in midpregnancy and at 36 weeks (or sooner if medical or obstetric complications eventuate).

5. Avoid delivery until maturity is indicated by amniotic fluid analysis.

6. Substitute regular insulin for half of the insulin lente, if labor and delivery are imminent.

7. Rupture the membranes and stimulate to induce labor at 36 to 37 weeks, if the gravida is a multipara and the cervix is favorable.

8. Effect a cesarean section during labor if

a. The cervix is unfavorable.

b. Severe preeclampsia or eclampsia, malpresentation, etc. complicate gestation.

c. Delivery within 12 hours is unlikely.

d. There is any evidence of fetal distress.

9. Choose an elective cesarean section if

a. The vertex is floating.

b. A breech is presenting.

c. The fetus is estimated to weigh more than 3,400 gm (7½ lb).

d. Complications ensue.

b. Neonate

Insist that a physician experienced in pediatrics be present at delivery, particularly to treat a compromised infant. (See Chapter 24.)

6. Prognosis

a. Mother

1. Maternal mortality of less than 0.2% is likely with adequate modern therapy.

2. Diabetic retinopathy and nephropathy usually increase during gestation.
   b. Offspring (Chapter 24)
      1. The fetal outcome is related to
         a. Severity of diabetes
         b. Occurrence of medical or obstetric complications
         c. Degree of prematurity at birth
      2. Even with current management, expect
         a. Perinatal mortality of 10% to 15%
         b. Anomalies in about 5%
      3. Neonates of diabetic mothers delivered vaginally may do better than those born by cesarean section.

ISOIMMUNIZATION— ERYTHROBLASTOSIS FETALIS

Erythroblastosis is a common hemolytic disease of the fetus and the newborn infant, the result of maternal isoimmunization to a fetal blood group antigen. Sensitization of the mother occurs promptly after an incompatible blood transfusion or after one or more pregnancies in which fetal erythrocytes have escaped into the maternal circulation. The mother produces antibodies that cross the placental barrier to cause agglutination and hemolysis of fetal red blood cells. Anti-A or anti-B (ABO) incompatibility is the most common, but sensitization to the Rh factor, anti-D, is the most severe.

Erythroblastosis complicates about one in 100 to 250 pregnancies, mostly of Caucasian women. Male and female offspring are affected with equal frequency. Sufficient fetal involvement may occur in half these pregnancies to warrant considering early delivery. Almost 15% of Caucasian, 2% to 3% of Negro, and 1% of Oriental women are Rh negative. Fortunately, sensitization occurs after mating with Rh-positive men in only about 5% of those susceptible. Erythroblastosis is often associated with premature delivery or perinatal death and can damage the central nervous system in survivors. The risk increases with Rh sensitization in each succeeding pregnancy, particularly if the father is homozygous for D in the rhesus group.

1. Pathogenesis, pathology, pathologic physiology
The antibodies produced by the gravida from a fetal blood group antigen introduced into her circulation tend to rise during pregnancy. The maternal antibody titer may or may not reflect the severity of fetal erythroblastosis, but at times the earlier the rise and higher the titer, the more serious the hemolytic disease of the fetus or neonate. A late or low rise in titer, however, may also accompany a severe disease.
   a. Fetus and newborn
      1. Degree of involvement of the fetus depends on
         a. Type and amount of antibody
         b. Duration of antigen-antibody interaction
      2. Rapid red cell destruction, hyperbilirubinemia, and anemia occur in utero; extramedullary erythropoiesis accompanies anemia. The elements involved in causing hemolyses are
         a. Incompatibilities in the ABO group (direct Coombs' test may be negative or weakly positive)
         b. Immunization against Rh_0 (D) in the rhesus group
         c. Sensitization against less common antigens such as c, E, K (Kell), and Fy^a (Duffy)
      The sensitization in the third category just given is due to the wide use of transfusions of blood containing antigens not present in the recipient and has been increasing in importance in recent years. A newborn infant with an

Rh-positive (Rh$_0$ (D)-positive) mother may therefore have erythroblastosis.
  b. Placenta
    The placenta often is large, boggy, and friable, with enlarged edematous villi. The degree of pathology is directly related to the extent of fetal disease.
  c. Gravida
    1. Hydramnios occurs in about half the hydrops fetalis cases.
    2. Premature labor is common.
    3. Soft tissue dystocia may complicate the delivery of a hydropic fetus.
    4. Additional fetal red blood cells may enter the maternal circulation at the time of separation and removal of the placenta.
2. Routine management of all pregnancies
  a. First visit
    1. Document blood group and Rh type.
    2. Screen blood serum for antibodies with the Hemantigen type screening test.
  b. At 28 to 36 weeks of gestation
    1. Repeat antibody screening test.
    2. If no antibody is demonstrated, no further studies are needed.
3. If antibody is demonstrated
  a. Obtain the gravida's serum for
    1. Identification of the antibody by testing with a known panel of red cells.
    2. Measurement of serum titer by antihuman globulin test.
  b. Perform amniocentesis after 23 weeks of gestation and repeat as indicated when
    1. Serum titer is over 1:8 or Rh antibodies are present.
    2. A previous infant had erythroblastosis.
Amniocentesis and the spectrophotometric measurement of the yellow pigment found in the amniotic fluid from *the degradation of fetal red blood cells have added new dimensions to the assessment of severe isoimmunization. Skilled interpretation of the spectrophotometric readings can identify a fetus likely to die if the pregnancy is allowed to continue to term.*
4. Technique of amniocentesis and spectrophotometry
  a. Locate the placenta. The ultrasonic B-scan is ideal. (See Figs. 18-1 and 18-2.)
  b. Have the patient void; check the fetal heart tone.
  c. Prepare with suitable antiseptic an area about 2 inches below and away from the gravida's midline and the back of the fetus.
  d. Raise a skin wheal and anesthetize a tract to the uterus with an appropriate local anesthetic.
  e. Perforate the amniotic cavity with a 20-gauge spinal needle behind the neck or on the small parts side away from the placenta, inserting the needle with one hand and holding the fetus away from the needle site with the other.
  f. Withdraw approximately 5 to 10 ml of fluid. If it is grossly bloody, obtain fluid from another puncture site.
  g. Centrifuge fluid for 10 minutes at 14,000 rpm and decant if it is cloudy or bloody; store in a dark bottle in the refrigerator; filter if the supernatant fluid is not clear. Centrifugation may be delayed up to 48 hours, while fluid is protected from light.
  h. Place clear fluid in a cuvette in a spectrophotometer and obtain at least fifteen optical density values from 350 to 700 mμ; plot these values on two-cycle semilogarithmic graph paper, using optical density as the ordinate and decreasing wavelength as the abscissa (Fig. 18-3).
5. Interpretation of the spectral absorption curve of the amniotic fluid

a. Three grades of severity
   1. A mildly affected fetus for which a term delivery is recommended
   2. A moderately affected fetus with a good chance of survival if delivered when physiologic maturity testing indicates fetal capability to survive outside the uterus
   3. A severely affected fetus which, if immature by physiologic maturity testing, may require an intra-uterine transfusion to avoid fetal death

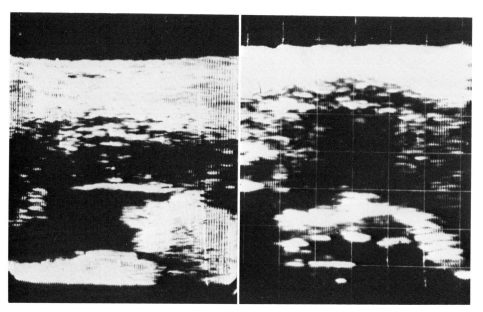

Fig. 18-1. Left, ultrasonogram showing a normal placenta on the anterior uterine wall. Right, ultrasonogram showing a hydropic placenta on the anterior uterine wall. (From Hoffbauer, H.: The antenatal diagnosis of fetal erythroblastosis. In Huntingford, P. J., Hüter, K., and Saling, E., editors: Perinatal medicine, Stuttgart, 1969, Georg Thieme Verlag.)

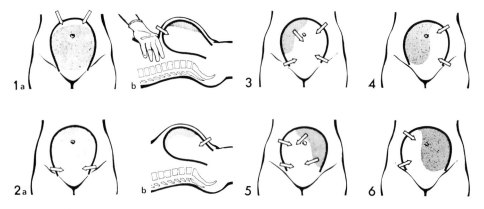

Fig. 18-2. Choice of a site for amniocentesis, depending on the position of the placenta. (From Hoffbauer, H.: The antenatal diagnosis of fetal erythroblastosis. In Huntingford, P. J., Hüter, K., and Saling, E., editors: Perinatal medicine, Stuttgart, 1969, Georg Thieme Verlag.)

b. Errors in interpretation
  1. False negatives—usually mild cases with no harm done
  2. False positives in a pregnancy with an Rh-negative fetus, indicating the possibility of a previous severely affected infant
6. Fetal transfusion
Fetal transfusion is indicated for the early treatment of marked degrees of

fetal isoimmunization (Liley's severely affected zone) prior to the thirty-second to thirty-fourth week of pregnancy. Once fetal hydrops has developed, however, intrauterine transfusion usually will not save the offspring. Intrauterine transfusion, generally every 7 to 10 days, is required to prevent fetal exodus before early delivery can be accomplished. Once the fetus is

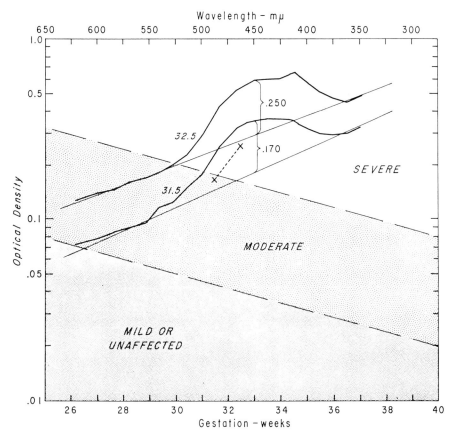

Fig. 18-3. Spectrophotometric analysis of amniotic fluid surrounding an erythroblastotic fetus. Amniocentesis was performed at 31½ and at 32½ weeks' gestation. The spectral absorption curve was obtained by plotting the optical densities at various wavelengths on two-cycle semilogarithmic graph paper. A tangential line joining the lowest portions of this curve approximates unstained amniotic fluid and is the base line for calculations. The difference between the involved and uninvolved curves is measured at 450 mμ. (Maximum absorption by bilirubin or bilirubin-like products occurs at 450 mμ.) This difference is plotted at the appropriate number of weeks' gestation, as illustrated by the dotted line. This case reveals rapid progression from moderate to severe disease. Under such conditions fetal death often is imminent; prompt delivery usually must be accomplished if gestational age will permit; otherwise, intrauterine fetal transfusion may be considered.

delivered, replacement transfusion and specific supportive measures are possible.

Fetal transfusion requires radiographically controlled percutaneous catheterization of the fetal peritoneal space. Packed red blood cells (O-negative blood) are then injected into the peritoneal cavity of the fetus. The erythrocytes soon pass into the fetal bloodstream. Techniques vary with local preference and equipment, but most are dependent on x-ray corroboration of the needle position. It is recommended that the procedure be performed only in specialized centers and by those experienced in the technique.

a. Preparation

1. The day before the fetal transfusion, blood is cross matched, amniocentesis is accomplished under sterile precautions, and meglumine diatrizoate (Renografin), 10 ml or its equivalent, is injected into the amniotic cavity. The object is amniography and a 24-hour fetal gastrointestinal series for target purposes.

2. The next day, supine anteroposterior and supine lateral films are made. The contrast medium should now be in the fetal intestine, and lead markers give surface landmarks in two planes. From these landmarks, the needle trajectory is determined.

b. Needle placement

With the patient under local anesthesia, the physician thrusts an 8-inch (No. 16), thin-walled, sharp, short-beveled, open-lumen needle through the abdominal and uterine wall into the fetal abdomen. It may rebound with the startled fetus, but it should not leak blood or amniotic fluid. A second pair of films should identify the tip of the needle in the fetal abdomen. About 5 ml of nitrous oxide or carbon dioxide is injected,

and a final lateral film is made. The gas bubble confirms the intraperitoneal position of the needle point. (If the needle is not placed properly, leave it for fetal fixation and as a guide for placement of a second needle.)

c. Catheter insertion

When the position of the needle tip is confirmed, polyethylene tubing (PE-60) about 38 to 40 cm in length is threaded through the needle, and the needle is removed. A dressing is applied to the mother's abdomen. A three-way stopcock is used to connect the catheter tubing from a bag of packed red cells and a 10 ml syringe. The latter is used to inject 50 to 150 ml of blood in 5 to 10 ml increments over a 2-hour period. Estimate the capacity of the fetal abdomen from the resistance to injection as it is filled. Transfusions are repeated every 7 to 10 days until delivery. Fetal hematopoiesis virtually stops; the majority of elements in the neonate's blood are transfused cells.

d. Maternal risks

Hemorrhage, infection, sensitization from a damaged placenta, and clotting derangements. (The estimated maternal complications are 2% to 3%.)

e. Fetal risks

Cardiac failure (overload), sepsis, radiation (less than pelvimetry), needle trauma, homologous serum jaundice. Estimated fetal loss is 10% to 15%. Fetal salvage approaches 50% overall but is lower in younger fetuses. Survival is rare if fetal hydrops has developed.

7. Management of the infant at delivery

a. Have available 1 unit of type O negative blood* low in anti-A and

---

*O-negative packed cells should be on hand for the severely involved fetus or one that has had fetal transfusions.

anti-B content and free of the antigenic blood group factor. Be certain this blood is compatible in a cross matching with the mother's serum. Use this blood if the infant is in need of an immediate partial exchange transfusion because of severe anemia.

b. Clamp the cord promptly.

c. Collect a tube of cord blood (allow clotting) for typing, Coombs' test, and blood serum bilrubin level determination. (See Chapter 23.)

d. Obtain a tube of oxalated cord blood for hemoglobin and smear for identification of immature red cell forms (nucleated red blood cells and spherocytes).

e. Place infant under radiant heat; observe for color, edema, and hepatosplenomegaly; support infant in general with full intensive care as indicated in Chapter 6.

8. Management of infants with severe hydrops fetalis

This disease signifying severe isoimmunization fortunately is becoming a rarity with improved prenatal management of the sensitized mother as well as Rh₀GAM prophylaxis. However, it has been reported in other conditions such as thalassemia, fetomaternal bleeding, congenital nephrosis, intrauterine atrial tachycardia, and diseases compromising liver function (e.g., syphilis, cytomegalovirus infection, toxoplasmosis).

a. Symptoms at birth

1. Severe anemia due to excessive hemolysis, leading to
   a. Cardiac decompensation
   b. Hypoxemia
2. Severe hypoproteinemia due to decreased protein synthesis, leading to
   a. Presence of edema at birth, giving infant a "Buddha" appearance
   b. Presence of fluid in abdominal and thoracic cavities, leading to
      (1) Distension of abdomen and elevation of diaphragm
      (2) Poor ventilation
3. Severe hypoxia and acidosis
4. Elevated central venous pressures

b. Treatment

The catastrophic mortality of 50% to 90% in these cases makes prompt treatment a necessity.

1. Closely monitor infant's ventilatory status, since assisted ventilation is needed in a large number of cases.
2. Place catheters in both umbilical vein and artery to monitor pressures in both inferior vena cava and aorta.
3. Aspirate fluid, if present, from peritoneal and thoracic cavities to ease ventilation of the infant.
4. Obtain arterial blood gas determinations and correct any acidosis, which frequently will aid in the correction of elevated central venous pressures.
5. Perform a partial exchange transfusion with packed O-negative red cells (Chapter 23) to bring the hematocrit within tolerable range (40% to 50%). Delay a 2-volume exchange until condition is stabilized.
6. Digitalize patient.
7. Attempt to achieve diuresis by slow (approximately 30 minutes) infusion of 1 gm/kg of salt-poor albumin.
8. Begin an infusion of 10% dextrose through catheters (total amount 60 to 80 ml/kg/24 hr).

9. Management of less affected infants after birth

a. Correct hypoalbuminemia and acidosis if present.

b. Give an early supply of carbohydrate—orally or parenterally, depending on infant's condition.

c. Anticipate needs for donor blood.

    d. Monitor infant's bilirubin and hematocrit levels every 4 to 6 hours.

    e. Place infant under phototherapy. Although this therapy will not affect hyperbilirubinemia drastically, in these cases it might diminish the number of potential exchange transfusions. For indications for and technique of exchange transfusion, see Chapter 23.

10. Management of infants with kernicterus
Kernicterus refers to the yellow staining of the brain tissue from the entry of unconjugated bilirubin. The resulting toxicity and injury to brain cells is responsible for neurologic damage and mortal hazard to newborn infants. An increase in the level of bilirubin increases the chance of kernicterus, but there is by no means a linear relationship. The amount of bilirubin unbound to albumin, the degree of acidemia, the fluid and caloric balance, the duration of exposure, and the degree of immaturity of the infant all determine the likelihood of the syndrome.

    a. Signs and symptoms

        1. Early signs and symptoms

            a. Refusal or regurgitation of feedings

            b. Depression of reflexes, particulary sucking, grasping, and the Moro reflex

            c. Increase in muscle tone

        2. Later signs and symptoms

            a. Opisthotonus and internal rotation and adduction of the arms

            b. Apnea and cyanosis

            c. Convulsions

        3. Residual findings in survivors

            a. Hypotonia and/or choreoathetosis

            b. Mental retardation

            c. Impaired eye movements, particularly supraversion

            d. Nerve type of hearing loss

    b. Prevention

An exchange transfusion will reduce the total body bilirubin level about 25%. Emergency exchange may be useful when the behavior of the infant suggests an early kernicterus.

11. Management of infants with ABO incompatibility
Sensitization of the infant's type A or B red blood cells with maternal anti-A or anti-B usually is a problem of less intensity when compared to Rh sensitization, although it certainly is more common. Sensitization to anti-A seems to occur more frequently. An increase in severity of fetal involvement with successive pregnancies, as in Rh sensitization, does not take place.

The infant may have a weakly positive direct Coombs' test at birth as well as a moderately elevated cord bilirubin level (less than 4 mg/100 ml).

Hyperbilirubinemia, if occurring, is usually mild and can be treated with phototherapy (Chapter 23); exchange transfusions are needed only in occasional cases. Slowly ongoing hemolysis may happen, however, and intermittent monitoring of hematocrit is advisable.

12. Prognosis

    a. Stillbirths and neonatal deaths from hemolytic disease occur in about one or two per 1,000 deliveries.

    b. If the newborn infant survives the first week, the outlook for survival is good. Exchange transfusion greatly reduces the occurrence of kernicterus and increases the likelihood of recovery.

13. Prevention

    a. Contradict the administration of incompatible blood or blood products.

    b. Human Rh immunoglobulin (Rho-GAM), 300 mg or more intramuscularly, given prior to the sensitization of the gravida will safely prevent hemolytic disease of the newborn (erythroblastosis). Unfortunately, Rho GAM will neither desensitize nor reduce the hazards of Rh incompatibility once sensitization has occurred. Isoimmunization is as yet irreversible, so that all women who have not been sensitized to this blood factor should receive Rh_0GAM prophylaxis less than 72 hours after delivery of an Rh-incompatible infant. Rh immunoglobulin should be given similarly after every abortion and Rh-positive gestation. Because human Rh immunoglobulin consists of gamma G globulin that can cross the placenta and damage the fetus, Rh_0GAM should not be administered to patients during pregnancy.

Certain preliminary laboratory studies must be accomplished before administration, so that scarce human Rh immunoglobulin will be given only to those who may benefit.

1. The parturient must be
   a. Typed and found compatible with the donor substance
   b. Rh (Rh_0 or D) negative and D^u negative
   c. Free of serum anti-Rh (Rh_0 or D) antibodies
2. Her neonate must be
   a. Rh (Rh_0 or D) positive and D^u positive
   b. Negative to a direct Coombs' test

THYROID DYSFUNCTION
Hyperthyroidism

Hyperthyroidism, either endogenous (goiter) or exogenous (excessive thyroid hormone administration), may complicate pregnancy and the puerperium seriously. Hyperthyroidism is related to an increased frequency of premature delivery, postpartum hemorrhage, and possibly toxemia of pregnancy; but it is not a cause of abortion or fetal anomalies. Nevertheless, overtreatment of the mother with antithyroid drugs may result in fetal hypothyroidism and deficient development, especially of the central nervous system. Treatment of the gravida with radioactive iodine at any time may cause irreparable damage to the fetal thyroid gland and gonads.

1. Treatment
   a. Insist on complete bed rest for observation and initial therapy of the mother.
   b. Obtain medical and obstetric consultation in severe cases.
   c. Prescribe Lugol's solution, 10 drops orally daily, to control mild to moderate toxic goiter.
   d. Thiouracil may be given instead of, or in addition to, Lugol's solution in more serious cases, but one should always add thyroxine, 0.2 to 0.4 mg daily (or equivalent concomitantly), to protect the fetus from hypothyroidism.
   e. Iodine suppression followed by subtotal thyroidectomy is the procedure of choice in many cases.
2. Prognosis
   a. The outlook for the mother is very good when a euthyroid status can be maintained.
   b. The fetus should do well, provided hypothyroidism or recurrent hyperthyroidism does not supervene.

Hypothyroidism

An extreme degree of hypothyroidism (myxedema) is associated with sterility; a less severe deficiency causes infertility, abortion, premature delivery, and congenital anomalies.

1. Clinical findings
   a. Signs
      1. Slight, generalized edema—puffiness of eyes, tightness of rings in the morning
      2. Dryness of skin, brittle nails, thinning of hair (notably eyebrows)
      3. Enlarged, soft thyroid gland
      4. Slow tendon reflexes
   b. Symptoms

1. Drowsiness, easy fatigue, vague arthralgia
2. Cold intolerance, decreased sweating
3. Weight gain, constipation

2. Laboratory studies in hypothyroidism during pregnancy
   a. Serum protein-bound iodine is below the normal range of 6 to 11 mg/100 ml.
   b. Serum butanol-extractable iodine is less than 4 to 6 mg/100 ml.
   c. Basal metabolism rate is most inaccurate in pregnancy.
   d. Radioactive iodine uptake by thyroid is dangerous to fetal thyroid unless in doses under 0.5 μCi.
   e. Radioactive triiodothyronine uptake by red blood cells is depressed by both hypothyroidism and pregnancy; therefore it is a poor test during gestation.

3. Treatment
   Give sodium L-thyroxine, 0.025 to 0.05 mg (¼ to ½ grain orally daily, or equivalent, for a week or two, depending on gestational age and need). If the mother is myxedematous, prescribe smaller doses. Gradually increase the dosage to 0.1 mg/24 hr or more, depending on response. Reduce dosage if irritability, tachycardia, fever, or diarrhea is present and otherwise unexplained.

4. Prognosis
   Prompt, adequate, continued supplemental thyroid hormone therapy will improve the likelihood of normal fetal growth and development. If therapy is considerably delayed or insufficient, irreparable mental and physical retardation will ensue.

   Reduction of perinatal casualty will result from judicious early delivery.

SELECTED REFERENCES

Adam, P. A. J., and Schwartz, R.: Diagnosis and treatment: should oral hypoglycemic agents be used in pediatric and obstetric patients, Pediatrics **42**:819, 1968.

Aickin, D. R., et al.: Urinary estriol excretion in pregnancies complicated by Rhesus immunization, Aust. N. Z. J. Obstet. Gynaecol. **12**:86, 1972.

Allen, S. T., Dubner, M. S., and Mockler, N. D.: Routine prenatal screening for atypical antibodies, Am. J. Obstet. Gynecol. **99**:274, 1967.

Bashore, R. A., and Lecky, J. W.: Intrauterine fetal transfusion in management of the Rh disease, Obstet. Gynecol. **38**:79, 1971.

Beard, R. W., and Roberts, A. P.: Asymptomatic bacteriuria during pregnancy, Br. Med. Bull. **24**:44, 1968.

Bowman, J. M., Friesen, R. F., Bowman, W. D., et al.: Fetal transfusion in severe Rh isoimmunization: indications, efficiency, and results based on 218 transfusions carried out on 100 fetuses, J.A.M.A. **207**:1101, 1969.

Carroll, R., MacDonald, D., and Stanley, J. C.: Bacteriuria in pregnancy, Obstet. Gynecol. **32**:525, 1968.

Connor, E. J.: Congenital malformations in offspring of diabetic mothers, Med. Ann. DC **36**:465, 1967.

Dowling, J. T., Appleton, W. G., and McColoff, J. T.: Thyroxine turnover during human pregnancy, J. Clin. Endocrinol. Metab. **27**:1749, 1967.

Farquhar, J. W., and Isles, T. E.: Hypoglycemia in newborn infants of normal and diabetic mothers, S. Afr. Med. J. **42**:237, 1968.

Gaither, D., and Clark, J. F. J.: Pregnancy and latent diabetes, J. Natl. Med. Assoc. **65**:139, 1973.

Goplerud, C. P., White, C. A., Bradbury, J. T., and Briggs, T. L.: The first Rh-isoimmunized pregnancy, Am. J. Obstet. Gynecol. **115**:632, 1973.

Gottesman, R. L., and Refetoff, S.: Diagnosis and management of thyroid disease in pregnancy, J. Reprod. Med. **11**:19, 1973.

Grimaldi, R. D.: Significance and management of abnormal oral glucose tolerance tests during pregnancy, Obstet. Gynecol. **32**:713, 1968.

Haeye, R. L.: The newborn infant of the diabetic mother, Penn. Med. **71**:68, 1968.

Hamilton, A. T., Paterson, P. J., and Breidalel, H. D.: Thyroidectomy during pregnancy, Med. J. Aust. **55**:431, 1968.

Hibbard, L., Thrupp, L., Summeril, S., Smale, M., and Adams, R.: Treatment of pyelonephritis in pregnancy, Am. J. Obstet. Gynecol. **98**:609, 1967.

Hofmeister, F. J., Schwartz, W. R., O'Leary, W. J., Stanhope, C. R., and Inman, J. E.: Decreasing the risk of fetomaternal transfusion at the time of delivery, Am. J. Obstet. Gynecol. **112**: 594, 1972.

Holt, E. M., Boyd, I. E., Dewhurst, C. J., Murray, J., Naylor, C. H., and Smitham, J. H.: Intrauterine transfusion: 101 consecutive cases treated at Queen Charlotte's Maternity Hospital, Br. Med. J. **3**:39, 1973.

Kaori, M., and Stelson, I.: Management of thyrotoxicosis in pregnancy: value of serial protein-bound iodine and Hamolski tests, Isr. J. Med. Sci. **5**:43, 1969.

Karlsson, K., and Kjellmer, I.: The outcome of diabetic pregnancies in relation to the mother's blood sugar level, Am. J. Obstet. Gynecol. **112**: 213, 1972.

Karnicki, J.: Results and hazards of prenatal transfusion, J. Obstet. Gynaecol. Br. Commonw. **75**: 1209, 1968.

Kincaid-Smith, P.: Bacteriuria and urinary infection in pregnancy, Clin. Obstet. Gynecol. **11**: 533, 1968.

Kitchen, W. H.: Neonatal mortality in infants receiving exchange transfusion, Aust. Pediatr. **6**: 30, 1970.

Leigh, D. A., Grüneberg, R. N., and Brumfitt, W.: Long-term follow-up of bacteriuria in pregnancy, Lancet **1**:603, 1968.

Liley, A. W.: Liquor amnii analysis in the management of pregnancy complicated by rhesus sensitization, Am. J. Obstet. Gynecol. **82**:1359, 1961.

Lunell, N. O., and Person, B.: Potential diabetes in women with large babies: a follow-up study, Acta Obstet. Gynecol. Scand. **51**:293, 1972.

Man, E. B., Reid, W. A., and Jones, W. S.: Thyroid function in human pregnancy. IV. Serum butanol extractable iodine drop with weight gain, Am. J. Obstet. Gynecol. **102**:244, 1968.

McFadyen, I. R., Eykyn, S. J., Gardner, N. H. N., Vanier, T. M., Bennett, A. E., Mayo, M. E., and Lloyd-Davis, R. W.: Bacteriuria in pregnancy. I. Prevalence and natural history, J. Obstet. Gynecol. Br. Commonw. **80**:385, 1973.

Misenhimer, H. R., and Kaltreider, D. J.: Preterm delivery of patients with decreased glucose tolerance, Obstet. Gynecol. **33**:642, 1969.

Niswander, K. R., Westphal, M. C., and Seekree, S.: Amniocentesis in management of the Rh problem, Obstet. Gynecol. **30**:646, 1967.

O'Sullivan, J. B., and Mahan, C. M.: Criteria for the oral glucose tolerance test in pregnancy, Diabetes **13**:278, 1964.

O'Sullivan, J. B., Charles, D., Mahan, C. M., and Dandrow, R. V.: Gestational diabetes and perinatal mortality rate, Am. J. Obstet. Gynecol. **116**:901, 1973.

Pedersen, J., Molsted, L., and Anderson, B.: Perinatal fetal mortality in 1245 diabetic pregnancies: secular trends 1946-1971 and variations according to the White and PBSP classifications, Acta Chir. Scand. (supp.) **433**:191, 1973.

Queenan, J. T.: Intrauterine transfusion: a cooperative study, Am. J. Obstet. Gynecol. **104**: 397, 1969.

Savage, W. E., Hajj, S. N., and Kass, E. H.: Demographic and prognostic characteristics of bacteriuria in pregnancy, Medicine **46**:385, 1967.

Smith, S. G., and Scragg, W. H., Jr.: Gestational diabetes, Obstet. Gynecol. **31**:228, 1968.

Spellacy, W. N., Buhi, W. C., Cohn, J. E., and Birk, S. A.: Usefulness of rapid blood glucose measurements in obstetrics: Dextrostix/reflectance meter system, Obstet. Gynecol. **41**: 299, 1973.

Taft, P.: Endocrine disease in pregnancy, Med. Hist. **1**:868, 1972.

Ursell, W., Brudenall, M., and Chard, T.: Placental lactogen levels in diabetic pregnancy, Br. Med. J. **2**:80, 1973.

Van den Bussche, G.: Bacteriuria in pregnancy, with special reference to pathogenesis and follow-up after delivery, S. Afr. J. Obstet. Gynecol. **6**:34, 1968.

Warrner, R. A., and Cornblath, M.: Infants of gestational diabetic mothers, Am. J. Dis. Child. **117**:678, 1969.

Werner, S. C.: Hyperthyroidism in the pregnant woman and the neonate, J. Clin. Endocrinol. Metab. **27**:1637, 1967.

Wong, S. W., Margolis, A. J., Westberg, J. A., and Johnson, P.: Intrauterine transfusion: fetal outcome and complications, Pediatrics **45**:576, 1970.

19

Respiratory emergencies

The dramatic adjustments occurring with the onset of ventilation at birth have been discussed (Chapter 6). It is not surprising that the main obstacle to survival is an unsatisfactory adaptation to the respiratory system. Five to ten percent of newborn infants have some respiratory difficulty, the incidence being inversely related to maturity of the infant. Pulmonary disorders are the main cause of neonatal deaths.

A general presentation of symptoms and management applying to many respiratory disorders will precede a specific discussion of main causes of ventilatory emergencies.

PRINCIPLES OF CARE FOR INFANTS WITH RESPIRATORY DISTRESS
Symptoms commonly observed
Tachypnea

A respiratory rate of over 60/min indicates tachypnea. Respiratory rates should be evaluated only when the infant is sleeping or resting. It is the most common sign of abnormal ventilation found in many respiratory disorders, as well as heart failure and early shock.

Intercostal retractions

Retractions of subcostal and intercostal tissues as well as the sternum demonstrate the infant's difficulty in stabilizing his thorax to improve lung inflation. This instability of the thoracic wall leads to increased excursion of the diaphragm, evident as abdominal protrusion during inspiration, the "seesaw" pattern of respiration. Retractions indicate inadequate filling of the lung with air, as in hyaline membrane disease (HMD), but also may result from obstructions of the upper airways.

Grunting

Typically seen in HMD, a "grunting" type of breathing is accomplished by the infant in an attempt to maintain maximum alveolar expansion and improve gas exchange by exhaling against a closed glottis. As the infant grunts, he emits a groaning sound at the onset of expiration.

Flaring of the nares

Flaring of the nares is an inspiratory widening of the nostrils. It is observed frequently in infants with significant respiratory distress.

Cyanosis

Cyanosis should be evaluated under bright daylight while the infant is quiet, or under fluorescent light. Central cyanosis is defined as a bluish discoloration of the mucous membranes and tongue, as well as the skin, and signifies arterial unsaturation. Cyanosis of pulmonary origin such as hypoventilation, diffusion difficulties, and ventilation/perfusion unevenness will be relieved by increasing the inspiratory oxygen concentration (F_{IO_2}). Failure of cyanosis to disappear while the infant is breathing pure oxygen indicates significant right-to-left shunts. Although more common in congenital heart disease, such shunting may accompany severe HMD, as well as persistence of the fetal circulation (primary pulmonary hypertension).

Blood gas changes

Hypoxemia (P_{aO_2} under 45 mm Hg) and respiratory acidosis (P_{CO_2} over 45 mm Hg) are frequently present. With increasing arterial oxygen unsaturation, metabolic acidosis will develop due to accumulation of lactic acid.

Respiratory depression or apnea

Respiratory depression manifested by shallow and irregular respiration interposed with prolonged apneic episodes and cyanosis is the most serious sign of impending catastrophe in the newborn. Its etiology may be pulmonary or nonpulmonary.

General management of respiratory distress

1. Initial care
   a. Place infant under radiant heat or in an isolette and maintain skin temperature between 97° and 98° F (36° and 36.5° C).
   b. Attach cardiorespiratory monitor.
   c. Administer sufficient oxygen with a hood to relieve cyanosis until blood gas results are obtained; then maintain P_{aO_2} between 45 and 70 mm Hg (or 35 and 45 when warmed heel capillary blood is used). Humidify O_2 if 40% or more is given. Ensure a patent airway, suction oropharynx as necessary, and ventilate with bag and mask if infant looks very critical or has apnea (consider intubation as discussed below).
   d. Insert an umbilical artery catheter (Chapter 7) if infant appears to be critically ill and/or requires significant oxygen (over 40%).
   e. Obtain x-ray films of chest and abdomen to ascertain diagnosis as well as verify correct catheter position.
   f. Monitor blood pressure with the Doppler method or via transducer from the arterial catheter. If the infant appears to be in shock, manage appropriately (Chapter 20).
   g. Administer parenteral fluids by peripheral vein or umbilical catheter.
   h. Obtain the following data on admission
      1. Weight, length, head circumference
      2. Hematocrit, hemoglobin
      3. Obtain blood type and cross matching for fresh whole blood
      4. Serum sodium, potassium, chloride, calcium, and bilirubin if infant appears jaundiced
      5. Blood gases, preferably from arterial blood
   i. Correct anemia if hematocrit is less than 45%; transfuse with fresh whole blood (10 ml/kg will raise hematocrit about 5%).
   j. Correct acidosis when necessary.
   k. Handle infant gently and maintain him in a position of comfort for easy breathing (shoulders may be raised slightly).
2. Continued care
   a. Monitor heart rate or heart and respiratory rates continuously until the infant's condition has sufficiently stabilized and apneic episodes no longer occur.
   b. Remove central catheters
      1. Arterial catheter—as soon as infant can be maintained in under 40% O_2 and his condition has sufficiently stabilized so that frequent arterial sampling for blood gases is no longer needed
      2. Central venous catheter—whenever pressure monitoring can be discontinued or this avenue is no longer needed for emergency support

Never leave a catheter in place solely for the purpose of administering fluids.

c. Observe serially the infant's hematocrit and avoid anemia. In continuing respiratory distress, maintain hematocrit above 40%.

d. Use a flow sheet for all blood gas results; F_{IO_2}, CPAP, or ventilator settings; laboratory data; etc; keep at the infant's bedside.

e. Monitor blood gases frequently, correct any acidosis promptly, and maintain normoxemia.

f. Carefully monitor intake and output, weigh infant daily, monitor serum electrolytes daily, and watch infant's nutritional state. Provide sufficient calories to prevent catabolism. During the acute phase of disease it is best not to feed the infant orally. Parenteral alimentation should be considered for prolonged care when gastrointestinal feeding is risky. Gastrointestinal feeding may be started as soon as condition stabilizes and the infant demonstrates good bowel motility. Nipple feeding or gastric or jejunal gavage will have to be considered, depending on the circumstances.

g. Be aware of the possibility of hyperbilirubinemia.

Oxygen therapy

Increased inspiratory oxygen concentrations are frequently needed in the management of respiratory disorders, after significant asphyxiation, during shock, etc. Although this therapy may be lifesaving to the infant, it is potentially dangerous and therefore requires skill in its administration.

Clinical assessment of hypoxia in a neonate is very inaccurate. Cyanosis may not necessarily mean hypoxemia as is the case in polycythemia. Conversely, an infant who appears to be noncyanotic may be hypoxic.

1. Administration of oxygen
   Although closed incubators allow increased oxygen concentrations to be offered, opening of portholes or side doors leads to a rapid drop of F_{IO_2}, subjecting infants with respiratory distress syndrome to an increased right-to-left shunt and possible profound hypoxia.
   a. Place the infant's head under a plastic hood and let the desired air/oxygen mixture flow through it at approximately 5 L/min (to prevent CO_2 accumulation). This method allows handling of the infant without disturbing inspired oxygen concentration. Care should be taken to maintain the temperature within the hood and the incubator at similar thermoneutral levels.
   b. Humidify oxygen if it is administered in concentrations in excess of 40%.
   c. Monitor oxygen concentration at least hourly for all infants who are not maintained in room air environment.

2. Sampling for blood gases
   Blood gas and pH determinations are usually obtained from an arterialized "heel stick" after thorough warming of a foot, from the aorta through an umbilical artery catheter, or from puncture of a radial or temporal artery.
   a. Heel-stick samples
      1. Advantages
         a. Samples can be obtained repeatedly for prolonged periods.
         b. Safety from complications associated with arterial catheters.
      2. Disadvantages
         a. P_{CO_2} up to 10 mm Hg higher in sick infants.
         b. P_{O_2} values above 45 mm Hg are significantly lower than arterial values. In fact, levels above 60 mm Hg may reflect dangerously high arterial levels—a factor to be considered in avoiding retrolental fibroplasia.

b. Aortic samples
 1. Advantages
    a. Accurate arterial values are obtained.
    b. Sampling can be done frequently without disturbing the infant.
 2. Disadvantages
    a. Complications from an aortic catheter are common enough to avoid this approach except in infants with moderate to severe respiratory distress.
    b. Right-to-left shunting through the ductus arteriosus leads to lower oxygen tension in postductal vessels. Occasionally, sampling from preductal sources (right temporal or radial artery) will offer a check on P_{aO_2} values in the retinal vessels.
c. Peripheral arterial samples
 1. Advantages
    a. Ability to obtain accurate preductal arterial values.
    b. Avoidance of central catheter.
 2. Disadvantage: repeated frequent sampling is difficult and often impossible.
d. Frequency of sampling
 1. When using oxygen concentrations of 35% or more, blood gas samples should be obtained at least every 4 to 6 hours.
 2. More frequent determinations are necessary during the acute stage of hyaline membrane disease.
 3. Infants requiring slightly increased oxygen concentrations for prolonged periods (extreme prematurity, Wilson-Mikity syndrome) require determination of their P_{aO_2} every 24 to 48 hours.
3. Complications of oxygen therapy
 a. Retrolental fibroplasia
    First reported in 1942, this disease will cause permanent partial or total blindness. Its occurrence is related to
    1. Immaturity of the infant's retina
    2. Oxygen tension in the arterial blood
    3. Duration of oxygen therapy
    The very immature infant with frequent apneic episodes is the most susceptible to this disease when given excessive oxygen concentration. An unphysiologically high oxygen tension for several hours may cause irreversible vasoconstriction of the retinal arteries, which may eventually lead to proliferation of new vessels through the retina and vitreous. Hemorrhage and retinal detachment follow.
    The precise level of oxygen tension and the time required to cause this disease vary with the maturity of the infant. Close monitoring of P_{aO_2} in all premature infants receiving supplemental oxygen, therefore, is of utmost importance. Arterial oxygen tensions should range between 45 and 70 mm Hg, and arterialized heel-stick tensions are more safely kept between 35 and 45 mm Hg.
    Repeated resuscitation of small premature infants with bag and mask for prolonged apnea should be done with the same concentration of oxygen they receive between episodes.
 b. Bronchopulmonary dysplasia (BPD)
    This disease was described by Northway and colleagues in infants with severe hyaline membrane disease treated with positive-pressure ventilators and high inspiratory oxygen concentrations. The disease resembles Mikity-Wilson syndrome in many ways. Symptoms include the following:
    1. Difficulty in weaning an infant with HMD from a positive-pressure respirator (frequently the first indication)
    2. X-ray changes (Fig. 19-1)
       a. The first findings of typical HMD may change to opacification of lung fields with oblitera-

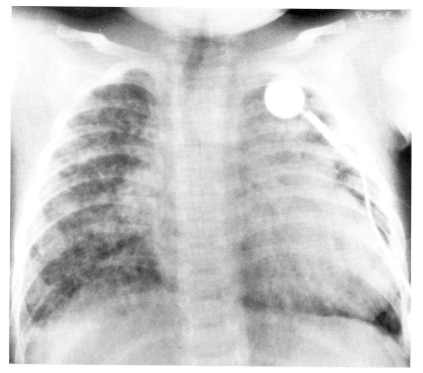

Fig. 19-1. Bronchopulmonary dysplasia after exposure to high concentrations of oxygen in conjunction with positive-pressure ventilation.

tion of heart border during the first week of life.

b. Between 10 and 20 days of age increasing coarse cystic changes are visible bilaterally.

c. These findings are persistent for weeks, gradually changing to emphysematous areas bilaterally with depression of diaphragms.

3. Increased or persistent tachypnea and labored respirations

4. Oxygen dependency for weeks

This disease has a mortality of 30% to 50%. Development of cor pulmonale and heart failure can complicate recovery. An important factor in the development of this disease seems to be the administration of oxygen in high concentrations (over 60%). Therefore, the minimal $F_{I_{O_2}}$ compatible with satisfactory oxygen tensions is recom-

mended. The high frequency of BPD in infants treated with positive-pressure respirators, in contrast to its virtual absence when negative-pressure respirators are used, may point to a more complicated etiology. Treatment is supportive only.

Treatment of acidosis

Treatment of acidosis is of importance to the infant's prognosis. When pH is normalized, pulmonary vascular resistance is lowered, leading to increased blood flow through the lung, improvement in myocardial contractility, and maintenance of cell metabolism.

1. Respiratory acidosis (P_{CO_2} over 45 mm Hg; normal, 35 to 40 mm Hg)

a. Caused by impaired elimination of CO_2 due to underventilation in relation to perfusion or ventilation of underperfused areas of the lung.

b. Treatment: If P_{CO_2} rises above 50 mm Hg, intermittent ventilation (5 to 10 minutes every 30 minutes) with bag and mask may be helpful. Rises of 10 mm Hg or more per hour, or P_{CO_2} over 65 mm Hg usually indicates the need for continuous assisted ventilation.

2. Metabolic acidosis
   a. Caused most often by hypoxemia and accumulation of lactic acid.
   b. A base deficit of more than 5 (see nomogram, Appendix H) should be corrected by the administration of alkali. Two types of alkali are used.
      1. Sodium bicarbonate ($NaHCO_3$), 1 ml = 1 mEq
         a. Advantage: readily available.
         b. Disadvantage: danger of hyperosmolality, hypernatremia, and elevation of P_{CO_2} in the absence of adequate ventilation.
      2. Tromethamine (THAM)
         a. Advantage: agent of choice in hypernatremic states.
         b. Disadvantage: may cause respiratory depression and/or hypoglycemia, also very hyperosmolar.
      We prefer $NaHCO_3$ for the correction of acidosis except when hypernatremia is present.
3. Dose of $NaHCO_3$ to be given
   a. Base deficit (mEq/L) × infant weight (kg) × 0.3 = mEq of $NaHCO_3$ to be given.
   b. In cases of severe asphyxiation, do not wait for a blood gas result, but give parenterally 2 to 4 mEq of $NaHCO_3$/kg of infant's weight.
4. Administration of $NaHCO_3$*
   a. Dilute with equal amounts of sterile water to lower osmolality.
   b. Infuse parenterally; to prevent tissue

damage, never infuse faster than 1 mEq/min. Avoid administration through improperly placed catheter.

RESPIRATORY FAILURE

Treatment of failing respirations in an infant with continuous transpulmonary distending pressure and/or assisted intermittent ventilation has become widely used in neonatal intensive care centers. Success of these techniques depends on the availability of a skilled neonatal team (physicians and nurses) and laboratory support throughout a 24-hour day.

1. Criteria for identifying respiratory failure
   a. Clinical criteria
      1. Severe apnea with bradycardia (under 100 beats/min) unresponsive to stimulation or intermittent ventilation with mask and bag
      2. Cyanosis in 60% oxygen or more
      3. Severe shock
   b. Blood gas criteria
      1. Significant acidosis (pH under 7.2) in spite of therapeutic measures as outlined above
      2. Hypoxemia (P_{aO_2} under 45 mm Hg) while infant is breathing high concentrations of oxygen (over 60%)
      3. Hypercarbia—P_{CO_2} rising more than 10 mm/hr or more than 65 mm Hg
2. Common causes of respiratory failure
   a. Pulmonary
      1. Hyaline membrane disease (HMD)
      2. Pneumothorax
      3. Bronchopulmonary dysplasia
      4. Wilson-Mikity syndrome
      5. Diaphragmatic hernia
   b. Nonpulmonary
      1. Severe septic shock
      2. CNS hemorrhage
      3. Hypothermia
      4. Analgesic or anesthetic drugs given to mother during labor and delivery

---

*Dose of $NaHCO_3$ should not exceed 8 mEq/kg/24 hr because of the relationship of hypernatremia and intracranial hemorrhage in neonates.

RESPIRATORY SUPPORT

1. *Continuous transpulmonary distending pressure*

   Alveolar collapse is inhibited or diminished by keeping a constant distending pressure at the end of each expiratory phase. The alveolar arterial oxygen difference diminishes. This effect leads to a higher P_{aO_2}, allowing reduction of inspired oxygen concentration to levels less toxic to the lung (50%).

   This concept was used first by Gregory and associates, who applied a continuous positive airway pressure (CPAP) in spontaneously breathing infants with HMD. Since then this method has become widely accepted.

   a. Methods used
      1. Continuous negative pressure (CNP)

         Alveolar collapse is inhibited by applying a constant negative pressure around the infant's body up to the neck by means of a small negative-pressure chamber. This method has proved successful. Access to the infant may be limited; however, intubation is not needed. Venous return to the heart is not diminished. Pressures of –5 to –8 cm H_2O are sufficient with milder disease; in more severe cases, pressures of –10 to –15 cm H_2O may be required.
      2. Continuous positive airway pressure (CPAP)

         Alveolar collapse is inhibited by applying a constant positive pressure to the infant's airway.

   b. Modes of CPAP
      1. Head chamber
         a. Advantage: intubation not needed.
         b. Disadvantages: suctioning infant's airway is difficult; neck seals frequently are leaking; gastric distention must be avoided by placement of orogastric tube.
      2. Mask CPAP
         a. Advantages: no need to intubate; easy to apply.
         b. Disadvantages: infants sometimes "fight" the mask; very small premature infants may tolerate it poorly; gastric distention has to be prevented by placement of orogastric tube; leaks occur at pressures of 8 to 10 cm H_2O.
      3. Nasal prongs (Argyle)
         a. Advantages: easy to apply; no need to intubate.
         b. Disadvantages: stabilization difficult at times; pressure swings significant and not always tolerated by infants needing higher pressures consistently. Gastric distention must be avoided by placement of orogastric tube.
      4. CPAP by intubation
         a. Advantage: pressure can be applied more consistently without variance or leakage problems.
         b. Disadvantage: intubation requires the skill and constant presence of an experienced team to avoid complications from this method (extubation, tube obstruction, faulty tube placement, etc.).

   In summary, any method leaves something to be desired, and the choice must be made according to personal belief and circumstances at the place where this therapy is used. Continuous transpulmonary distending pressure without intubation has the advantage of greater safety to the patient and should be the preferred mode whenever possible.

   c. We apply CPAP to any infant who
      1. Has HMD and, while breathing spontaneously, requires more than 60% O_2 to maintain P_{aO_2} above 45 mm Hg.

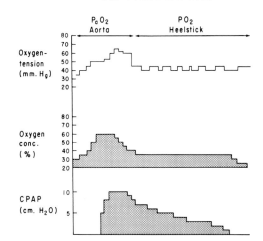

RDS treated with CPAP

Fig. 19-2. Increasing amounts of ambient oxygen were required to raise arterial oxygen tension to acceptable values (50 mm Hg). CPAP was introduced to avoid administration of high concentrations of oxygen to this preterm infant, thereby maintaining the oxygen tension at a lower F_{IO_2}. As the infant recovered, first the oxygen concentration and then the CPAP were reduced gradually, maintaining oxygen tension in an acceptable range.

2. Has HMD and demonstrates very deep retractions while in 45% O_2 or more.

3. Is very immature and has frequent apnea that cannot be treated adequately by stimulation or occasional bagging. Stabilization of alveoli may help in this case.

d. Method (Fig. 19-2)

1. Start with the same O_2 concentration used before CPAP was initiated.

2. Air-oxygen mixture should be warmed and humidified if more than 40% oxygen is given or the infant is intubated.

3. Gas flow from the nebulizer through the CPAP equipment should be between 4 and 6 L/min.

4. Set pop-off valve at 20 to 30 cm H_2O for safety.

5. Apply initial pressure of about 5 cm H_2O (1 mm Hg = 1.3 cm H_2O)

6. Increase pressures by 2 to 3 cm H_2O until P_{aO_2} is at least 45 to 50 mm Hg (maximal pressure 10 to 15 cm H_2O).

7. Monitor blood pressure frequently. Significant transmission of transpulmonary pressure may impede venous return and cause hypotension. It usually can be corrected with prompt administration of volume expander (see the discussion on shock, Chapter 20). If this measure does not improve the blood pressure, CPAP may have to be limited to lower pressures.

8. Every 30 minutes inflate infant's lungs several times to prevent CO_2 accumulation and to sigh the infant's lungs.

9. As infant improves, P_{aO_2} may rise significantly. Maintain normal oxygen tensions by decreasing O_2 concentration gradually in 5% to 10% increments until less than 40% is administered (blood gases may be needed as often as every 30 minutes).

10. At this point the CPAP can be lowered gradually by increments of 1 to 2 cm.

11. When pressure of 2 cm or less is reached, place infant's head under plastic hood, giving the same amount or 10% more oxygen than before; observe carefully, and monitor blood gases.

e. Complications
   1. Hypotension
   2. Pneumothorax
      As long as pop-off valves are utilized, this possibility should be kept to a minimum. (For management of pneumothorax, see p. 227.)

f. Conditions in which positive-pressure insufflation is hazardous

1. Diaphragmatic hernia with hypoplastic lung
2. Meconium aspiration before thorough tracheal aspiration
3. Tracheoesophageal fistula, with lower esophageal segment connecting to trachea
4. Intestinal obstruction

2. *Assisted ventilation*

Except as a short-term emergency measure, the prolonged use of ventilators for neonates should be reserved for intensive care centers, where continuous team care can be given. Indications for assisted ventilation were outlined previously, but they do vary somewhat among institutions.

a. Type of ventilator

The purpose of this chapter will not be to describe assisted ventilation in detail, since this technique can be taught better under actual circumstances in an intensive care setting. Many types are available, and preference depends on the opinion of the user.

1. Negative-pressure ventilators (e.g., Air-Shields)
   a. Advantages: no intubation necessary; bronchopulmonary dysplasia rarely seen as complication.
   b. Disadvantages: difficulty in caring for the infant and in ventilating small premature infants; irritation of skin by neck seal; cooling of infant.
2. Positive-pressure ventilators
   a. Volume-controlled ventilators
   b. Flow- or pressure-controlled ventilators
      (1) Advantages: can be used with or without the use of endotracheal tubes; easy accessibility to the patient; small infants can be ventilated more efficiently.
      (2) Disadvantage: higher incidence of bronchopulmonary dysplasia.
3. Positive-pressure ventilation using bag and mask
   a. Advantage: patient is not intubated.
   b. Disadvantage: large number of highly trained nurses needed for this mode of ventilation when used over prolonged periods.

Our experience is limited to the use of the positive-pressure ventilators with the Bourns and Baby-Bird ventilators. We use oroendotracheal tubes (Portex Z-79 or Shiley, size 2.5 to 4 mm in diameter). A tight fit should be avoided; an infant weighing less than 1,500 gm will accept a tube size of 3 mm (2.5 mm in the very small infant).

b. Intubation
1. Place infant in supine position, neck straight and extended.
2. Ventilate infant with bag and mask for 1 minute, using 100% oxygen.
3. Insert endotracheal tube (Chapter 6). If unsuccessful after 30 seconds, or if infant has bradycardia, ventilate again for 1 or 2 minutes and repeat procedure.
4. Place endotracheal tube 1 to 1.5 cm below the vocal cords.
5. Auscultate over both sides of thorax while ventilating the infant through endotracheal tube, assuring equal ventilation of both lungs.
   a. If no breath sounds are audible, endotracheal tube is not in trachea.
   b. If no breath sounds can be heard over the left chest, endotracheal tube may be in right primary bronchus; retract tube until breath sounds are audible equally on either side.

6. Secure tube with following procedure:
   a. Place tincture of benzoin on upper lip.
   b. Fasten butterfly-shaped piece of Elastoplast over benzoin on upper lip.
   c. With No. 4-0 silk, place sutures through either side of tube and Elastoplast, and tie in place.
   d. Secure tube, in addition, by placing narrow strips of tape around the tube and across cheek bilaterally.
7. Obtain chest x-ray films to assure proper position of tube (tip approximately 1.5 cm above carina, about T_2).

c. Placing on ventilator
1. Set on control mode initially.
2. Use a respiratory rate of approximately 50/min and sufficient pressure or volume to see adequate chest expansion.
3. Obtain blood gases frequently (e.g., every 15 to 30 minutes) in early phase of care to determine appropriate F_{IO_2} respiratory rate rate and pressures required. Arterial oxygen tension should be maintained between 45 and 70 mm Hg, and P_{CO_2} between 35 and 45 mm Hg; acidosis should be corrected promptly.
4. Warm and humidify air-oxygen mixture.
5. Adjust respirator settings so that infant does not breathe out of phase with the ventilator.
6. If inspiratory oxygen concentration of more than 40% is required, use positive end expiratory pressure (PEEP) to allow the lowest possible F_{IO_2}.

d. Weaning from respirator
1. As infant improves, preparation for weaning may be accomplished by the following measures:

   a. Gradually reduce oxygen concentration by 5% to 10% increments until less than 40% is tolerated.
   b. If PEEP is used, reduce pressure by 1 to 2 cm increments to a pressure of 2 cm.
2. Actual weaning may proceed (depending on type of ventilator used, maturity of infant, etc.), by one of the following measures:
   a. Place infant gradually on CPAP.
   b. Adjust respirator to an "assist" mode on which the infant triggers the respirator. Once this is tolerated, disconnect the respirator and place the infant under a plastic hood with same F_{IO_2} used before.
   c. Gradually reduce respiratory rate to the lowest rate (Baby-Bird) and then allow infant to breathe spontaneously.

e. Extubation
1. Should be undertaken only when
   a. Infant tolerates spontaneous breathing in hood for at least 12 hours, and blood gases are normal.
   b. Gastric contents are aspirated.
   c. Team supervision is assured after extubation.
2. Procedure of extubation
   a. Suction airways and ventilate infant for several minutes.
   b. Cut sutures; loosen tape.
   c. Withdraw tube while holding maximum inflation of chest, using the anesthesia bag.
   d. Place infant in an oxygen environment 10% higher than that used before extubation.
   e. Assure proper humidification of inspired air.
   f. Continue chest physiotherapy and intermittent suctioning of the nasopharynx.

f. Airway care during intubation (to be done every 1 to 2 hours)
  1. All suctioning must be done under sterile precautions (sterile gloves, catheters, solutions).
  2. Ventilate infant for 1 to 2 minutes.
  3. Give physiotherapy to all parts of infant's chest, starting with percussion, followed by vibration.
  4. Instill 0.25 to 0.5 ml of sterile normal saline solution into infant's trachea.
  5. Insert catheter into endotracheal tube as deep as possible.
  6. Begin suction while drawing back the catheter from endotracheal tube, taking no more than 5 to 10 seconds.
  7. Ventilate infant for 1 to 2 minutes.
  8. Repeat suctioning, turning head from one side to the other on subsequent suctions.
  9. Change infant's position at intervals (every 1 to 2 hours) to assure adequate ventilation of all parts of the lung.
g. Complications of intubation
  1. During intubation
    a. Placement in esophagus is indicated by lack of chest movement and increasing abdominal distention.
    b. Placement below carina is indicated by unequal breath sounds and hypoxia.
    c. Traumatic placement may result in injury to hypopharynx, vocal cords, and trachea.
    d. A disproportionately small tube for the size of the trachea will lead to insufficient respiratory exchange.
    e. Accidental extubation is due to improper fixation of tube.
    f. Tube obstruction is caused by insufficient humidification or warming of inspired gas as well as by insufficient care in tracheal suctioning.
  2. After intubation
    a. Edema of laryngeal area may cause increasing respiratory distress.
    b. Subglottic stenosis or stricture may occur.

CAUSES OF RESPIRATORY DISTRESS IN THE NEONATE
Hyaline membrane disease, or respiratory distress syndrome (RDS)

The onset of respiratory distress in the first few hours of life, followed by the familiar expiratory grunt first noted after 3 to 6 hours of age, is generally indicative of hyaline membrane disease. The name refers to the pink-staining fibrinoid deposits that line the alveolar ducts, which are observed at autopsy examination. The precise mechanism of formation is obscure, but the disease, with its interference with alveolar ventilation, is responsible for as many as 20,000 infant deaths each year in the United States. From 20% to 30% of those with the established disease die. Affected males have nearly double the mortality of female infants.

1. Associated factors
  a. Insufficient surfactant production associated with prematurity
  b. Asphyxiation during labor and delivery, further diminishing surfactant
  c. Presence of acidosis, hypoxemia, hypovolemia, and hypothermia
2. Pathophysiology
  Diminished surfactant production in lung parenchyma causing progressive alveolar collapse, as well as stressful circumstances such as hypoxemia, acidosis, and shock, leads to vasoconstriction of the pulmonary arteries and pulmonary hypoperfusion. The following events apparently occur:
  a. Reduction in lung compliance (lung stiffness) and thus an increase in the work of breathing—these changes reduce alveolar ventilation and further decrease gaseous exchange.

b. Right-to-left shunts—these may occur outside the lungs at ductus arteriosus or foramen ovale sites; additionally, intrapulmonary shunts have been shown to bypass the alveoli.

c. Effusion of plasma through the capillary walls, with fibrin deposits (hyaline membranes) in the alveoli and alveolar ducts—this leads to airway obstruction and further compounds the problem.

Many other factors have been implicated, including elevated circulating catecholamines, bradykinin deficiency, and disseminated intravascular clotting.

3. Gross and microscopic pathology

  a. Gross changes observed in *infants dying of this disease*

    1. Resorption atelectasis with distended terminal bronchioles

    2. Lung sections resembling liver in color and consistency

  b. Microscopic findings

    1. Pink-staining fibrinoid deposits adjacent to the aerated portions of the terminal bronchioles and alveolar ducts (hyaline membranes)

    2. Pulmonary vascular engorgement, often with frank hemorrhage

4. Clinical features

  a. Moderately severe cases

    1. Gradual increase in respiratory rate (over 60/min)

    2. Intercostal retraction

    3. Expiratory moan or grunt, sternal and costal retraction, flaring of alae nasi

    4. Fine rales heard at end of inspiration, with reduced air interchange

    5. Foam appearing in the mouth and on the lips (pulmonary edema)

    6. Cyanosis without oxygen addition

    7. Baby inactive, assuming a frog-like position

  b. Severe cases

    1. Hypotonia, hypotension, peripheral edema

    2. Cyanosis, requiring higher concentrations of oxygen to clear

    3. Apneic periods

Survival is indicated by a gradual improvement in respiratory symptoms and blood gas values. Complications include sepsis, pulmonary and cerebral hemorrhage, kernicterus, hypoglycemia, and pneumothorax.

5. Laboratory observations

Changes in blood gas and pH determinations are not specific for hyaline membrane disease and are frequently abnormal, but they serve as an important guide to the seriousness and progress of the disease.

  a. Falling pH (under 7.25)

  b. Rising P_{CO_2} (over 55 mm Hg)

  c. Falling P_{aO_2} (under 45 mm Hg)

6. Chest x-ray examination (Fig. 19-3)

  a. A reticulogranular pattern of the lung can be expected, or opacification of both lung fields in severe cases.

  b. The radiolucent bronchial airway (air bronchogram) extends beyond the heart border because of the air-filled bronchial tree outlined by opacified perihilar areas.

7. Management

  a. Offer initial and continued care (p. 213).

  b. Maintain arterial oxygen tension between 45 and 70 mm Hg (35 to 45 mm Hg arterialized capillary blood).

  c. Correct acidosis.

  d. Use CPAP if infant is hypoxic in 60% oxygen or more.

  e. Place on ventilator if CPAP trial is not successful, the infant becomes apneic, or P_{CO_2} rises.

  f. Expect recovery to take anywhere from one to several weeks, depending on severity of disease.

  g. Delay oral feeding. Consider parenteral alimentation after first few days of glucose infusions. We prefer the delay of gastric feedings until

    1. Respiratory rate is less than 60/min.

    2. Infant does not require assisted ventilation and has been extubated

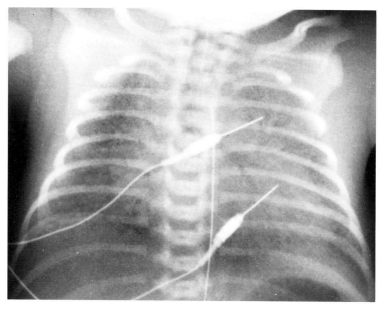

Fig. 19-3. Reticulogranular pattern of lung fields in hyaline membrane disease (idiopathic respiratory distress syndrome).

for 24 hours (exceptions are long-term respirator cases).

3. Infant shows functioning gastrointestinal tract (no distention, normal bowel sounds, etc.).

8. Sequelae

Survival in severe cases is compatible with later normality, but there is a possibility of later neurologic complication and pulmonary fibrosis, even with diligent care.

9. Prevention

   a. Delay delivery when possible until 39 weeks have elapsed, or until the L/S ratio or the rapid surfactant test is mature—unless the risks to the infant of prematurity are less hazardous than the complications of pregnancy.

   b. Give optimum care at delivery with prompt resuscitation, amelioration of metabolic acidosis, and avoidance of hypovolemia and chilling.

Apnea of prematurity

Apnea is primarily an extension of periodic breathing in the immature infant with his decreased sensitivity to carbon dioxide and oxygen. When apnea persists beyond 10 seconds, bradycardia is likely and if respirations do not resume in another 20 seconds, cyanosis will develop, accompanied by asphyxia. (See also the discussion on monitoring for apnea, Chapter 7.)

Approximately 30% of infants less than 32 weeks (1,750 gm) at birth have apneic periods, and nearly all infants of less than 30 weeks' gestation. Other causative factors include the following:

1. Temperature variations—above and below thermoneutral level (skin temperature, 97° F or 36° C)
2. Airway obstruction by mucus, etc.
3. Vasovagal response to feedings
4. Hypoglycemia, hypocalcemia
5. Sepsis or meningitis
6. Intracranial hemorrhage or cerebral defect
7. Hyaline membrane disease

Management

1. Monitor respiration and heart rate. Heart rate monitoring alone may be

sufficient, since bradycardia follows apnea in most cases. Some infants, however, may have a fixed heart rate during apnea, so that monitoring of respiration also becomes necessary.

2. Prevent dehydration and temperature irregularities that might increase the frequency of apnea.

3. Treat apnea in its early stages by gentle stimulation.

4. Suction nasopharynx if cyanosis persists, and resuscitate infant with bag and mask if there is no response to stimulation, using the same air-oxygen mixture administered to the infant before resuscitation. Avoid hyperoxemia by careful monitoring of infant's P_{aO_2}.

5. Consider intubation or the use of nasal prongs with a continuous transpulmonary distending pressure (1 to 4 cm H_2O), which acts as a "lung stabilizer" for infants with frequent apnea. This procedure is particularly useful when the infant does not tolerate repeated bag and mask ventilation.

Meconium aspiration syndrome

Fetal aspiration, in which meconium-contaminated amniotic fluid and other particulate matter enter the lungs, is probably the result of hypoxia in utero, accompanied by increased fetal respiratory activity. These events may occur either gradually, as in placental insufficiency with chronic fetal distress, or abruptly from any sudden interruption of maternal-fetal oxygen transport, as occurs with cord prolapse or placental separation.

1. Pathophysiology: foreign materials present in the lungs will do the following:
   a. Prevent complete expansion of the lungs after delivery
   b. Hinder resuscitation
   c. Impair air exchange, with an increased chance of respiratory and metabolic acidosis

2. Pathologic anatomy: examination of the lungs on microscopic section may show the following:
   a. A deposit of packed squamous or epithelial cells, vernix, and lanugo in the alveoli
   b. Aspirated meconium in the bronchial tree, with chemical pneumonitis

3. Clinical and x-ray findings
   a. Signs of respiratory distress from aspiration may include
      1. An increase in inspiratory effort and tachypnea
      2. Medium to gross rales resulting from aspirated debris in the bronchi
   b. X-ray films of the lung fields usually reveal
      1. Hilar infiltration, with fan-shaped atelectatic areas (Fig. 19-4)
      2. Lobular emphysema from air trapping, with the possibility of pneumothorax
      3. An isolated lobe of atelectasis (occasionally)

4. Complications
   a. Development of pneumothorax from check-valve obstruction in the airway
   b. Pneumonia

5. Prevention and treatment
   a. Deliver the infant promptly when signs of fetal asphyxia occur.
   b. Offer careful resuscitation, including
      1. Intubation and aspiration if obstructive material is present (Tenacious meconium may have to be removed by tracheal lavage with normal saline solution, followed by suctioning.)
      2. Avoidance of positive pressure until the airway is cleared
      3. Aspiration of the stomach of a meconium-stained infant
   c. Offer full intensive care: monitor blood gases, give oxygen if needed, correct acidosis, humidify air/oxygen mixture.
   d. Administer antibiotics if infant is in continued respiratory distress.

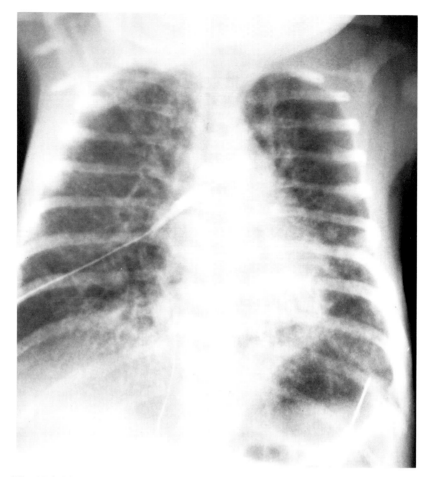

Fig. 19-4. Meconium aspiration syndrome associated with severe respiratory distress.

Pneumothorax and pneumomediastinum

Trapped air outside the lung parenchyma is not infrequently discovered on x-ray examination in the newborn period. Such infants may or may not have symptoms of respiratory distress. Over half the reported cases are found in low birth weight infants. The majority of cases spontaneously resolve without specific treatment. The discovery of emphysema (a frequent prelude to pneumothorax) or the presence of minimal pneumothorax or pneumomediastinum requires close observation. The prompt awareness of any increase in the accumulation of air outside the lung, par-ticularly under pressure (tension pneumothorax), can be lifesaving.

1. Etiology and pathogenesis
   a. Occasionally due to excessive positive pressure used in resuscitation
   b. A common complication of positive-pressure ventilation
   c. Often associated with partial bronchial obstruction (ball-valve effect)
2. Steps in development
   a. Overdistention of distal air sacs (emphysema)
   b. Rupture of these sacs and escape of air into the interstitial spaces, with extension down the vascular sheath

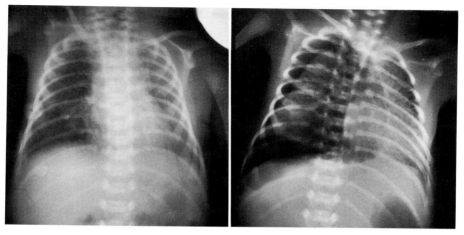

Fig. 19-5. Emphysema of the right lung (left radiograph), which has developed into a serious tension pneumothorax in the right film.

into the mediastinum (pneumomediastinum)

c. Rupture of air into the pleural spaces

3. Clinical signs of pneumothorax, particularly under tension
   a. Increasing tachypnea
   b. Rapid development of cyanosis
   c. Increased anteroposterior diameter of the chest
   d. Shift of apical cardiac impulse
   e. Hyperresonance to chest percussion
   f. Abdominal distention from depressed diaphragm
   g. Falling blood pressure

4. Diagnosis made from x-ray examination of chest (Fig. 19-5)
   a. Pneumothorax is indicated by
      1. Areas of free air outlining the partially collapsed lung
      2. No evidence of bronchial markings beyond the border of the collapsed lung
      3. Depression of the diaphragm on the affected side
   b. Pneumomediastinum is indicated by
      1. Free air surrounding cardiac silhouette
      2. "Sail sign" of floating thymus lifted off heart by air

5. Management
   Diagnosis of a pneumothorax or pneumomediastinum demands continuous observation of the infant by an experienced team. Although many cases with pneumothorax will resolve with conservative treatment, a substantial percentage become life-threatening when there is tension and thus require immediate aspiration of air or chest tube.
   a. Support infant with oxygen if needed.
   b. Monitor and observe infant carefully for increased respiratory distress.
   c. In case of acute emergency (severe distress, suspected tension pneumothorax), aspirate accumulated air in pleural space with 21-gauge needle connected to a three-way stopcock and syringe (Chapter 7).
   d. For severe respiratory distress due to pneumothorax and any tension pneumothorax, insert catheter (Fr 12 or 14) into fourth intercostal space, midaxillary line; connect to continuous suction of 10 to 20 cm H_2O. Since an air leak in the lung commonly seals after 24 hours, an underwater seal may be sufficient from then on. Remove the catheter if there is no reaccumulation of air after clamping tube.

e. Pneumomediastinum is usually treated by supportive measures only.

Transient tachypnea of newborn, or type II-RD

Transient tachypnea occurs primarily in mature infants with no specific antenatal events, although maternal sedation and delivery by cesarean section may be associated factors. Its incidence has been reported to be up to 30% of all cases of respiratory distress. The pathogenesis appears to be the delayed absorption of fetal lung fluid trapped in the interstitial spaces and engorged periarterial lymphatics (insufficient fall in pulmonary vascular pressure). The outcome is invariably favorable after a course of several hours to several days.

Differentiation from hyaline membrane disease or aspiration syndromes is usually easy because of its mild, self-limited course and different-appearing chest x-ray film.

1. Clinical features
   a. Elevated respiratory rates (up to 120/min) in the absence of significant retractions or rales
   b. Occasionally cyanosis in room air; always relieved with additional oxygen
   c. Blood gas determinations that tend to improve to near normal by 6 hours, in contrast to hyaline membrane disease
2. Chest x-ray examination
   a. May demonstrate prominent hilar markings with peripheral streaking, suggesting fluid engorgement
   b. Possible slight overaeration of lungs
3. Management
   a. Close observation with monitoring of vital signs
   b. Oxygen to prevent the appearance of central cyanosis
   c. Support with parenteral fluids during symptomatic stages

Pulmonary hemorrhage

Pulmonary hemorrhage is a nonspecific disorder with many possible causes. It may be found in as many as 10% of autopsies performed on premature infants, infants who were small for dates, or stillborns. Asphyxia appears to be a common denominator. The association with hyaline membrane disease suggests that red blood cells as well as fibrin may escape from the capillaries. Disseminated intravascular coagulation has recently been suspected. Cold injury, infection, and hypothrombinemia due to vitamin K_1 deficiency have been suspected as factors.

1. Clinical signs
   a. Bloody froth in the mouth or nose after a sudden cyanotic episode
   b. Chest retraction, tachypnea, and cyanosis
2. Treatment
   a. General supportive care, including antibiotics and vitamin K_1, is indicated.
   b. Any clotting defect may be responsive to transfusion of fresh whole blood or plasma.

Pulmonary dysmaturity

This disease, first described by Wilson and Mikity in 1960, occurs in small premature infants, usually after the first week of life. Etiology is obscure and not necessarily related to oxygen therapy. The disease resembles bronchopulmonary dysplasia (Fig. 19-1), in which infants have been subjected to high O_2 concentrations while on a positive-pressure ventilator for severe RDS. Mortality is approximately 30%.

1. Clinical features
   a. Tachypnea, mild retractions, occasionally apnea
   b. Elevated P_{CO_2} in severe cases and hypoxemia in room air
   c. Reduced functional residual capacity and vital capacity
   d. Bilateral diffuse coarse cystic changes and hyperaeration of lung fields, revealed by chest x-ray films
   e. Symptoms that increase in severity over several weeks and gradually improve after several months

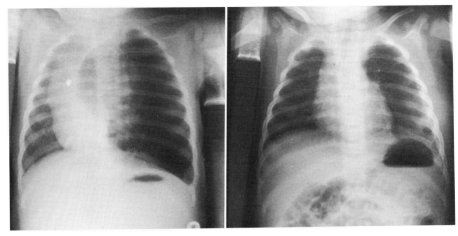

Fig. 19-6. Lobar emphysema with depressed diaphragm and displaced mediastinum (left film). After lobectomy, the lung has returned to its normal position.

 f. Hyperaeration of lung base during recovery phase, demonstrated by x-ray films (Cystic changes disappear gradually, and x-ray films will appear normal between 6 months and 2 years of age.)

 g. Cor pulmonale, a complicating factor in some severe cases

2. Management
 a. Administration of oxygen if necessary to prevent hypoxemia
 b. General supportive measures

Respiratory distress and congenital anomalies of the respiratory tree

Congenital anomalies of the respiratory tree are infrequent individually, but this group should be considered when respiratory difficulty has its onset in the birth room. Respiratory effort accompanied by cyanosis, sometimes with wheezing, choking, or gasping, and excessive mucus requires a definitive investigation of the airway and its structures. Lesions may be intrinsic or may encroach on the respiratory passage or lung parenchyma from without. A lateral x-ray film of the airway as well as an anteroposterior x-ray film of the chest is mandatory as an emergency procedure. Fluoroscopy of the esophagus with barium swallow and angiography at times may be warranted. The following is a partial list of such defects*:

 1. Choanal atresia
 2. Tracheal or laryngeal stenosis, or webs
 3. Mediastinal masses
 4. Congenital lung cysts and lobar emphysema (Fig. 19-6)
 5. Agenesis and hypoplasia of the lungs
 6. Esophageal atresia with or without tracheoesophageal fistula
 7. Diaphragmatic hernia
 8. Malformation of the great vessels, including vascular ring
 9. Phrenic nerve and vocal cord paralyses

---

*A more definitive approach can be found in these valuable books: Avery, M. E., and Fletcher, B. D.: The lung and its disorders, ed. 3, Philadelphia, 1974, W. B. Saunders Co.; Caffey, J.: Pediatric x-ray diagnosis, ed. 6, Chicago, 1972, Year Book Medical Publishers, Inc.

SELECTED REFERENCES

Ackerman, B. D., Stein, M. P., Sommer, J. S., and Schumacher, M.: Continuous positive airway pressure applied by means of a tight-fitting face mask, J. Pediatr. **85:**408, 1974.

Adamson, T. M., Hawker, J. M., Reynolds, E. O. R., and Shaw, J. L.: Hypoxemia during recovery from severe hyaline membrane disease, Pediatrics 44:168, 1969.

Auld, P. A. M.: Oxygen therapy for premature infants, J. Pediatr. **78:**705, 1971.

Avery, M. E., and Fletcher, B. D.: The lung and its disorders, ed. 3, Philadelphia, 1974, W. B. Saunders Co.

Brumley, G. W.: The critically ill child: the respiratory distress syndrome of the newborn, Pediatrics 47:758, 1971.

Chernick, V., and Reed, M. H.: Pneumothorax and chylothorax in the neonatal period, J. Pediatr. 76:624, 1970.

Chernick, V., and Vidyasagar, D.: Continuous negative chest wall pressure in hyaline membrane disease: one year experience, Pediatrics 49:753, 1974.

Daily, W. J. R., Belton, H. M., Sunshine, P., and Smith, P. C.: Mechanical ventilation of newborn infants. III. Historical comments and development of a scoring system for the selection of infants, Anesthesiology 34:119, 1971.

Daily, W. J. R., Klaus, M., and Meyer, H. B. P.: Apnea in premature infants: monitoring, incidence, heart rate changes, and an effect of environmental temperature, Pediatrics 43:510, Part I, 1969.

Daily, W. J. R., and Smith, P. C.: Mechanical ventilation of newborn infants. V. Five years' experience, Anesthesiology 34:132, 1971.

DeLeon, A. S., Elliott, J. H., and Jones, D. B.: The resurgence of retrolental fibroplasia, Pediatr. Clin. North Am. 17:309, 1970.

Duc, G.: Assessment of hypoxia in the newborn, Pediatrics 48:469, 1971.

Esterly, J. R., and Oppenheimer, E. H.: Massive pulmonary hemorrhage in the newborn. I. Pathologic considerations, J. Pediatr. 69:3, 1966.

Finnegan, L. P., McBrine, C. S., Steg, N. L., and Williams, M. L.: Respiratory distress in the newborn, Am. J. Dis. Child. 119:212, 1970.

Gregory, G. A., Gooding, C. A., Phibbs, R. H., and Tooley, W. H.: Meconium aspiration in infants: a prospective study, J. Pediatr. 85:848, 1974.

Gregory, G. A., Kitterman, J. A., Phibbs, R. H., Tooley, W. H., and Hamilton, W. K.: Treatment of the idiopathic respiratory distress syndrome with continuous positive airway pressure, N. Engl. J. Med. 284:1333, 1971.

Gruber, H. S., and Klaus, M.: Intermittent mask and bag therapy: an alternative approach to respiration therapy for infants with severe respiratory distress, J. Pediatr. 76:194, 1970.

Helmrath, T. A., Hodson, W. A., and Oliver, T. K., Jr.: Positive pressure ventilation in the newborn infant: the use of face mask, J. Pediatr. 76:202, 1970.

Hobel, C. J., Oh, W., Hyvarinen, M. A., Emmanouilides, G. C., and Erenberg, A.: Early versus late treatment of neonatal acidosis in low birth weight infants: relation to respiratory distress syndrome, J. Pediatr. 81:1178, 1972.

Hodgman, J. E., Mikity, V. G., Tatter, D., and Cleland, R. S.: Chronic respiratory distress in the premature infant, Pediatrics 44:179, 1969.

Hunt, C. E.: Capillary blood sampling in the infant: usefulness and limitations of two methods of sampling compared with arterial blood, Pediatrics 51:501, 1973.

Johnson, J. D., Malachowski, N. C., Grobstein, R., Welsh, D., Daily, W. J. R., and Sunshine, P.: Prognosis of children surviving with the aid of mechanical ventilation in the newborn period, J. Pediatr. 84:272, 1974.

Kattwinkel, J., Fleming, D., Cha, C. C., Fanaroff, A. A., and Klaus, M. H.: A device for administration of continuous positive airway pressure by the nasal route, Pediatrics 52:131, 1973.

Krauss, A. N., Klain, D. B., and Auld, P. A. M.: Chronic pulmonary insufficiency of prematurity, Pediatrics 55:55, 1975.

Krauss, A. N., Levin, A. R., Grossman, H., and Auld, P. A. M.: Physiologic studies on infants with Wilson-Mikity syndrome, J. Pediatr. 77:27, 1970.

Nelson, N. M.: Compromised convalescence from hyaline membrane disease, Pediatrics 44:158, 1969.

Northway, W., Rosan, R. C., and Porter, D.:

Pulmonary disease following respirator therapy, N. Engl. J. Med. **276**:357, 1967.

Reynolds, E. O. R., Robertson, N. R. C., and Wigglesworth, J. S.: Hyaline membrane disease, respiratory distress, and surfactant deficiency, Pediatrics **42**:758, 1968.

Rigatto, H., and Brady, J. P.: Periodic breathing and apnea in preterm infants, I and II, Pediatrics **50**:202, 1972.

Rowe, S., and Avery, M. E.: Massive pulmonary hemorrhage in the newborn. II. Clinical considerations, J. Pediatr. **69**:12, 1966.

Russell, G., and Cotton, E. K.: Effects of sodium bicarbonate by rapid injection and of oxygen in high concentration in respiratory distress syndrome of the newborn, Pediatrics **41**:1063, 1968.

Schapiro, R. L., and Evans, E. T.: Surgical disorders causing neonatal respiratory distress, Am. J. Roentgenol. **114**:305, 1972.

Simmons, M. H., Adock, E. W., Bard, H., and Battaglia, F. C.: Hypernatremia and intracranial hemorrhage in neonates, N. Engl. J. Med. **291**:6, 1974.

Smith, P. C., and Daily, W. J. R.: Mechanical ventilation of newborn infants. IV. Technique of controlled intermittent positive-pressure ventilation, Anesthesiology **34**:127, 1971.

Stahlman, M. E., Hedvall, G., Dolanski, E., Faxelius, G., Burko, H., and Kirk, V.: A six-year follow-up of clinical HMD, Pediatr. Clin. North Am. **20**:433, 1973.

Stern, L.: The use and misuse of oxygen in the newborn infant, Pediatr. Clin. North Am. **20**:447, 1973.

Thibeault, D. W., Grossman, H., Hagstrom, J. W. C., and Auld, P. A. M.: Radiological findings in the lungs of premature infants, J. Pediatr. **74**:1, 1969.

Usher, R.: Reduction of mortality from respiratory distress syndrome of prematurity with early administration of intravenous glucose and sodium bicarbonate, Pediatrics **32**:966, 1963.

20

Cardiovascular emergencies

Cardiac failure, cyanosis, and cyanotic episodes, and shock are outlined in this section. (Cardiovascular adjustments of the infant at birth were discussed in Chapter 6.)

ANATOMIC AND PHYSIOLOGIC VARIATIONS IN THE PREMATURE INFANT

1. Blood vessels
   a. Capillary walls are thin and easily damaged by increased hydrostatic pressure and asphyxia.
   b. Elastic supportive tissue is reduced.
   c. The ductus arteriosus may remain patent for many weeks after birth.
2. Heart rate patterns
   a. Normally beween 130 and 140 beats/min when the infant is at rest
   b. May rise to 180 beats/min when the infant is restless or crying
   c. Drops under 110 beats/min when the infant is cool, acidotic, or hypoxic
3. Heart murmurs
   Although a heart murmur may signify congenital heart disease and requires a base-line work-up (electrocardiogram and chest x-ray examination), most murmurs in the first few days of life represent delays in physiologic closure of the fetal circulatory channels.

CYANOSIS AND CYANOTIC EPISODES

Most cyanotic conditions of the newborn infant are associated with respiratory fail-ure or distress—conditions discussed under the respiratory system. The presence of a blue or dusky hue during the first few days of life is brought to the attention of the physician most often by the experienced nurse. The causes of this usually unexpected appearance vary from the trivial to the serious. If central cyanosis can be ascertained, a plan of diagnosis must be carried out.

The normal infant may require 10 to 20 minutes to be relieved entirely of central cyanosis after the birth process, whereas the prematurely born may continue to have an O_2 tension of under 40 mm Hg without cyanosis because of the high level of fetal hemoglobin. Thus the color of the mucous membranes is not as helpful as an index of the oxygen tension, a measure of its availability to the tissues. *Peripheral cyanosis* may persist in the newborn for days and usually is due to a cold environment, a high hematocrit value, ecchymosis from local venous obstruction (cord around the neck), hypovolemic shock with peripheral vasoconstriction, or generalized ecchymosis of an arm or leg from bruising.

Central cyanosis

1. Etiologic factors (excluding respiratory pathology)
   a. Central nervous system. Breathing is likely to be slow and shallow, with reduced ventilation and lowered P_{aO_2}.
      1. Intracranial hemorrhage or abnormality

2. Meningitis or meningoencephalitis
3. Perinatal asphyxia and shock
4. Narcosis from maternal medication
  b. Metabolic factors. Breathing may be irregular.
    1. Hypoglycemia (cardiomegaly)
    2. Tetany
  c. Congenital heart disease. Breathing may be rapid, but it is not distressed unless the infant is in heart failure.
    1. Right-to-left shunt and diminished pulmonary blood flow without heart failure, for example, tetralogy of Fallot, pulmonary atresia, tricuspid atresia. Breathing is deep and slightly increased in frequency.
    2. Congenital heart disease with heart failure.
  d. Polycythemia. The heart may be enlarged. Reduce hematocrit value by a partial exchange transfusion with fresh frozen plasma if it is over 70% to avoid neurologic sequelae.
  e. Shock and sepsis. Hypovolemia and septic shock lead to intense vasoconstriction and can be associated with central as well as peripheral cyanosis.
  f. Methemoglobinemia. Lavender-colored blood that does not turn red on exposure to air is diagnostic.
2. Diagnostic observations and procedures
  a. Observe the baby for breathing pattern.
  b. Auscultate the heart, determine liver size and check peripheral pulses.
  c. Obtain x-ray film of the chest and an electrocardiogram.
  d. Obtain hematocrit, blood glucose, and serum calcium levels.
  e. Perform an analysis of blood gases, including the arterial oxygen tension.
  f. Consider spinal tap and study for sepsis.

CARDIAC FAILURE

Heart failure may simulate disorders of other organs or systems, and other disease entities may present with some of the clinical signs of heart failure. The closer to the time of birth its appearance is recognized, the more critical its nature. Clinical deterioration or failure to improve within 12 hours of treatment usually is an indication for cardiac catheterization and angiocardiography.

1. Incidence—7 to 8/1,000 live births (0.7% to 0.8%)
2. Pathogenesis
  a. Structural heart disease (most common cause) because of errors of embryogenesis in the first 2 months of gestation, for example, transposition of the great vessels, hypoplastic left heart
  b. Myocarditis due to invasion of the heart by viral organisms, for example, Coxsackie B viruses, or infection from bacterial sepsis or its toxins
  c. Respiratory disease with increased vascular resistance, such as hyaline membrane disease or pneumonia
  d. Polycythemia or circulatory overload in overtransfusion or twin-to-twin transfusion
  e. Anemia, as with hydrops fetalis
  f. Arrhythmias due either to congenital heart block (less than 80 beats/min) or to paroxysmal atrial tachycardia (180 to 300 beats/min)
  g. Miscellaneous conditions, including glycogen storage disease, hypertension, and endocardial fibroelastosis
3. Clinical features
  a. Common signs are tachypnea (60 to 100 respirations/min at rest), tachycardia (150 to 180 beats/min at rest), fatigue or difficulty with feeding, enlarging liver (3 to 5 cm below the costal margin), and pulmonary rales or rhonchi.
  b. Less common signs are systemic edema, elevated venous pressure, inappropriate sweating, a gallop rhythm, and pulsus alternans.
  c. Chest x-ray film often discloses enlargement of the heart (cardiothorac-

ic index of over 75%), changes in cardiac contour, or diminished or engorged pulmonary vasculature.

    d. Electrocardiogram may indicate hypertrophy of one or more chambers, abnormalities of the mean QRS axis, and rhythm disturbances.

4. Noncardiac diseases simulating heart failure

    a. Cardiomegaly of hypoglycemia in the newborn

    b. Central cyanosis with heart murmurs in respiratory disease, for example, idiopathic respiratory distress

    c. Liver enlargement from specific conditions such as fetal viral invasion, galactosemia, or neuroblastoma

    d. Tachypnea from metabolic acidosis or minor pulmonary disorders, for example, transient tachypnea of the newborn

    e. Peripheral edema observed in "late edema of the premature infant," hypoalbuminemic states, and lymphedema

    f. Factitious cardiomegaly from an apparent wide mediastinal shadow altered by a chest deformity or an x-ray film taken during expiration

5. Management

    a. Offer intensive care, with skin temperature maintained at 97° ± 1° F (36° C), oxygen concentration between 30% to 35%, ECG monitoring, and an inclined plane position (head raised at an angle of 10° to 20°).

    b. Digitalize patient (for dosage, see Appendix E). Observe for

        1. Bradycardia (discontinue digitalis when the heart rate is under 100 beats/min)

        2. Signs of heart block, multiple ectopic beats

        3. Hypokalemia

    c. Maintain fluid and nutritional support.

    d. Consider diuretics, for example, furosemide (Lasix), 1 mg/kg of body weight, intramuscularly or intravenously.

    e. Obtain consultation for consideration of early cardiac catheterization, angiocardiography, and possible surgery.

SHOCK

Shock in a neonate presents a major emergency requiring prompt detection and treatment. It may be defined as a state of severe circulatory failure in which cardiac output does not meet tissue requirements.

1. Causes of shock

    a. Hypovolemic shock resulting from severe blood loss secondary to rupture of umbilical cord, abruptio placentae, twin-to-twin transfusion, etc. (See Chapter 23.)

    b. Septic shock in overwhelming infections

    c. Cardiogenic shock, organic heart disease leading to severe failure

    d. Shock from inappropriate or excessive use of CPAP or PEEP

    e. Asphyxial shock

    f. Shock from metabolic causes, such as hypoglycemia and adrenal insufficiency

2. Recognition of shock

    a. Tachycardia

    b. Tachypnea

    c. Pallor (especially after blood loss)

    d. Poor filling of blanched skin, indicating poor tissue perfusion

    e. Metabolic acidosis

    f. Decreasing urinary output

    g. Hypotension (See Fig. 20-1 for range of normal blood pressure.)

3. Management of shock

    a. Place infant in an isolette or radiant warmer, keeping skin temperature at 97° F.

    b. Monitor the infant's heart rate, as well as arterial and, if possible, venous pressure, urinary output, and blood gases.

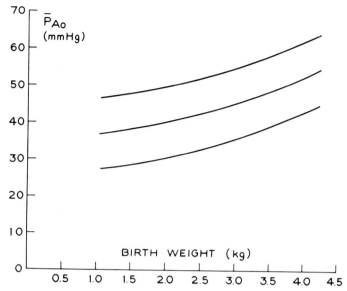

Fig. 20-1. Parabolic regression (middle line) and 95% confidence limits (top and bottom lines) of mean aortic blood pressure by birth weight in normal newborn infants during 2 to 12 hours of life. (From Kitterman, J. A., Phibbs, R. H., and Tooley, W. H.: Pediatrics 44:959, 1969.)

c. Offer oxygen and assisted ventilation if needed to prevent hypoxemia.

d. Begin blood volume expansion, giving blood or Plasmanate, 5 to 10 ml/kg of body weight intravenously over 2 to 5 minutes (an alternative is normal saline solution, 5 to 10 ml/kg of body weight, and albumin, 1 gm/kg). Repeat these amounts if necessary, depending on arterial or central venous pressures.

e. Correct metabolic acidosis by administering sodium bicarbonate; continue to monitor blood gases as a measure of effectiveness of therapy.

f. Consider infusion of isoproterenol (in cases of severe nonimproving vaso-constriction dosage is 0.1 to 0.5 µg/kg/min). Closely observe patient for cardiac arrhythmia.

g. Administer antibiotics if sepsis is suspected as the cause of shock (agents such as gentamicin or kanamycin may have to be slowly infused parenterally to be effective).

h. Digitalize patient if needed.

SELECTED REFERENCES

Lees, M. H.: Heart failure in the newborn infant, J. Pediatr. 75:139, 1969.

Lees, M. H.: Cyanosis of the newborn infant, J. Pediatr. 77:484, 1970.

Nadas, A. S., and Tyler, D. C.: Pediatric cardiology, ed. 3, Philadelphia, 1972, W. B. Saunders Co.

21

Gastrointestinal emergencies

SYMPTOMS COMMONLY ENCOUNTERED WITH GASTROINTESTINAL EMERGENCIES

Early intrauterine function of the gastrointestinal tract of the fetus can be observed by 14 weeks of fetal life when dye injected into the amnion is swallowed and concentrated in the intestinal tract. Bile is formed in the liver as early as 12 weeks of gestational age. When passed into the intestines, the bile gives meconium its distinctive color. Desquamated cells from the skin and intestinal wall, along with intestinal juices, help to compose this gelatinous and sticky substance.

The swallowing of amniotic fluid and its absorption into the fetal circulation, with part being excreted back into the amnion as urine, is a process that helps to maintain the delicate balance in fluid homeostasis between fetus, mother, and amnion.

Anatomic and physiologic variations in the premature infant

1. The sucking reflex is often too weak to handle offered feedings.
2. The cardiac sphincter is lax and intestinal mobility depressed, leading to easy regurgitation and delay in evacuation of meconium from the intestinal tract.
3. Gastric acid and intestinal enzymes may be insufficient for complete digestion and absorption.

4. Gastric capacity may not be sufficient to meet caloric and fluid requirements of the infant.
5. First stool—meconium passage is delayed several days in some, and in the absence of distention no special attention is necessary.

Gastrointestinal function is easily upset and may reflect a problem in biochemical homeostasis, disease, or mechanical obstruction in the infant. Prompt diagnosis is necessary to prevent the development of further malfunction and clinical deterioration. A differential diagnosis of variations in gastrointestinal behavior during the neonatal period is offered to facilitate early diagnosis.

Vomiting

1. Irritative vomiting (first few days of life) from
   a. Excessive mucus swallowed during the birth process
   b. Mucus produced by the neonate, perhaps the result of asphyxial injury to the mucous membranes in chronic fetal distress; seen particularly with severe dysmaturity
2. Feeding intolerance from
   a. Overfeeding by gavage, too rapid feeding by nipple, or underfeeding with aerophagia
   b. Urging of milk when the infant is reluctant to suck
   c. Improperly prepared formula

3. Infections due to enteric pathogenic organisms or parenteral infection, including that of the urinary tract
4. Central nervous system irritation, for example, edema, hemorrhage, malformation, and particularly meningitis, with projectile vomiting at times
5. Intestinal obstruction, the signs of which are distention and/or green bile-stained vomitus
6. Esophageal obstruction, the signs of which are choking with mucus, immediate regurgitation of feedings, cardioesophageal relaxation (chalasia), or achalasia (esophageal spasm)
7. Metabolic causes, as in tetany, infants of toxemic mothers, hypoglycemia
8. Miscellaneous causes include
   a. Maternal drug addiction
   b. Gastrointestinal allergy
   c. Inborn errors of metabolism, for example, phenylketonuria, galactosemia
   d. Adrenogenital syndrome

Abdominal distention with or without ileus

Causes of abdominal distention include the following:

1. Overfeeding (with delay in peristaltic activity)
2. Constipation (including meconium plug syndrome)
3. Bacterial gastroenteritis and nonspecific necrotizing enterocolitis
4. Systemic bacterial infection, particularly from *Escherichia coli*
5. Metabolic disorders, for example, hypocalcemia, hyperkalemia, hypermagnesemia
6. Autonomic nervous system imbalance as a result of asphyxia or shock
7. Intestinal obstruction
8. Tracheoesophageal fistula when the lower esophageal segment connects with the tracheal lumen
9. Urinary tract obstruction, for example, polycystic kidneys, hydronephrosis
10. Pneumoperitoneum from rupture of the stomach or intestine and release of free gas—occasionally due to dissection of air from pneumomediastinum into abdomen
11. Fluid accumulations—edema, blood, urine, or chyle
12. Tumor growths, cysts, or hydrocolpos
13. Hepatosplenomegaly

Diarrhea

An increased number of small stools (six to eight daily) is not significant unless they have a water ring of 2 to 4 cm in diameter. Causes of diarrhea are as follows:

1. Nonspecific factors such as food intolerance (check stool for glucose with Clinistix),* overfeeding, parenteral infection, or short gut syndromes
2. Specific epidemic diarrhea
3. Enterocolitis

Epidemic diarrhea

Epidemic diarrhea, which is a potent cause of nursery epidemics, results in a high mortality. Premature and debilitated infants are especially susceptible. The incubation period is from 1 to 3 days. Sporadic cases may occur.

1. Pathogenesis
   Pathogenic *Escherichia coli* contracted from the mother at delivery or from an infected infant in the nursery is the usual agent; however, a number of other bacterial and viral organisms have been identified as causes. The organisms responsible are not always pathogenic to mature individuals, but the premature

---

*Newborn infants may have an easily acquired depression in disaccharide absorption (lactose, maltose, and sucrose) from a temporary reduction in their respective enzymes. Insult to the intestine, especially in diarrheal states, can result in disaccharidase deficiency, particularly in the lactose component. Simple sugars such as glucose are preferred for the carbohydrate used in the feedings given through the recovery phase of such an illness. Lactose intolerance has often been found to superimpose itself on an existing diarrhea, with further delay in recovery.

or debilitated infant may not resist them.

2. Clinical features
   a. Refusal of feedings
   b. Frequent watery stools
   c. Dehydration with occasional shock and pallor
   d. Vomiting and/or distention
3. Diagnosis
   Depends on stool culture and differentiation of pathogens by typing and/or fluorescent-antibody methods
4. Treatment
   a. Infants with suspected or cultured epidemic diarrhea
      1. Give parenteral antibiotics, for example, kanamycin.
      2. Discontinue feedings and start giving intravenous fluids.
      3. Isolate such infants from the nursery area.
   b. Infants in the same nursery with those of 4a or asymptomatic carriers of pathogenic organisms
      1. Give neomycin, 50 to 100 mg/kg four times daily by mouth, for 7 to 10 days.
      2. Repeat cultures every 2 to 3 days.
      3. Isolate these babies in the nursery.
      4. Close the nursery to new admissions until repeat cultures are negative.

Constipation

Infrequent passage of stool is of concern only when distention is present or the stool is overfirm. Any distention requires careful investigation, but simple firm stools may be relieved by a change in feeding, the injection of a half-normal saline solution (about 5 to 10 ml) into the rectum, or the insertion of a small piece of glycerin suppository. Causes of constipation are muscular hypotonia (seen in mongolism and hypothyroidism), dehydration, feeding of homogenized milk, congenital obstruction or stenosis of the intestine, and aganglionosis of the colon (Hirschsprung's disease).

GASTROINTESTINAL SURGICAL EMERGENCIES

Serious congenital anomalies are found in 1% to 2% of all infants at birth. About a fourth are surgically correctable and usually involve obstruction of the gastrointestinal tract. Although specific anomalies of the gut are infrequent and in the range of one for every 2,000 to 5,000 births collectively, they are frequent enough to justify a definitive search in the birth room (Chapter 6), particularly in infants with a reduced birth weight.

1. Signs of intestinal obstruction
   a. *Maternal hydramnios.* Amniotic fluid may accumulate because of an imbalance in its circulation caused by mechanical interruption in high intestinal or esophageal obstruction in the fetus. This prevents the fluid swallowed by the fetus from being absorbed through the gut into the maternal circulation.
   b. *Excessive gastric aspirate.* Fluid (clear or green stained) obtained from the stomach in excess of 15 to 20 ml indicates possible intestinal obstruction.
   c. *Bile-stained vomitus.* Since this sign does not occur in the normal infant, such an occurrence indicates intestinal obstruction until proved otherwise. Exceptions are swallowed amniotic fluid contaminated with meconium and a relaxed pyloric sphincter in the very prematurely born infant.
   d. *Abdominal distention.* This early postnatal sign is the result of accumulation and delay in the passage of swallowed air. In high intestinal obstruction the abdomen may be scaphoid. Paralytic ileus may distend the abdomen similarly and can be the result of infection, asphyxia, or shock.
   e. *Obstipation.* This later sign is more significant if the infant is distended or the meconium is abnormal in color and consistency.

2. Diagnostic procedures
   a. Specific physical examination includes the following:
      1. Carefully palpate abdomen for masses (volvulus), doughy intestinal loops (meconium ileus), and scaphoid abdomen (diaphragmatic hernia)
      2. Digitally explore the anus to demonstrate imperforate anus, meconium plug syndrome, or the "white meconium" of intestinal atresia.
      3. Pass a soft Fr 10 radiopaque catheter into the stomach. Failure of the catheter to pass into the stomach indicates esophageal obstruction, and the catheter will demonstrate the level of obstruction on x-ray film. Note the quantity and color of stomach contents.
   b. Radiograph of the abdomen. Gas patterns (contrast material may not be indicated) on an upright x-ray film may indicate the level of an intestinal obstruction as follows:
      1. Air extending as far as the pyloric end of the stomach indicates a pyloric web.
      2. Air extending to the second portion of the duodenum ("double-bubble") suggests duodenal atresia, annular pancreas, or incomplete intestinal rotation.
      3. Air extending to midgut indicates jejunal or ileal obstruction.
      4. Minute bubbles of air intermixed with meconium in intestinal loops (ground-glass appearance) suggest meconium ileus.
      5. Distention of gas in the colon supported by a dilated bowel in the flank area indicates the possibility of aganglionic megacolon, meconium plug syndrome, or imperforate anus.
      6. Free air in the abdomen (pneumoperitoneum) signifies gastrointestinal perforation.
   c. A barium enema may indicate
      1. Microcolon (small intestinal obstruction)
      2. Malrotation of the intestine (ectopic position of cecum)
      3. Hirschsprung's disease, by the identification of a narrowed zone leading into a dilated colon. Barium must be diluted and injected in minimal quantity, or this clue will be obscured by an overriding dilated opaque bowel pattern. A later film will show delayed evacuation of barium and occasionally the ragged ulcers of enterocolitis.

3. Initial treatment of specific surgical diseases
   All infants suspect for gastrointestinal emergencies should have full supportive care, gastric suction, prompt x-ray examination and, when a surgical condition is likely, full team care, including a pediatric surgeon.
   a. When full facilities for care are not present
      1. Transfer the infant immediately for diagnosis to a regional pediatric center (Chapter 11).
      2. Do minimal diagnostic procedures.
      3. Supply environmental warmth, sufficient oxygen, correction of acidosis, and aspiration equipment, with nasogastric tube in place.
   b. When facilities are adequate
      1. Start administering parenteral fluids promptly before surgery is begun.
      2. Select an experienced anesthesiologist.
      3. Prevent heat loss in the operating room.
      4. Replace significant blood loss, but use fresh frozen plasma if the hemoglobin level is over 12 to 13 gm (hematocrit value of 50%), when indicated.
      5. Limit surgical procedures to justifi-

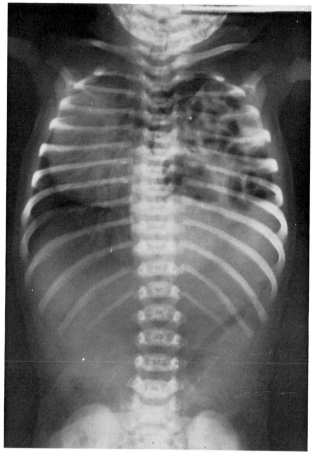

Fig. 21-1. Diaphragmatic hernia in which early recognition and prompt surgery resulted in survival.

able requirements, in keeping with the size and physiologic state of the infant.

Diaphragmatic hernia (Fig. 21-1)

Herniation typically occurs through the posterolateral portion of the diaphragm or the foramen of Bochdalek. Left-sided herniation occurs more frequently than right-sided involvement.

1. Symptoms
   a. Respiratory distress
   b. Increased anteroposterior diameter of chest
   c. Scaphoid abdomen
   d. Cyanosis
   e. Bowel sounds in chest (not always present)
2. Diagnostic aid: x-ray film of chest and abdomen, demonstrating opacified hemithorax (at birth) or gas-filled bowel in hemithorax (after birth)
3. Management
   a. Maintain gastric drainage for deflation of the gastrointestinal portion residing in the lung cavity (especially important during air transport to a surgical center)
   b. If assisted ventilation is required, it must be done by experienced personnel via an endotracheal tube only. One should remember that the lungs

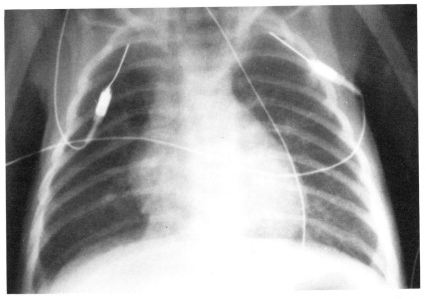

Fig. 21-2. Esophageal atresia with tracheoesophageal fistula. Note dilated and air-filled upper atretic segment of esophagus clearly outlined by its increased radiolucency.

are frequently hypoplastic and susceptible to alveolar rupture.

  c. Start correction of acidosis with NaHCO$_3$.

  d. Call pediatric surgeon.

Esophageal atresia with tracheoesophageal fistula (Fig. 21-2)

Among all varieties of esophageal atresia, the one accompanied by a fistula connecting the lower segment of the esophagus with the trachea occurs far more frequently. Absence of a fistula is evident in the lack of air in the intestinal tract on x-ray film.

1. Symptoms

  a. Excessive mucus

  b. Choking and cyanotic episodes

  c. Hoarse cry

  d. Regurgitation and possible aspiration of first feeding

2. Diagnostic aids

  a. Failure of a Fr 8 or 10 radiopaque catheter to enter the stomach. To ensure that the catheter is not coiled in esophageal pouch, listen over stomach for air injected through tube; check pH for acidity.

  b. Chest x-ray film taken with a radiopaque catheter in the esophagus reveals that tip of catheter lies coiled in dilated air-filled upper pouch of atretic esophagus.

3. Initial management

  a. Maintain esophageal suction through a double lumen-sump catheter.

  b. Keep the infant in an inclined plane position with his head up to avoid gastric reflux and spillage of esophageal pouch secretions into the lung passages.

  c. Place on parenteral feedings.

  d. Call pediatric surgeon.

Necrotizing enterocolitis

Necrotizing enterocolitis (NEC) is an often fatal disease that involves an inflammatory process of the gastrointestinal tract and is frequently complicated by intestinal perforation. NEC has been reported to occur in up to 5% of all admissions to neonatal intensive care units and up to

25% in infants less than 1,300 gm at birth. The etiology has not been clearly identified.

1. Associations with NEC
   a. Immaturity
   b. Hypoxia (asphyxia, patent ductus arteriosus, mesenteric ischemia)
   c. Hypertonic feedings
   d. Excessive feedings
   e. Sepsis (bacteria entering injured mucosa)
2. Warning signs of NEC
   a. Onset of repeated apneic episodes
   b. Poor skin color
   c. Abdominal distention
   d. Palpable loops of bowel
   e. Repeated gastric residuals of more than 2 ml before feeding
   f. Stool positive to guaiac
3. Serious signs on x-ray films
   a. Persistent dilated loops of bowel
   b. Bowel-wall edema
4. Convincing signs on x-ray films
   a. Pneumatosis intestinalis, portal air
   b. Pseudo-obstructive pattern
   c. Evidence of perforation (free air under diaphragm on upright abdominal x-ray film)
5. Initial management
   a. Prompt discontinuation of gastrointestinal feeding with nasogastric decompression
   b. Substitution of parenteral alimentation
   c. Surgery when indicated
6. Problems in later management
   a. Prolonged requirements for parenteral nutrition to allow healing of gastrointestinal tract
   b. Frequency of short gut syndrome after significant bowel resection, often leading to gastrointestinal intolerance to feeding because of malabsorption
   c. Strictures on healing
7. Prevention
   In very immature or seriously ill infants the following recommendations may keep the incidence of NEC to a minimum:
   a. Caution in the introduction and rate of increase in parenteral feeding (Consider temporarily substituting parenteral alimentation.)
   b. Feeding of iso-osmolar milks initially (20 calories/30 ml or less—MCT oil added to feedings will aid in caloric support)
   c. Prevention of distention from high-volume feedings

Miscellaneous conditions

1. Intestinal obstruction
   a. Maintain gastric suction.
   b. Replace fluid losses.
   c. Observe for abdominal calcification as the result of intrauterine perforation and meconium peritonitis.
2. Omphalocele or gastroschisis
   a. Cover exposed viscera with warm sterile saline packs.
   b. Maintain gastric suction.
3. Hirschsprung's disease (aganglionic megacolon)
   a. Consider in any newborn with distention
   b. Have a competent radiologist perform an examination.
   c. Be prepared to have a colostomy performed.
4. Incarcerated or strangulated hernia
   The incidence of inguinal hernia is in-

creased in both male and female premature infants. Unrelieved incarceration can produce strangulation and signs of intestinal obstruction. An infant whose fussiness is unrelieved by feedings should be examined for hernia.

a. Apply gentle steady pressure on the hernial mass with one hand while the legs are held partly elevated with the other; have the infant suck on a nipple if possible.

b. If this fails, sedate, apply cold packs, and after an appropriate rest, attempt again (rarely is an incarceration irreducible).

c. Operate if gangrene from strangulation is suspected.

d. Repair any hernia that continues to annoy the baby, even if his weight is as low as 2 kg.

e. Warn the mother whose child has an uncomplicated hernia of the need for prompt consultation in the event of any later discomfort or swelling.

SELECTED REFERENCES

Holt, S. A., and Friedland, G. W.: Neonatal necrotizing enterocolitis, West. J. Med. **120:** 110, 1974.

Hopkins, G. B., Gould, V. E., Stevenson, J. K., and Oliver, T. K., Jr.: Necrotizing enterocolitis in premature infants, Am. J. Dis. Child. **120:** 229, 1970.

Leonidas, J. C., Krasna, J. H., Fox, H. A., and Broder, M. S.: Peritoneal fluid in necrotizing enterocolitis: a radiological sign of clinical deterioration, J. Pediatr. **82:**672, 1973.

Silverman, W. A., Sinclair, J. C., and Scopes, J. W.: Regulation of body temperature in pediatric surgery, J. Pediatr. Surg. **1:**321, 1966.

Talbert, J. L., Felman, A. H., and DeBusk, F. L.: Gastrointestinal surgical emergencies in the newborn infant, J. Pediatr. **76:**783, 1970.

22

Central nervous system emergencies

Neuromuscular development of the fetus is a continuous process. By 28 weeks of gestation the premature infant has developed most of the basic reflex responses, although they are often too weak for functional purpose. Response to sound may be observed. Before term is reached the infant has achieved highly integrated reflex patterns. Such responses may be governed without inhibition or control of the cerebrum, and the cortex may not yet function at a conscious level. Soon after 38 weeks of postmenstrual age has been reached, and at term in the newborn infant, the infant may show meaningful response to visual stimuli. An awareness can be observed in the tracking of the eyes in response to a moving face at a distance of 20 cm. A social smile will often follow at about the first month of corrected age (accounting for the number of weeks of prematurity). Basic reflexes are gradually suppressed as cortical responsiveness increases.

In the prematurely born infant, neurologic development appears to continue unabated as would have occurred in the intrauterine environment, unless adversely affected by critical events.

Sensory stimulation from incubator motors, bright lights, circulating air, and at times cool mist sprays may cause hyperactivity of the infant in the first days of life. Whether harm is induced is not known, but such an abnormal environment is in distinct contrast to the relative sensory isolation and protection found in the warm and dark confines of an intrauterine fluid compartment.

ANATOMIC AND PHYSIOLOGIC VARIATIONS IN THE PREMATURE INFANT

1. Anatomy
   a. Gyri of the cerebral cortex are less developed and convoluted than in the term infant.
   b. Cerebrospinal fluid volume appears to be proportionately increased over that of the fetus or the term infant. This may explain the widened area (over 2 cm) of reflected light on transillumination of the premature infant's skull, even after 40 weeks of postmenstrual age has been reached.
2. Electroencephalogram
   With increasing immaturity the following are seen:
   a. Waves of lessening amplitude and decreasing frequency
   b. An increasing latency of wave response to photic and acoustic stimulation
   c. Less superimposed activity, even when injury or abnormality has occurred
3. Behavior (early)
   a. Jerky movements of the extremities, with arms and legs held in an extended manner

b. Frequent movement, although much time is spent in sleep

c. Muted cry and facial grimacing

4. Examination
   a. Decreased tonus to the point of flaccidity in the markedly immature infant
   b. Suppression in reflex behavior
   c. Development of ankle clonus after 1 month of age in many infants

SIGNS OF CENTRAL NERVOUS SYSTEM DISORDERS
Seizures and hyperactivity

Convulsions in the newborn are common and indicate central nervous system dysfunction. In the very premature infant, signs of cerebral irritation may be absent because of the relative lack of development function. Signs of apnea and cyanosis only may occur. Most seizures occur in the first week of life, with a peak incidence on the second day.

1. Etiologic factors
   a. Perinatal asphyxia
      Fetal asphyxia with profound anoxia is the most serious and common cause of seizures, usually manifested in the first 48 hours of life. Fetal bradycardia and late deceleration patterns accompanied by acidosis are indicative of fetal asphyxia and provide justification for considering an emergency cesarean section. Asphyxia tends to potentiate metabolic disorders, which may be convulsants in themselves.
   b. Intracranial hemorrhage (more common in breech delivery and cephalopelvic disproportion)
   c. Developmental malformations, for example, cerebral agenesis, porencephalia
   d. Cerebral infections, for example, bacterial meningitis, transplacental viral invasion with meningoencephalitis (cytomegalovirus disease, rubella, herpes simplex)

   e. Hypocalcemia (serum calcium usually under 7 mg/100 ml)
   f. Hypoglycemia (serum glucose under 10 to 15 mg/100 ml)
   g. Miscellaneous factors
      1. Hypernatremia (over 148 mEq/L), hyponatremia (under 125 mEq/L), and hypomagnesemia (under 1 mEq/100 ml)
      2. Inborn errors of metabolism, for example, galactosemia, maple syrup urine disease, pyridoxine deficiency
      3. Hyperviscosity (hematocrit value over 75%)
      4. Narcotic withdrawal after maternal addiction
      5. Kernicterus (bilirubin encephalopathy)
      6. Congenital heart disease
      7. Uremia
      8. Local anesthetic agents given to mother

2. Management (emergency)
   a. Place the neonate in an incubator with oxygen supplementation.
   b. Obtain blood for glucose, calcium, sodium, potassium and BUN and start intravenous glucose infusion.
   c. Monitor the heart and/or respiratory rate.
   d. Perform a spinal tap.
   e. Infuse slowly the following solutions in turn intravenously (with an appropriate lag period) for observation of symptomatic relief:
      1. A 25% glucose solution, 2 to 4 ml
      2. A 10% calcium gluconate solution, 1 to 2 ml/kg of body weight
      3. A 50% solution of magnesium sulfate, 0.1 to 0.2 ml/kg of body weight
   If convulsive behavior continues
   f. Control convulsions with phenobarbital sodium, 10 mg/kg intramuscularly. Repeat in 20 minutes if the infant is still convulsing. After seizures are controlled, continue administering

phenobarbital at approximately 5 mg/ kg of body weight daily.

   g. Arrange an electroencephalogram and consider additional diagnostic procedures.

3. Prognosis

   a. Overall mortality is approximately 30% (higher in preterm).

   b. Intact survival occurs in less than 50% of survivors. Approximately half of those with sequelae have further seizures.

   c. The earlier the convulsion in relation to birth, the more serious the prognosis.

   d. Subarachnoid hemorrhage is less serious than intraventricular bleeding.

   e. Hypocalcemic convulsions have the most favorable outcome.

   f. Cerebral malformations have the worst outcome.

   g. Encephalographic tracings demonstrating periodic paroxysmal activity, multifocal discharges, or depressed tracings have a generally poor outlook.

Lethargy and hypotonia (depressed or absent obligatory reflexes)

An inactive premature infant with a decrease in muscle tone over that expected for his maturity may have been hurt. A change from active to inactive status deserves immediate attention because of the possibility of infection. A lethargic infant is slow to arouse, but one with irritability is slow to relax. Etiology is often similar to those conditions producing hyperirritability states and includes the following:

1. Brain injury from hemorrhage, asphyxia, or developmental defect
2. Infection, particularly meningitis
3. Fatigue from excessive handling
4. Hypoglycemia
5. Fluid and electrolyte imbalance, for example, metabolic acidosis, dehydration, hyponatremia
6. Myasthenia gravis

Hydrocephalus and microcephalus

Head measurements (often neglected) should be recorded at birth and charted longitudinally on a growth graph (Fig. 7-3). Thus a base line is established for determination of the rate of growth. Any measurement above or below 2 SD from the mean for the infant's gestational age is suspect for abnormality. Infants who have suffered fetal undernutrition or malnutrition may have a head circumference well below the 3rd percentile and yet develop normally, particularly if growth of the head accelerates into the usual channels of growth during the first year. Relative macrocephaly in comparison with other measurements is common in the low birth weight infant because of the tendency for preferential brain growth. Seldom is such a head measurement above the mean for the gestational age.

1. Hydrocephalus

Evidence of an early increase in size suggests hemorrhage, inflammation, or congenital hydrocephalus. Later increase in size suggests obstruction of cerebral spinal fluid flow or simply the effects of fluid accumulation from sodium retention or hypoproteinemia. Observe infant for

   a. Fullness or bulging fontanel (seen also in vitamin A excess and during tetracycline therapy)

   b. Early unlapping of the cranial sutures,* which normally overlap in the premature infant at birth and stay thus for the first 3 to 4 weeks of life

   c. Excessive head growth (more than 1.2 cm/wk for a 3-week period)

   d. Asymmetric or extensive transillumination

---

*Infants severely undernourished during fetal life may show spreading of sutures on the basis of "catch-up" growth in brain cell size with optimum postnatal nutrition. A separated sagittal suture at birth is seen in severely undergrown and dysmature infants who have suffered from insufficient calcium deposition.

2. Microcephaly (injured or maldeveloped brain), suggested by
   a. Continued overlapping sutures after 4 weeks of age
   b. Longitudinal growth in head circumference under 0.70 cm/wk (preterm)
   c. Head size proportionately less than length

Behavioral changes

Vomiting, apnea and cyanosis, persistent asymmetry of movements or reflexes, and retraction of the head are signs indicating central nervous system abnormality.

DIAGNOSTIC PROCEDURES

1. Blood sample for glucose, calcium, phosphorus, and magnesium levels; blood gas and pH determinations
2. Urine sample for galactosuria and aminoaciduria
3. Spinal tap and subdural taps (For technique and usual findings, see p. 104.)
4. Transillumination (p. 105)
5. Electroencephalogram, which may show the following abnormal tracings:
   a. Localized electrical focus (least serious abnormality)
   b. Multiple focal discharges
   c. Periodoic paroxysmal discharge
   d. Flat tracings

INTRACRANIAL HEMORRHAGE AND ANOXIC INJURY

Central nervous system injury during the period of labor and delivery is a serious hazard not only as a major cause of mortality but also in its relationship to later mental retardation and neurologic deficit in the survivors. These effects may be from anoxia or trauma or both. Direct injury to the spinal cord and tears in the supportive structure of the brain lead to subdural hemorrhage primarily in the full-term infant. Paraventricular, intraventricular, and subarachnoid hemorrhages are more common in the premature infant and more likely the result of anoxia. The dam-

age to the central nervous system from anoxia alone, even without gross hemorrhage, is incalculable, and such damage can occur long before delivery, as well as in the neonatal period.

1. Pathogenesis
   a. Asphyxia before and after birth
   b. Vein rupture within the infant's head from the stress of delivery, with an increase in intravascular pressure
   c. Mechanical injury from obstetric manipulation
   d. Coagulation defects
2. Clinical signs
   a. Irritability and seizure activity
   b. Lethargy and poor feeding
   c. Irregular respirations and apnea and cyanosis
   d. Pallor and excessive jaundice
3. Diagnosis
   a. Fullness of the fontanel and/or sagittal suture spread
   b. Bloody spinal fluid with xanthochromia
   c. Subdural accumulation of blood
   d. Falling hematocrit value
4. Treatment
   a. Remove any excess accumulation of subdural bloody fluid; if fontanel is full after the spinal tap, perform subdural taps.
   b. Treat any coagulation defect; give fresh frozen plasma or blood.

MENINGITIS

The preterm infant is four times more susceptible to meningitis (one in 250 born) than the term infant. The presence of sepsis, debility, or any change in clinical behavior must alert the physician to this possibility. Readiness to perform spinal fluid examination on infants suspected of such infection is the only hope of reducing the morbidity and the high mortality from this disease.

In the early weeks of life bacterial organisms are predominantly gram-negative coliform types, particularly of the K_1 antigen strains. *Listeria monocytogenes, Pseudomonas* organisms, and group B streptococci are occasionally encountered.

1. Suggestive symptoms and signs
   a. Lethargy and/or irritability with occasional seizures
   b. Rise or fall in temperature
   c. Pallor or grayness of the skin
   d. Disinterest in, or spitting up of, feedings
   e. Apnea and cyanosis
   f. Sagittal suture spread, with or without a full fontanel
   g. Other signs of infection, for example, hepatosplenomegaly, jaundice
2. Diagnosis dependent on spinal fluid examination
   a. Culture 0.5 to 1 ml of the fluid on a chocolate agar slant in a carbon dioxide jar, in addition to the routine cultures.
   b. Do a cell count from the second tube.
   c. Spin down 1 to 2 ml of the fluid and make several smears of sediment for a Gram stain and possible fluorescent antibody study, particularly if there is a pleocytosis (occasionally there may be bacteria without an increase in cells).
   d. Determine the glucose level—under

20 mg/100 ml suggests bacterial infection or systemic hypoglycemia.
3. Management (Chapter 9)
   a. Administer gentamicin and ampicillin while waiting for substantiation of infection by culture.
   b. Give full intensive care.
4. Prognosis
   Intact survival is unlikely in neonatal meningitis unless the diagnosis is made early and treatment effective. Mortality is in the general area of 30%, with well over half the survivors demonstrating some residual neurologic change.

SELECTED REFERENCES

Amiel, C.: Intraventricular hemorrhages in the premature infant, Biol. Neonate **7**:57, 1964.

Gary, O. P., Ackerman, A., and Fraser, A. J.: Intracranial hemorrhage and clotting defects in low birth weight infants, Lancet **1**:545, 1968.

McInerney, T. K., and Schubert, W. K.: Prognosis of neonatal seizures, Am. J. Dis. Child. **117**: 261, 1969.

Rose, A. L., and Lombroso, C. T.: Neonatal seizure states: a study of clinical, pathological, and electroencephalographic features in 137 full-term babies with a long-term follow-up, Pediatrics **45**:404, 1970.

Towbin, A.: Central nervous system damage in the human fetus and newborn infant, Am. J. Dis Child. **119**:529, 1970.

23

Hematologic emergencies

ANEMIA

Pallor, although a common sign of asphyxia or illness, usually is due to anemia (often secondary to blood loss) occurring before, during, or after delivery.

A hematocrit reading taken after birth is a valuable base-line measurement in potential blood loss. The initial value is usually higher than the cord level, depending on the volume of placental transfusion and the degree of sludging in the tissues (stasis usually from chilling). Any fall in hematocrit value in the first few hours of life is an indication of acute blood loss.

1. Early anemia
   a. Causes
      1. Blood loss before or during birth is usually due to
         a. Fetomaternal transfusion
         b. Occult bleeding from tearing of aberrant fetal vessels leading from the cord to the placenta (velamentous insertion of the cord)
         c. Placental tearing or membrane laceration (placenta previa, vasa previa, respectively)
         d. Placenta transection at cesarean section
         e. Twin-to-twin transfusion (parabiotic twins)
         f. Rupture of spleen or tear of capsule of liver
      2. Blood loss after birth can occur from
         a. Holding of the infant above the level of placenta with cord unclamped
         b. Birth trauma with loss of blood into the infant's own body spaces, for example, intracranial hemorrhage, multiple cephalohematoma, and subcapsular hemorrhage of the liver
         c. Slipped tie from cord stump
         d. Coagulation defects from insufficient clot-forming factors such as thromboplastin and prothrombin, which are synthesized in the liver and dependent on vitamin K for production
         e. Thrombocytopenia from maternal platelet antigen sensitization
         f. Coagulation defects produced by maternal ingestion of drugs such as coumarin
      3. Hemolytic diseases include
         a. Erythroblastosis fetalis
         b. Spherocytosis and congenital nonspherocytic hemolytic anemia
         c. Drug-induced disorders such as may be caused by vitamin K analogs given in excess to the mother or the infant
         d. Glucose-6-phosphate dehydrogenase deficiency and other red blood cell enzyme defects

b. Treatment
   1. Transfuse
      a. Immediately after birth if the neonate is pale, hypotonic, and shocked
      b. During the first 24 hours if the infant's hematocrit value is below 30% to 35% (10 to 12 gm of hemoglobin, higher levels for distressed infants). Infants with RDS should be transfused at levels of less than 45% (hemoglobin under 14 gm/100 ml)
      c. Toward the end of the first week if the hematocrit value is below 25% to 30% (8 to 10 gm of hemoglobin)
   2. Do serial hematocrit readings
      a. Every 60 minutes for suspected blood loss, since a measurable progressive fall (from plasma dilution) indicates blood loss and the possible necessity of transfusion
      b. Every other day after exchange transfusion until stabilized
2. Delayed anemia
   a. Causes
      1. Physiologic anemia of prematurity (after the age of 4 weeks)
         a. The premature baby begins life with a hemoglobin level comparable to that of the term infant. The postnatal fall is exaggerated by a
            (1) Greater percentage of body growth
            (2) Somewhat shorter red blood cell life-span
            (3) Delay in onset of erythropoiesis
         b. The more immature premature will show an hematocrit value fall to as low as 20% to 25% (6 to 8 gm of hemoglobin) by 6 to 7 weeks of age. At this time a rapid increase in reticulo-

cytes checks this fall, raising the total hemoglobin mass, and finally the hemoglobin level itself.
      2. Infection
      3. Blood loss (chronic)
      4. Insufficient exogenous iron, usually after 2 months of age
      5. Vitamin E deficiency
   b. Treatment and prevention
      1. Administer 2 mg/kg elemental iron orally daily for prevention of iron-deficiency anemia by 2 months of age.
      2. Give 20 to 30 mg elemental iron orally daily for treatment of iron-deficiency anemia.
      3. Provide 25 IU of Aquasol E daily to preterm infants under 1,500 gm.

POLYCYTHEMIA

Polycythemia is diagnosed in the first week of life when the *venous** hematocrit is over 65% or hemoglobin is over 22 gm/100 ml. The symptoms reported below may not occur but are usually the result of hyperviscosity of blood with decreased flow.

1. Associations
   a. Hypervolemia from excessive placental transfusion, fetomaternal transfusion, or twin-to-twin transfusion
   b. Increased erythropoiesis resulting in a high amount of hemoglobin and occurring in small-for-dates infants, those with dysmaturity, and those who have chronic fetal distress
2. Symptoms (indicating hyperviscosity)
   a. Lethargy
   b. Poor feeding
   c. Hyperbilirubinemia
   d. Cardiac decompensation
   e. Grunting respirations (hypervolemia)

*Hematocrit and hemoglobin values may differ significantly, depending on the source of the sample; heel-stick values usually are 5% to 10% higher than "central" samples obtained through a catheter or by venipuncture.

f. Cyanosis

g. Seizures

3. Management

    a. Perform partial exchange transfusion (approximately 20 ml/kg) with fresh frozen plasma for infants with *venous** hematocrit over 70%.

    b. Treat similarly infants with hematocrit over 65% having any of the above symptoms.

    c. Lower hematocrit into the range of 55%.

PETECHIAL AND ECCHYMOTIC HEMORRHAGES
Thrombocytopenia

The clinical expression of thrombocytopenia in the neonate is dramatic and extensive. Unlike the occasional petechiae visible on the scalp and face of an otherwise normal infant after vaginal delivery, petechial hemorrhages of thrombocytopenia are visible over the entire body. Platelets are usually below 50,000/mm³ and are often less than 10,000/mm³.

1. Associations

    a. Overwhelming infections (e.g., cytomegalovirus infection, rubella, toxoplasmosis, herpes virus infection, and bacterial sepsis)

    b. Severe erythroblastosis fetalis

    c. Platelet depletion after repeated exchange transfusions

    d. Maternal drugs inducing thrombocytopenia in the fetus (e.g., thiazides)

    e. Autoimmune thrombocytopenia

    f. Congenital leukemia

    g. Disseminated intravascular coagulation

2. Management

Besides specific treatment, such as antibiotics in sepsis, platelet transfusions may reduce the bleeding tendency.

---

*Hematocrit and hemoglobin values may differ significantly, depending on the source of the sample; heel-stick values usually are 5% to 10% higher than "central" samples obtained through a catheter or by venipuncture.

Transfusions are advisable if platelet count is under 10,000/mm³. Complete exchange transfusion with freshly drawn whole blood is another alternative in such cases.

Disseminated intravascular coagulation

Disseminated intravascular coagulation (DIC) is a relatively common disorder in the newborn in which the equilibrium between microclot formation and destruction in the vascular system is disturbed. Thrombocytes are rapidly removed from the circulation, leading to a bleeding diathesis.

1. Causes

    a. Overwhelming infections, viral and bacterial

    b. Respiratory distress syndrome

    c. Shock associated with other disorders

2. Clinical signs

    a. Increased bleeding tendency (e.g., from heel-sticks)

    b. Bleeding from umbilicus, trachea, or gastrointestinal tract

3. Diagnostic aids

The consumption of clotting factors in DIC leads to abnormalities in the coagulation system. The disorder should be strongly suspected if the following associations are found:

    a. Decreased numbers of platelets

    b. Evidence of red blood cell damage on smear (e.g., schistocytes)

    c. Prolonged partial thromboplastic time

    d. Prolonged prothrombin time

    e. Fibrinogen deficiency

    f. Evidence of fibrin-degradation products

4. Management

    a. Therapy should be directed against the primary cause (sepsis, shock, etc.).

    b. The use of repeated exchange transfusions with fresh heparinized blood may be preferable to heparinization (100 mg/kg/4 hr) of the infant.

    c. Platelet transfusions may aid in decreasing the bleeding tendency when the infant's thrombocyte count is under 10,000/mm³.

Vitamin K deficiency

The ability of a neonate to synthesize and utilize vitamin K is dependent on gestational as well as chronologic age. Lack of vitamin K or impaired liver function leads to impaired synthesis of factors II, VII, IX, and X and to increasing bleeding tendency in a neonate evident in a prolonged prothrombin time. The prothrombin time normally is prolonged during the first 3 to 4 days in term infants and the first 10 to 14 days in preterm infants.

1. Causes
   a. Antibiotic treatment eliminating the normal gastrointestinal flora
   b. Diarrhea and malabsorption
   c. Deficient intake of vitamin K when the infant is fed with certain commercial milks
   d. Lack of vitamin K supplementation during prolonged parenteral fluid therapy
2. Management
   Administer vitamin K_1 (not vitamin K analogs, which may cause hyperbilirubinemia), 0.5 to 1 mg, after birth to every neonate; also administer when vitamin K deficiency is suspected at these times.

HYPERBILIRUBINEMIA

Bilirubin is one of the breakdown products of hemoglobin from hemolyzed red blood cells. During fetal life, bilirubin is cleared through the placenta. Jaundice in the newborn is most often caused when normally formed bilirubin overwhelms the conjugation system in its glycuronyl transfer into a water-soluble form suitable for excretion by the liver. If untreated, 10% to 20% of the prematurely born will have a peak bilirubin level greater than 15 mg/100 ml at 4 to 7 days of age and will be at risk of kernicterus.

1. Conditions associated with increased bilirubin levels

a. Factors influencing hemolysis
   1. Physiologic factors
      a. Rate of blood cell destruction (1% to 1.4%/24 hr, depending on the percentage of fetal hemoglobin—each gram yields 35 mg of bilirubin)
      b. Degree of immaturity of the liver
      c. Amount of additional blood received from the placenta
   2. Erythroblastosis fetalis
   3. Enclosed hemorrhage, for example, cephalhematoma, ecchymosis from bruising (breech delivery), ingestion of placental or maternal blood with melena
   4. Congenital red blood cell abnormality with hemolysis (spherocytosis)
   5. Congenital enzyme deficiency, that is, glucose-6-phosphate dehydrogenase deficiency, hexokinase deficiency, galactosemia
   6. Drug-induced hemolytic anemia mediated through an enzyme deficiency, that is, vitamin K analog to mother or infant
   7. Infection-induced hemolysis
b. Factors delaying or interfering with bilirubin conjugation into the soluble or "direct" form
   1. Metabolic factors such as asphyxia, hypoglycemia, hypothermia, or decreased thyroid activity
   2. The maternal steroid pregnane-3-alpha, 20 beta-diol, a normal hormone in the mother excreted in human milk
   3. Drugs, for example, novobiocin
   4. Familial nonhemolytic icterus (Crigler-Najjar syndrome)
c. Factors that compete or interfere with the albumin-binding site for bilirubin, thus making free bilirubin available for cerebral entry
   The infant is thus at increased risk of kernicterus at lower levels of serum bilirubin

1. Metabolic acidosis
2. Drugs such as long-acting sulfa drugs, salicylates, tranquilizers
3. Free fatty acids
4. Hyperosmolarity
5. Low albumin levels

    d. Factors that lead to impaired excretion of conjugated bilirubin and cause delayed jaundice

Water-soluble conjugated or direct bilirubin is not encephalotoxic and does not enter brain tissue. Many physicians subtract the "direct" bilirubin from total bilirubin in judging the need for exchange transfusion, particularly after the fourth day of life.

    1. Hepatitis caused by viral, bacterial, protozoal, or toxic agents
    2. Biliary duct obstruction (congenital or due to inspissation); malformation of bile canaliculi

2. Diagnostic approach to unexpected jaundice
    a. Complete family and pregnancy history, including breast feeding as well as physicial examination
    b. Capillary blood for "direct" and "indirect" bilirubin level
    c. Peripheral smear for evidence of red blood cell immaturity and variations in morphology
    d. Coombs' test and Hemantigen screen; blood typing of mother and baby
    e. Observation and appropriate cultures for suspected infection
    f. Special tests for enzyme deficiencies and galactosemia when indicated

3. Phototherapy

Light therapy reduces peak serum levels of unconjugated bilirubin as much as 25% to 50%. This is of significant importance, since there is convincing evidence that a serum bilirubin level below the traditional "20 mg/100 ml of safe level" can be toxic to human brain cells, particularly in the acidotic premature infant.

Lamps emitting a high percentage of light, of approximately 450 mμ, are the most effective. By phototherapy, bilirubin is photooxidized to biliverdin, then to secondary yellow pigments, and finally to colorless and presumably nontoxic compounds. The precise intensity of illumination to be used in phototherapy is inexact but can be better expressed in quantity of radiant power for specific wavelengths (milliwatts/cm^2 or flux) than footcandles. The energy drop-off of the various lights available on the market differs considerably. Although long-lasting special blue lamps have a more efficient output of energy in the desired wavelengths, their color makes evaluation of cyanosis in an infant difficult. For this reason we prefer the less effective Vita-Lite tubes, which also have a good energy output for about 1,000 hours but create a more natural light.

Continuous exposure of the unclothed infant to fluorescent white light generally is recommended. The eyes should be protected from the light rays to prevent corneal and retinal damage. There is little question that phototherapy has reduced markedly the number of infants who have required exchange transfusions. After 10 years' use, significant evidence is lacking to indicate that the potential benefits do not far outweigh the possible hazards.

    a. Indications
    1. Very premature infants who show bruising, at first sign of jaundice
    2. Preterm infants who may have had asphyxia, at first sign of jaundice
    3. Preterm infants with a bilirubin level over 10 mg/100 ml, term infants with a bilirubin level over 15 mg/100 ml, or infants who show jaundice in the first 24 hours of life while undergoing a diagnostic work-up
    4. Infants with hyperbilirubinemia who have known sepsis and hemolytic disease and who are under clinical control

5. Infants with severe hyaline membrane disease

b. Observations to be made on infants receiving phototherapy
   1. Determine bilirubin level every 12 hours (degree of bilirubinemia cannot be estimated from skin color) and 12 hours after discontinuance of phototherapy (rebound effect).
   2. Monitor infant's temperature frequently.
   3. Perform hematocrit reading during and after phototherapy for unexpected anemia.

c. Advantages
   1. Markedly limits the number of primary exchange transfusions in nonspecific hyperbilirubinemia and decreases the number of secondary exchanges in erythroblastosis
   2. Reduces the chance of kernicterus in some premature infants who are at greater risk with lower serum values of bilirubin
   3. Shortens the period in which bilirubin determinations are necessary

d. Hazards
   1. The suppression of jaundice may limit an important sign of sepsis, hemolytic disease, or hepatitis.
   2. Higher levels of bilirubin than are suggested by skin color may be present.
   3. Although the bilirubin rise in mild erythroblastosis may be controlled, hemolysis continues and may be followed by unrecognized anemia.
   4. Damage to the retina may occur without eye protection.
   5. An increase in the infant's body temperature may require adjustments in incubator control.
   6. Dehydration from increased evaporation through skin.
   7. Thermistors in incubators equipped with a Servo-Control should be screened from direct radiation.
   8. Plastic shields should protect infants in radiant warmers.

EXCHANGE TRANSFUSION

1. Indications for exchange transfusion
   a. Immediate exchange (usually a partial exchange) for infants with severe erythroblastosis who suffer from anemia (hematocrit value under 30%), shock, and edema.
   b. Early exchange for infants with a

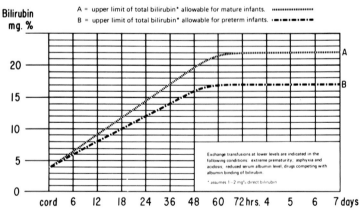

Fig. 23-1. Guide for predicting the need for exchange transfusion on basis of rate of rise and peak levels of bilirubin.

positive Coombs' test and occasionally for those with an ABO incompatibility who have the following findings in addition

1. Cord bilirubin of at least 4 mg/100 ml
2. Jaundice developing in the first 6 hours
3. Hemoglobin less than 12 gm (hematocrit value of 40%) at birth
4. Marked reticulocytosis (over 7%)

A reduced hemoglobin value or an increase in immature red blood cell forms is supportive evidence but is not diagnostic of hemolytic disease of the newborn.

c. Criteria for late exchange transfusion on the basis of unconjugated (indirect) serum bilirubin values

By plotting bilirubin estimations longitudinally as in Fig. 23-1, one can predict the peak of the curve and the infant's need for therapy (phototherapy or exchange transfusion).

No longer is 20 mg/100 ml a precise and safe level for maintaining an upper limit for the bilirubin level. Each infant's treatment must be considered individually. The risk of brain damage is dependent on the degree of prematurity, the amount of unbound bilirubin, the level of acidosis, and the state of hydration and nutrition.

Measurement of the bilirubin-binding capacity of the plasma is of value for the determination of the risk of kernicterus and the need for exchange. Unfortunately, too few centers have defined its precise clinical relationship, and therefore its practicality for most hospitals remains uncertain.

d. Immediate and early exchange transfusions are performed to
   1. Increase the amount of hemoglobin.
   2. Remove a significant number of sensitized cells.

e. Later exchanges are aimed at the removal of free unbound indirect bilirubin for the prevention of kernicterus (p. 208).

2. Type of blood used
   a. Fresh blood less than 48 hours old to assure optimal red blood cell survival.
   b. Blood that contains no antibody to the infant's red blood cells, that is, Rh-negative blood for infants with Rh-positive red blood cells, or blood containing little or no anti-A or anti-B for infants with an ABO incompatibility ("low" titer type) blood, or red cells of the infant's type resuspended in fresh A-B plasma.
   c. Blood with an appropriate hematocrit level, that is, packed or slightly packed cells for infants who are anemic.

3. When the bilirubin level is excessive (usually over 20 mg/100 ml)
   a. Give 1 gm/kg of salt-poor albumin 60 minutes before the exchange.
   b. Follow the exchange with the same therapy—1 gm binds 16 mg of bilirubin. *Warning:* An increase in venous pressure may be a contraindication because protein has a hyperosmolar effect and expands blood volume.

4. Technique of exchange transfusion
   a. Add 10 ml of $NaHCO_3$ (1 ml = 0.9 mEq) or 10 millimoles of 1.2 molar tromethamine (THAM) to each unit of ACD blood when the infant is in a precarious metabolic state. One unit of tromethamine (36 gm) + 250 ml of 5% glucose = 1.2 molar solution (8 ml = 9.6 millimoles).
   b. Use heating coil for warming blood to body temperature.
   c. Prevent cooling of infant during the procedure, preferably by placing him under radiant heat.

d. Restrain adequately infant's extremities

e. Place a radiopaque catheter into an umbilical vessel (Chapter 7), assuring proper position (thoracic inferior vena cava, thoracic aorta, aortic bifurcation) by obtaining x-ray films.

f. Attach 3-way stopcock and syringe to proximal end of catheter (disposable exchange transfusion sets contain all necessary attachments).

g. Monitor pressures (central venous or arterial) keep venous pressures between 5 and 12 cm H_2O. Keep arterial pressures in normal range (Chapter 20).

h. At the beginning of the exchange, obtain blood from catheter for hematocrit and bilirubin determinations.

i. Keep an accurate record during the exchange transfusion, noting each successive amount of blood removed and replaced, vital signs of infant, and drugs given.

j. Monitor infant's cardiac rate and electrocardiogram (if possible) continuously.

k. Observe respirations and skin color, as well as the color of the withdrawn blood.

l. Maintain the infant's blood temperature and oxygen requirements.

m. Inject 0.5 ml of calcium gluconate, diluted with saline solution, slowly after each 100 ml of blood is exchanged.

　1. Calcium lessens general irritability and irregularity of the heart.

　2. Too rapid an injection slows the heart.

n. Exchange at least 170 ml of blood/kg of body weight.

o. Consider hypoglycemia in erythroblastosis and screen with the Dextrostix test, if the baby's condition is less than excellent.

p. Obtain blood for determination of hematocrit and bilirubin levels at the end of procedure. Consider preparing a new unit of blood for a possible repeat exchange

5. Complications of exchange transfusions

a. Heart failure from hypervolemia or hypovolemia

b. Bradycardia or cardiac arrest from low pH of donor blood (acidosis), hyperkalemia (old blood), rapid injection of calcium, or faulty catheter position

c. Hypocalcemia from citrate binding

d. Hypothermia and increased blood viscosity from cold blood or external chilling

e. Air emboli entering the heart from air leaks in the system or suction through the catheter when a negative venous pressure develops on sudden inspiratory effort

f. Thrombotic emboli entering the pulmonary vein

g. Sepsis from an infected cord stump or contaminated equipment

h. Intensification of hypoglycemia (Be prepared to give 5 ml of 20% glucose, followed by a glucose infusion.)

i. Thrombocyte depletion after repeated exchange transfusions

Although the above complications may be encountered as infrequently as in 1% of exchange transfusions, their occurrence varies with the experience of the team preparing this procedure and therefore should be undertaken by persons thoroughly familiar with this technique.

OTHER METHODS OF LOWERING BILIRUBIN LEVELS

Therapy with phenobarbital has been advocated on the principle that hepatic enzyme induction is enhanced by increasing Y and Z protein synthesis, which will raise bilirubin uptake into the hepatocyte. The slowness of action, however (approximately 2 weeks), limits the usefulness of this drug for most cases of neonatal hyperbilirubinemia.

Administration of agar similarly is of little

value, and trials comparing either agar or phenobarbital with phototherapy still prove the latter to be significantly more effective.

SELECTED REFERENCES

Amiel, C.: Intraventricular hemorrhages in the premature infant, Biol. Neonate **7**:57, 1964.

Behrman, R. E., Brown, A. K., Currie, M. R., Hastings, J. W., Odell, G. B., Schaffer, R., Setlow, R. B., Vogl, T. P., and Wurtman, R. J.: Preliminary report of the committee on phototherapy in the newborn infant, J. Pediatr. **84**:135, 1974.

Cremer, R. J., Perryman, P. W., Richards, D. H.: Influence of light on the hyperbilirubinemia of infants, Lancet **1**:1094, 1958.

Dallman, P. R.: Iron, vitamin E, and folate in the preterm infant, J. Pediatr. **85**:742, 1974.

Gary, O. P., Ackerman, A., and Fraser, A. J.: Intracranial hemorrhage and clotting defects in low birth weight infants, Lancet **1**:545, 1968.

Giunta, F., and Rath, J.: Effect of environmental illumination in prevention of hyperbilirubinemia of prematurity, Pediatrics **44**:162, 1969.

Goldman, H. I., and Amadio, P.: Vitamin K deficiency after the newborn period, Pediatrics **44**:745, 1969.

Hathaway, W. E., Mull, M. M., and Pechet, G. S.: Disseminated intravascular coagulation in the newborn, Pediatrics **43**:233, 1969.

Klein, R. M.: Shedding light on the use of light, Pediatrics **50**:118, 1972.

Lucey, J., Ferreiro, M., and Hewitt, J.: Prevention of hyperbilirubinemia of prematurity by phototherapy, Pediatrics **41**:1047, 1968.

Maurer, H. M., Shumway, C. N., Draper, D. A., and Hossaini, A. A.: Controlled trial comparing agar, intermittent phototherapy, and continuous phototherapy for reducing neonatal hyperbilirubinemia, J. Pediatr. **82**:73, 1973.

Pierson, W. E., Barrett, C. T., and Oliver, T. K., Jr.: The effect of buffered and non-buffered ACD blood on electrolyte and acid-base homeostasis during exchange transfusion, Pediatrics **41**:802, 1968.

Silberberg, D. H., Johnson, L., and Ritter, L.: Factors influencing toxicity of bilirubin in cerebellum tissue culture, J. Pediatr. **77**:386, 1970.

Sisson, T. R. C., Kendall, N., Glauser, S. C., Knutson, S., and Bunyaviroch, E.: Phototherapy of jaundice in newborn infants. I. ABO blood group incompatibility, J. Pediatr. **79**:904, 1971.

Stiehm, E. R., and Clatanoff, D. V.: Split products of fibrin in the serum of newborns, Pediatrics **43**:770, 1969.

24

Metabolic emergencies

The premature infant is less able to maintain physiologic homeostasis than is the full-term infant. Nevertheless, in the absence of stress, the immature infant may control body chemistry within very narrow ranges. An exception is in hydrogen ion control. Pulmonary and kidney function have a limited reserve in their capacities for this function. Respiratory and metabolic acidosis may often occur.

The kidneys are anatomically deficient in their complement of glomeruli and tubular components until after 35 weeks of gestational age. In addition to a limitation in the excretion of acid, the premature infant is handicapped in the ability to concentrate and dilute, clear urea, and excrete phosphate when he is faced with heavy feeding loads or stressed by fluid restrictions.

Many enzyme systems of the immature infant are developed only in proportion to gestational age, for example, the conjugation of bilirubin, the regulation of blood glucose, and the metabolization of tyrosine. Nevertheless, these enzymatic and organ systems, faced with the challenge of early extrauterine life, may mature in advance of their biologic time clock.

TRANSIENT HYPOGLYCEMIA OF THE NEWBORN

Early hypoglycemia (first 3 days of life) is a blood glucose level under 30 mg/100 ml in term infants and 20 mg/100 ml in low birth weight infants. This disorder prevails among preterm infants and especially those suffering from intrauterine growth retardation. Symptomatic hypoglycemia is a preventable syndrome and may damage as many as 5,000 infants born each year in the United States. Persistent hypoglycemia is rare.

1. Incidence
   a. About 5% to 10% of low birth weight infants have hypoglycemia.
   b. Two to 3/1,000 of all infants born may have symptomatic hypoglycemia.
2. Pathogenesis
   a. Decreased rate of entry of glucose into the blood, usually from insufficient glycogen and fat stores, for example, in infants, who are premature, dysmature, the smaller twin, or born of toxemic mothers
   b. Increased rate of removal of blood glucose, which occurs in the following conditions:
      1. Asphyxial conditions, including primary apnea and cerebral injury
      2. Hypothermia
      3. Hyaline membrane disease (breathing effort and asphyxia)
      4. Hypermetabolism (the undergrown infant with increased cell numbers per unit of weight)
   c. Interruption of glucose infusions
      1. During exchange transfusions
      2. During blood transfusions
      3. Infiltration or discontinuance of infusion (rebound hypoglycemia)
3. Signs

a. Irritability, tremors, eye-rolling, seizures, and coma
b. Apnea and cyanosis
c. Listlessness and poor feeding

4. Diagnosis

Blood glucose determinations (checked) are below 20 mg/100 ml in low birth weight infants and 30 mg/100 ml in term infants. The glucose level will drop 18 mg/100 ml/hr in a specimen not processed properly. In order to obtain accurate results, analyze specimen at once or do one of the following to stabilize the glucose content:
a. Place sample in ice.
b. Centrifuge off red blood cells.
c. Add sodium fluoride.

5. Management

a. Give 2 to 4 ml/kg of a 25% glucose solution intravenously.
b. Continue infusion of 10% to 15% glucose solution at 80 ml/kg/24 hr.
c. Add 2 to 3 ml of 10% calcium gluconate and 2 to 3 mEq of sodium chloride/100 ml of infused fluid.
d. Feed the infant when he is asymptomatic.
e. Reduce parenteral glucose gradually after blood glucose levels have remained over 50 mg/100 ml and feedings have been established (never reduce infusion abruptly, or a hypoglycemic reaction may result).
f. Give hydrocortisone, 5 mg/kg of body weight, or ACTH (4 units every 12 hours), if blood glucose fails to rise above 30 mg/100 ml after 6 hours or if symptoms of hypoglycemia persist.
g. Monitor therapy with longitudinal blood glucose determinations.

6. Prevention

a. Identify these groups of infants at birth susceptible to hypoglycemia:
1. Undergrown and/or undernourished infants (below the 10th percentile of the Lubchenco grid [Fig. 3-3])
2. Premature infants, particularly those under 2,000 gm at birth or suffering from hyaline membrane disease
3. Infants subjected to fetal distress and asphyxia during labor and delivery
4. Infants born after prolonged gestation, especially those showing signs of dysmaturity (peeling of skin with loss of subcutaneous fatty tissue)
b. Test these infants by means of the Dextrostix method at 2, 8, 16, 24, 48, and 72 hours of age; more frequent tests are needed if levels are in the low range (under 50 mg/100 ml). If Dextrostix shows barely perceptible blue coloration or no color (indicating a level around or below 25 mg/100 ml), confirm this result by obtaining a blood sample for determination of glucose level by the laboratory. Manage confirmed levels of under 30 mg/100 ml for term and preterm infants by parenteral administration of glucose.
c. Offer early feeding (at 2 hours of age) to infants at risk for hypoglycemia and continue feeding at 3-hour intervals, preferably with a 24-calorie/30 ml formula after the first feeding of 10% dextrose has been tolerated (p. 188).

HYPOGLYCEMIA OF INFANTS WITH ERYTHROBLASTOSIS FETALIS

Erythroblastosis fetalis, for reasons not known, is accompanied by hyperplasia of the islands of Langerhans in the pancreas, and hypoglycemia is observed on occasion. Hyperinsulinemia similar to that in the infant of a diabetic mother apparently is the cause of hypoglycemia that typically occurs on the first day of life or after an exchange transfusion with citrated blood. The incidence of hypoglycemia is higher in infants with more severe disease.

1. Treatment
   Confirmed hypoglycemia should be managed as previously suggested.
2. Prevention
   a. Monitor blood glucose by Dextrostix, as suggested for infants of diabetic mothers.
   b. Feed infants early and frequently to ensure good caloric and carbohydrate intake.
   c. Ensure constant glucose infusion during, and especially several hours after, an exchange transfusion with citrated blood to prevent rebound hypoglycemia.

INFANTS OF MOTHERS WITH DIABETES (IDM) AND "GESTATIONAL DIABETES"

The failing competence of the placenta often observed after 36 weeks of gestation adds a factor of fetal deprivation to some infants, not to mention the chance of fetal death (Chapter 18).

1. Complications
   The increased morbidity and neonatal mortality are based on the following complications:
   a. Hyaline membrane disease, the most important complication, may have its genesis in the increased exposure to intrauterine asphyxia, the method of delivery (cesarean section in preterm infants), and a disordered metabolic state. Tachypnea, not always due to hyaline membrane disease, is recognized in as many as 50% of infants of diabetic and prediabetic mothers. Delayed maturation of the fetal lung (in Class A, B, and C diabetic mothers) is another factor explaining the occurrence of hyaline membrane disease in infants delivered close to term.
   b. Hypoglycemia due to temporary hyperinsulinism (a response of the normal fetal pancreas to the higher maternal glucose level; infants of mothers whose glucose levels during the last 2 months of pregnancy were maintained in the normal range have less hyperinsulinism) should be suspected in
      1. Infants of diabetic mothers
      2. Infants of mothers with gestational diabetes
      3. Infants oversized for their gestation or having the appearance of an "IDM," that is, soft skin, abundance of subcutaneous fatty tissue, and round "tomato" face, as well as being large for gestational age
   More than 50% of IDMs have hypoglycemia, a fall in blood glucose levels below 30 mg/100 ml. Up to 10% of all infants have symptoms of hypoglycemia, tremors, apnea and cyanosis, and seizures. Usually blood glucose levels return to normal by 8 hours of age, but persistent hypoglycemia may continue with fetal malnutrition.
   c. Lethal congenital anomalies occur in 2% to 3% of all infants of diabetic mothers.
   d. Hypocalcemia and hypomagnesemia, with a symptomatology indistinguishable from hypoglycemia, may occur.
   e. Hyperbilirubinemia, hyperkalemia, and hyperphosphatemia may be seen.
2. Treatment
   a. Have competent assistance at delivery.
   b. Resuscitate the infant promptly, with maintenance of warmth, support of blood volume, and correction of metabolic acidosis.
   c. Offer full incubator care, regardless of the infant's weight.
   d. Feed 10% glucose every 2 hours times 3, then formula if tolerated.
   e. Screen hourly with Dextrostix for 8 hours, then every 4 hours until 24 hours of age.
   f. A confirmed serum glucose level be-

low 30 mg/100 ml requires administration of parenteral glucose.

g. Offer continuous parenteral infusion of 10% to 15% dextrose (80 ml/kg/24 hr) to any infant whose mother has established diabetes and who suffered from asphyxia during labor and delivery or shows signs of respiratory distress. Continue infusion until infant has sufficient oral intake; then gradually taper rate of infusion.

HYPERGLYCEMIA

Hyperglycemia indicates a serum glucose level over 125 mg/100 ml. This not infrequent disorder usually is transient. Because glucose easily enters the brain, generalized swelling and possible damage may occur. Hyperglycemia also will lead to osmotic diuresis secondary to glycosuria, and dehydration may ensue.

1. Factors associated with hyperglycemia
   a. Extreme prematurity
      The immature infant in the first few days of life frequently demonstrates intolerance to rapid infusion of dextrose solutions. Because of increased insensible water loss, these infants often require large amounts of parenteral fluid to avoid excessive weight loss. Infusions of over 0.4 gm/kg/hr (i.e., 100 ml of 10% glucose/kg/24 hr) may not be metabolized by the immature infant in this early period.
   b. Severe stress (e.g., septic shock or severe RDS with shock)
      Transient hyperglycemia not infrequently accompanies these diseases and normally improves as the primary condition is controlled.
   c. Rapid infusion of dextrose solution
      As infants are treated for dehydration or shock, and fluids are administered rapidly, hyperglycemia may result, especially when 10% dextrose is used.
2. Treatment

If hyperglycemia is observed, reduce glucose load by decreasing the rate of glucose infusion or the concentration of glucose solution administered.

3. Prevention
   a. Check urine glucose every 4 to 8 hours with Clinistix.
   b. Perform Dextrostix test if 1+ or more.
   c. Reduce glucose load if blood glucose values exceed 130 mg/100 ml.
   d. Limit glucose infusion rate to 0.3 to 0.4 gm/kg/hr in the small preterm infant in the first days of life.

HYPONATREMIA

Hyponatremia indicates a serum sodium level under 125 mEq/L. It produces damage to the central nervous system due to an increase in brain volume.

1. Factors associated with hyponatremia
   a. Asphyxiation or severe RDS due to inappropriate secretion of antidiuretic hormone (ADH), with loss of sodium in the urine
   b. Water intoxication
   c. Certain oliguric states
   d. Diarrhea
   e. Adrenal insufficiency
   f. Treatment of the mother with low-salt diets and diuretics
2. Symptoms
   a. Lethargy
   b. Apneic episodes
   c. Shock
3. Treatment
   a. Over a 6- to 24-hour period administer a quantity of sodium in mEq equal to 60% × kilograms of body weight × mEq of the serum sodium deficit below 135 mEq/L.
   b. Recheck the serum sodium level.
   c. Limit fluid intake if inappropriate secretion of ADH is suspected.

HYPERNATREMIA

Hypernatremia indicates a serum sodium level over 148 mEq/L and is dangerous because it causes a shift of water away from the brain (since sodium does not cross readily into the central nervous system). This leads to pressure differences within the system, causing dilatation and possible rupture of capillaries in the brain. Occasionally this condition leads to acute tubular necrosis.

1. Etiology
   a. Excessive sodium administration, especially of sodium bicarbonate during resuscitation and treatment of acidosis
   b. Insufficient fluid administration
   c. Dehydration due to increased insensible water loss of the small preterm infant or to hyperthermia or diarrhea
2. Symptoms
   a. Lethargy
   b. Extreme irritability on stimulation
   c. Seizures
3. Treatment
   a. Reduce serum sodium values slowly (24 to 48 hours).
   b. Replace any fluid deficit (over 10% of body weight) with as much as 100 ml/kg of 5% glucose containing 4 mEq/kg of NaCl in the first 24 hours. Plain glucose solution encourages brain edema and cerebrovascular complications.
   c. Gradually reduce volume and electrolytes to approximately maintenance requirements (125 to 170 ml/kg/24 hr, with 2 to 3 mEq/kg/24 hr of sodium, potassium, and chloride on the basis of serial electrolyte determinations).

HYPOCALCEMIA

Approximately 30% of preterm infants weighing less than 2,000 gm at birth have serum calcium levels of less than 7 mg/100 ml before 48 hours of age.

1. Factors predisposing infants to hypocalcemia
   a. Relative hypoparathyroidism caused by suppressed function of the fetal parathyroid from transferred maternal parathyroid hormone

This function improves gradually after birth.
   b. Decreased renal capacity for phosphorus excretion
   This handicap is accentuated with increased phosphorus loads, such as in infants who are fed cow's milk. Phosphorus retention depresses serum calcium levels, leading to the classical neonatal tetany seen at 6 or 7 days of life.
   c. Preterm delivery, rendering the infant deficient in calcium
   Sluggish response of parathyroid activity and renal immaturity are accentuated.
2. Factors further adding to the risk of hypocalcemia
   a. Stress such as asphyxia, which tends to cause increased corticosteroid and thyrocalcitonin release, which may result in lowered serum calcium
   b. Treatment of acidosis with bicarbonate, which tends to decrease the ionized portion of serum calcium
   c. Exchange transfusions with citrated blood, temporarily causing binding of serum calcium with citrate
   d. Low calcium intakes, especially seen in prolonged parenteral infusion if insufficient calcium is given
3. Symptoms commonly observed
   a. Twitching of extremities
   b. Jitteriness, especially during handling of infant
   c. High-pitched cry
   d. Seizures
   e. Prolonged Q-T segment on electrocardiogram
4. Diagnosis
   a. Serum calcium level under 7 mg/100 ml (3.5 mEq/L)
   b. Corresponding rise in serum phosphorus to over 8 mg/100 ml
5. Treatment
   a. Symptomatic infants or infants not receiving oral feedings should receive 1 to 2 ml/kg of 10% calcium gluconate, slowly intravenously. (Con-

tinued requirements may range between 2 and 5 ml/kg/24 hr for several days.)

  b. Nonsymptomatic infants receiving oral feedings: Offer calcium gluconate or calcium lactate, 1 to 3 gm daily in divided doses. Therapy may have to be continued from several days to 2 or 3 weeks and gradually discontinued.

6. Prevention

   Addition of calcium gluconate 3 ml/100 ml of dextrose infusion given to high-risk infants from the first day of life while monitoring serum calcium levels will lessen the incidence of hypocalcemia.

HYPOMAGNESEMIA

1. Blood serum levels are under 1 mEq/L.
2. Incidence is infrequent.
3. Associations are newborns undergoing exchange transfusion (citrate-binding), infants of diabetic mothers, and those who are small for dates.
4. Symptoms are irritable behavior extending into tetany and indistinguishable from hypocalcemia.
5. Suspect when serum calcium levels are low but phosphorus levels are normal.
6. Treat with 0.2 ml/kg of a 50% solution of magnesium sulfate intramuscularly.

HYPERMAGNESEMIA

1. Blood serum levels are over 5 mEq/L.
2. Incidence is infrequent.
3. It is found in infants whose mothers were treated with MgSO₄ for toxemia.
4. The symptoms are profound central nervous system depression with a decrease in sensitivity of motor end plates.

SELECTED REFERENCES

Altstatt, L. B.: Transplacental hyponatremia in the newborn infant, J. Pediatr. 66:985, 1965.

Barrett, C. T., and Oliver, T. K., Jr.: Hypoglycemia and hyperinsulinism in infants with erythroblastosis fetalis, N. Engl. J. Med. 278:1260, 1968.

Battaglia, F. C., Prystowsky, H., Smisson, C., Hellegers, A., and Bruns, P. D.: Fetal blood studies. XIII. The effect of the administration of fluids intravenously to mothers upon the concentrations of water and electrolytes in plasma of the human fetuses, Pediatrics 25:2, 1960.

Campbell, M. A., Ferguson, I. C., Hutchinson, J. H., and Kerr, M. M.: Diagnosis and treatment of hypoglycemia in the newborn, Arch. Dis. Child. 42:353, 1967.

Clarke, P. C. N., and Carre, I. J.: Hypocalcemic hypomagnesemic convulsions, J. Pediatr. 70:806, 1967.

Cornblath, M., Joassin, G., Weisskopf, B., et al.: Hypoglycemia in the newborn, Pediatr. Clin. North Am. 13:905, 1966.

Dweck, H. S., and Cassady, G.: Glucose intolerance in infants of very low risk weight, Pediatrics 53:189, 1974.

Feldman, W., Drummond, K. N., and Klein, M.: Hyponatremia following asphyxia neonatorum, Acta Paediatr. Scand. 59:52, 1970.

Finberg, L.: Hypernatremic dehydration in infants, N. Engl. J. Med. 289:196, 1974.

Griffiths, A. D.: Association of hypoglycaemia with symptoms in the newborn, Arch. Dis. Child. 43:688, 1969.

Lipsitz, P. J., and English, I. C.: Hypermagnesemia in the newborn infant, Pediatrics 40:856, 1967.

Lubchenco, L. D., and Bard, H.: Incidence of hypoglycemia in newborn infants classified by birth weight and gestational age, Pediatrics 47:831, 1971.

Pildes, R. S., Cornblath, M., Warren, I., Page-El, E., di Menza, S., Merritt, D. M., and Peeva, A.: A prospective controlled study of neonatal hypoglycemia, Pediatrics 54:5, 1974.

Raivio, K. O., and Osterlind, K.: Hypoglycemia and hyperinsulinemia associated with erythroblastosis fetalis, Pediatrics 43:217, 1969.

Simmons, M. A., Adcock, E. W., Bard, H., and Battaglia, F. C.: Hyponatremia and intracranial hemorrhage in neonates, N. Engl. J. Med. 291:6, 1974.

Tsang, R. C., Chen, I., Hayes, W., Atkinson, W., Atherton, H., and Edwards, N.: Neonatal hypocalcemia in infants with birth asphyxia, J. Pediatr. 84:428, 1974.

Tsang, R. C., Light, I. J., Sutherland, J. M., and Kleinman, L. I.: Possible pathogenic factors in neonatal hypocalcemia of prematurity, J. Pediatr. 82:423, 1973.

25

Growth and development of the preterm infant

THE PRETERM INFANT
Growth

Growth of the preterm infant dramatically slows from the fetal rate.
1. Weight
   a. Birth weight loss averages 10% to 15% for all weight groups. The low weight is reached at 4 to 6 days of age.
   b. Birth weight is regained in 1 to 3 weeks, depending on maturity and nutritional intake.
   c. Infants suffering fetal undernutrition lose less weight and regain their birth weight more rapidly—especially if they are fed early, they lose no weight at all.
   d. By 40 weeks of postmenstrual age,* body weight is as much as 1,000 gm below that expected had the infant been delivered at term. This discrepancy may be reduced by early feedings.
2. Length
   a. Growth in length slows in the first week of extrauterine life.
   b. Growth at the fetal rate in body

length is resumed about the third week of life if adequate nutrition is available (more than 1 cm/wk).
   c. By 40 weeks of postmenstrual age the very premature infant can be as much as 3 to 5 cm shorter than an infant born at term.
3. Head circumference
   a. A similar lag occurs in the rate of head growth. During the first few days of life many infants' heads will decrease approximately 0.5 cm in circumference, with an accompanying overlapping of the sagittal suture.
   b. The later weekly increment of growth increase is often as much as 0.9 to 1.1 cm. Increase in head size at a rate above 1.2 cm/wk suggests hydrocephalus.
   Not infrequently the rate of head growth of the preterm or small-for-dates infant will surpass that projected for the fetus and for the infant of normal gestation. This temporarily more rapid increase in size, as well as a slight separation of the sutures, may be confused with hydrocephalus. However, the rate of head growth is seldom over 1.3 cm/wk. An increase in transillumination may be noted, along with pitting pedal edema. Salt excess and/or low protein intake may

---

*Postmenstrual age refers to the combined gestational period (fetal) and postnatal age. As in the measurement of gestational age, the time is reckoned from the first day of the last menstrual period. Conception occurs approximately 2 weeks later, a date seldom known.

be responsible for this "pseudo-hydrocephalus," but head growth by 2 months of corrected age will resume an appropriate channel for head size.

4. Cellular growth

Much interest has focused on growth as a function of cell size and/or numbers. Cell division is more active during intra-uterine life, and then gradually slows after birth, depending on the organ system. Each system has its own biologic time clock for growth. Severe limitation in nutrition may reduce cell numbers as well as cell size. Cellular division and growth in the brain is critical before and after birth, and although knowledge of long-term effects of undergrowth in the human fetus and neonate is limited, adequate nutrition should be offered whenever possible during this period.

Development

1. Neuromuscular development
   a. Neurologic development of the pre-term infant appears to keep pace with that of his fetal counterpart in utero, assuming that neither severe limitation in nutrition nor cerebral injury has occurred.
   b. The following longitudinal observations help to establish the infant's postmenstrual age and, in retrospect, substantiate gestational age at birth.
      1. Nipple sucking may be adequate for emptying a bottle by 32 to 33 weeks of postmenstrual age and sufficient for taking all feedings by 33 to 34 weeks.
      2. The infant, in response to elicitation of the Moro reflex, will exhibit an extension of arms, followed by some flexion response, during the thirty-fifth week.
      3. The tonus of the neck muscles may be sufficiently developed so that
         a. At 36 weeks the wakeful infant can hold the head firmly on arm traction.
         b. At 37 weeks the infant can raise the head from the mattress momentarily in the prone position.
      4. After 38 weeks the infant will fix the eyes on the observer's face and follow its movements; in addition the infant will have a vigorous cry, maintain body temperature, and have regular respiration.
      5. After 40 weeks the infant will turn the head in following an object.
2. Enzymatic and organ development

   Early birth and subsequent physiologic demands may cause some functions to mature early, such as
   a. Kidney and gastrointestinal efficiency
   b. Enzymatic conjugation of bilirubin, regulation of glucose metabolism, and metabolization of tyrosine
   c. Immunologic responses
3. Ossification (see p. 32 for appearance of centers in fetal life)

   Ossification centers (on x-ray film) follow a prescribed pattern in their appearance and are useful when present to indicate the level of maturity. Delay in their development and time of appearance occurs in
   a. Immature infants—distal femoral epiphyses may not appear until after 40 weeks of postmenstrual life, in contrast to the usual fetal appearance at 36 to 37 weeks of gestation (2 to 3 mm in diameter).
   b. Malnutrition—the smaller of dissimilar-sized, single-ovum twins invariably has the late-appearing epiphyses.

Neurologic and intellectual deficits

The factors that influence mortality of the fetus and neonate must also increase the chance of problems in the survivor. In general, the lower the birth weight, the greater the incidence of later handicaps. One third to one half of infants weighing under 1,500 gm have been reported to have moderate to severe problems. Although it is likely that fetal asphyxia, trauma, and delay in resuscitation are primarily responsible for most later handicaps, it is now clear that other factors must be considered, including the following:

1. Developmental defects
   a. Greater incidence of anomalies
   b. Relative infertility of some mothers
   c. Poor pregnancy experience, often a continuum of reproductive wastage
2. Postnatal insults that may result from
   a. Delay in instituting nutritional requirements
   b. Biochemical changes, for example, hypoglycemia, hyperbilirubinemia, acidosis
   c. Later asphyxia from complications of early birth, for example, hyaline membrane disease, pneumonia, prolonged apneic periods
3. Low social environment with
   a. Cultural impoverishment
   b. Substandard feeding habits
   c. Increased likelihood of genetic inadequacy
   d. Poor physical and intellectual nurturing and stimulation

Nevertheless, asphyxia is the usual common denominator and carries a substantial but often unpredictable burden for the infant, depending on its severity, duration, and the resistance of the infant (maturity and nutritional state). Prolonged hypoxia can produce definite cerebral lesions (periventricular leukomalacia). However, severe asphyxia per se before or after birth may leave the brain unscathed.

In the monkey, less than 10 minutes of complete postnatal anoxia apparently does little in the way of physical damage to the brain or later behavior. A longer period of anoxia increases the chance of damage, with the certainty of permanent change after 15 minutes of apnea. In human studies, effects from apnea observed after birth are difficult to interpret, since an unknown period of asphyxia is likely to have been present prior to birth.

The complications and problems of infants who were small for dates or oversized at birth are discussed in Chapter 17. The smaller preterm infants, particularly those who weigh under 2,000 gm at birth, will be discussed in this chapter. In addition to these groups, other newborns at risk have a considerably increased chance of impairment in later development. They also require careful longitudinal observations. This miscellaneous group includes infants with (1) fetal asphyxia, prolonged resuscitation, or low Apgar scores; (2) suspected or diagnosed intracranial birth injury; (3) severe respiratory distress or sepsis; (4) neonatal convulsions, irritability or lethargy, and inattention to sound or visual stimuli; (5) suspected or diagnosed congenital malformations, hereditary disease, or fetal infection; and (6) families with serious social or mental health problems.

THE SMALLER PRETERM INFANT

The quality of survivors in the last 5 years or so appears to have improved over the gloomy outlook reported in the past for the very prematurely born infants. The following factors have probably contributed:

1. Identification of fetal distress and appropriate management of the pregnancy to reduce the incidence of fetal asphyxia
2. Regionalization of care in specialized centers
3. More adequate provision of fluids, glucose, and electrolytes from the time of birth
4. Improved temperature control
5. Use of physiologic monitoring
6. Ventilatory assistance

Intellectual development

A reduced intellectual ability of children who were prematurely born in the past is well known, and the more immature at birth, the greater the likelihood of a deficit.

The relationship of prematurity to complications of pregnancy that contribute to asphyxial damage, the greater susceptibility to trauma of the early born, and the delays in feeding and metabolic support may be the factors primarily responsible. The increased frequency of women with a lower socioeconomic background to bear preterm infants and the cultural impoverishment that may be present also play a role in these intellectual deficits. Inadequate school performance may be noted even when intelligence is in the normal range. Nevertheless, there appears to be a definite improvement in the later intellectual functions of the preterm infant who has been supported by full intensive care methods throughout the perinatal period.

Neurologic deficits

In the past, nearly 40% of patients enrolled in cerebral palsy clinics were infants of low birth weight. Over 75% of children with spastic diplegia were born early. Longitudinal osbervations of infants who were very premature at birth have demonstrated in the past that approximately 10% to 15% have some degree of cerebral palsy. However, mental retardation and speech deficiency are not the rule in these children.

The incidence of cerebral palsy and other neurologic defects has been reduced in recent years to about 5%, which suggests improvement in the care of the preterm infant.

The following observations suggest cerebral palsy:
1. History of difficulty in sucking or swallowing
2. Gradual increase in extension tone, such as
   a. Extension of head when ventrally suspended
   b. Resistance to dorsiflexion of feet
   c. Difficulty in sitting alone
   d. Adductor spasm on abduction of legs
   e. Toe walking with tightening of heel cords

3. Asymmetry of movements, particularly in hand action and fisting
4. Hyperreflexia with sustained clonus
5. Hypotonia with increased range of motion

Vision and hearing

Strabismus has occurred in the past in 10% to 15% of the lower weight groups of ex-preterm infants. Refractive errors likewise are more common. Retrolental fibroplasia, caused by oxygen excess, is almost exclusively a disorder of the smaller preterm infant. This condition is on the increase even though largely preventable.

Hearing impairment occurs in 1% to 5% of these infants, either singly or with other defects; however, ototoxic drugs as well as viral invasion may play a part in pathogenesis. Again, the incidence of these defects is probably much lower today in the modern neonatal center.

Behavior disorders

Incoordination, distractibility, a short attention span, and emotional instability, often referred to as "minimal brain syndrome," are observed occasionally. Lack of confidence, shyness, and overdependence may be recognized. Some of these variations may reflect subtle injury to the central nervous system, whereas others may stem from the parents' overconcern for, or at times rejection of, the infant.

Nevertheless, the great majority of preterm infants, regardless of size at birth, are remarkably well adjusted and normal in behavior. The fact of their prematurity may be used as an excuse for variations of behavior not uncommon in the general school population.

Health and illness

Preterm infants have greater risk of infectious disease in the first year of life. The number of their hospital admissions for severe respiratory disease is several times that of mature control infants. Un-

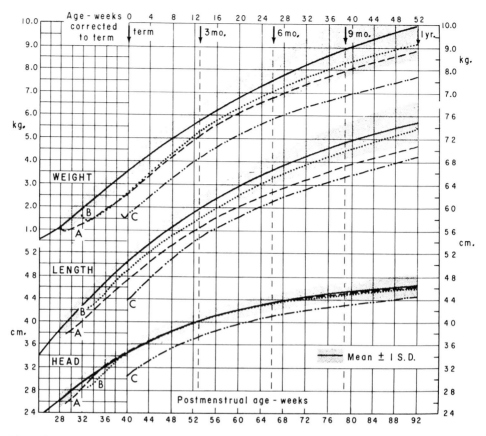

Fig. 25-1. Mean growth curves of three groups of low birth weight infants plotted in three parameters. Very premature (**A**) and moderately premature (**B**) infants are both appropriate in size for gestation; full-term infants are severely undergrown (**C**). (From Babson, S. G.: J. Pediatr. **77**:11, 1970.)

explained crib deaths are two to three times more common in the preterm than in the term infant.

Physical growth

Despite a more optimistic prognosis generally, the growth lag suffered by preterm infants at birth may never be made up entirely. Nearly all longitudinal studies indicate a continued difference in height and weight as compared with standard populations. Nevertheless, caution must be used in such evaluations because prematurity data include children who may show reduced growth as a result of (1) central nervous system injuries or deficiencies, (2) sub-

optimal nutrition, and (3) low birth weight from intrauterine growth retardation.

After exclusion of the seriously handicapped, we must conclude that prematurely born children do not differ importantly from their siblings in later growth.

Fig. 25-1 demonstrates growth through the first year of life in three groups of low birth weight infants in weight, length, and head circumference, corrected for gestational age. Infants in group A were small and premature, those in group B were moderately premature and also appropriate in size, and those in group C were all under 2,000 gm and born at term.

Curves for length and weight in these

low birth weight infants parallel but remain below the curves of growth considered normal for the fetus and infant; those in the undersized group of infants were reduced the most.

Head circumference in the groups of preterm infants, after an initial lag, increases at an accelerated rate, so that their growth curves may approach or temporarily surpass the expected mean curve for fetal growth. Thereafter, head circumference follows the expected pattern observed in normal infants.

In the undergrown infant, head circumference at birth is usually reduced proportionately to length. The curve for head size appears to approach that seen in infants of normal size, but the difference existing at birth is only partly reduced.

THE LARGER PRETERM INFANT

The larger preterm infant is not immune to asphyxial insults that can result from subtle birth trauma or the asphyxia associated with hyaline membrane disease. Lubchenco and colleagues have reported an increased chance of intellectual deficiency, and yet Stahlman has found a satisfactory outcome in such infants requiring assisted ventilation. The potential prognosis should be good, however, if infants undergoing early labor are supplied with optimal medical and nursing care during the entire perinatal period.

CHILD ABUSE

The low birth weight infant who was prematurely born is three times more likely to be subjected to physical and emotional abuse and neglect than the average infant. Insufficient attention to nutritional requirements and the practice of poor hygiene are not uncommon. The following associations may intensify child abuse:

1. Prolonged separation of mother and infant directly after birth
2. Warnings by family friends and physi-

cians of the possibility of death or defect if the infant should live
3. Occurrence of an unplanned, unwanted pregnancy
4. Stressful intrafamily relationships

The physician and nurse should be aware of these factors surrounding birth and the possibility that the infant might become subconsciously or overtly rejected. Child neglect can be reduced if the perinatal team will do the following:

1. Stress the positive and optimistic side to women with a pregnancy at risk.
2. Prepare the mother for the possibly frightening exposure to an intensive care nursery.
3. Have mother and father enter the nursery after appropriate instruction and touch their infant as soon after birth as possible. This necessary binding with eye-to-face contact may overcome a tenuous maternal tie.
4. Explain reasons for each type of equipment, for example, bilirubin lights, eye protection, monitor attachments.
5. Continue to maintain contact with parents during and after the hospital stay.
6. Interview parents of high-risk neonates during the hospital stay for possible stressful states. The social worker and public health nurse are often necessary members of the professional team in the alleviation of problems contributing to the instability of the family unit.

LONGITUDINAL ASSESSMENTS

The frequency of sequelae seen in the prematurely born and the growth-retarded infant, as well as in those at risk for other reasons, requires careful serial observations for early identification of handicapping defects. The examination should include the following:

1. Growth measurements and their plotting in relation to gestational age

2. Developmental screening such as the Denver Developmental Screening Test[*]

3. Neurologic examination, especially for tonus, reflex behavior, vision, eye muscle coordination, hearing, and sound production, including speech development

A favorable course in later development may be anticipated (although it is by no means a certainty) by a positive response to the following observations at the period of time indicated.

1. At time of discharge from the hospital (usually between 37 and 40 weeks of postmenstrual age, gestation plus postnatal age)
    a. Holds head parallel with body on arm traction and raises head in the prone position
    b. Cries vigorously with hunger
    c. Follows observer's face with eyes at 39 to 40 weeks
       In addition, the infant should be gaining well in weight, and have a satisfactory neurologic exam, including an acceptable and symmetric transilluminated area over the skull[†] and a normal-appearing retina.

2. At 6 months of corrected age (postnatal age less weeks of prematurity) An infant born at 27 weeks of gestational age (13 weeks early) must have reached 9 months of postnatal age to have a corrected age of 6 months.
    a. Grasps objects well that are held in different locations
    b. Transfers them from hand to hand
    c. Sits with support
    d. Laughs responsively
    e. Differentiates people

3. At 12 months of corrected age the infant
    a. Pulls self to a standing position and takes a few steps with support
    b. Says a few meaningful words
    c. Has a well-developed pincer grasp in obtaining and eating small bits of food

Motor delay must always be interpreted with caution, particularly in children who were extremely premature. Also, signs of increased tone through 6 months of postnatal age may not be significant. Some delay can be compatible with later normality. The following signs, however, are prejudicial to it: (1) history of difficult feeding, (2) irritability, (3) hypertonia with stiffening of body, and (4) hypotonia.

Gross changes in neurologic behavior require multidisciplinary examinations (speech, intelligence, hearing, vision, etc.), since several areas of handicapping are likely. Complete care includes counseling of parents, arrangements for remedial care, planning for education, and utilization of appropriate physician and paramedical personnel and public health facilities, together with the crippled children's services.

Children who demonstrate minor deviations from accepted standards of development or who show variations in behavior pattern (short attention span, clumsiness, etc.) may need much more attention than they often get. In these situations the family should receive continued and interested support from the physician, and the child should have encouragement, particularly in the area of self-worth.

SELECTED REFERENCES

Amiel-Tison, C.: Cerebral damage in full-term newborn. Aetiological factors, neonatal status, and long-term follow-up, Biol. Neonate **14:** 234, 1969.

Babson, S. G.: Growth of low birth weight infants, J. Pediatr. 77:12, 1970.

Churchill, J. A., Masland, R. L., Naylor, A. A., and Ashworth, M. R.: The etiology of cerebral palsy in preterm infants, Dev. Med. Child Neurol. **16:** 143, 1974.

[*]W. K. Frankenburg and J. B. Dodds, University of Colorado Medical Center.

[†]See Chapter 22. This often neglected examination can frequently detect gross disease. Mature infants do not show more than 1 to 2 cm of reflected light, but the infant who was immature at birth may show normally up to 4 cm of reflected light.

Davies, P. A., and Davis, J. P.: Very low birth weight and subsequent head growth, Lancet 11:1216, 1970.

Davies, P. A., and Tizard, J. P. M.: Very low birth weight and subsequent neurological defect, Dev. Med. Child Neurol. 17:3, 1975.

Drillien, C. M.: Complications of pregnancy and delivery, Ment. Retard. 1:280, 1969.

Drillien, C. M.: Later development and follow-up of low birth weight babies, Pediatr. Ann. 1: 44, 1972.

Eaves, L. C., Nuttal, J. C., Klonoff, K., and Dunn, H. G.: Developmental and psychological test scores in children of low birth weight, Pediatrics 45:9, 1970.

Francis-Williams, J., and Davies, P. A.: Very low birth weight and later intelligence, Dev. Med. Child Neurol. 16:709, 1974.

Grunnet, M. L., Curless, R. G., Bray, P. F., and Jung, A. L.: Brain changes in newborns from an intensive care unit, Dev. Med. Child Neurol. 16:320, 1974.

Lubchenco, L. O., Bard, H., Goldman, A. L., Coyer, W. E., McIntyre, C., and Smith, D. M.: Newborn intensive care and long-term prognosis, Dev. Med. Child Neurol. 16:421, 1974.

Lubchenco, L. O., Delivoria-Papadopoulos, M., Butterfield, L. J., French, J. H., Metcalf, D., Hix, I. E., Danick, J., Dodds, J., Downs, M., and Freeland, E.: Long-term follow-up studies of prematurely born infants. I. Relationship of handicaps to nursery routines, J. Pediatr. 80: 501, 1972.

Lubchenco, L. O., Delivoria-Papadopoulos, M., and Searls, D.: Long-term follow-up studies of prematurely born infants. II. Influence of birth weight and gestational age on sequelae, J. Pediatr. 80:509, 1972.

Minkowski, A., Larroche, J., Vignaud, J., Dreyfus-Brisac, C., and Saint-Anne Dargassies, S.: Development of the nervous system in early life. In Falkner, F. F., editor: Human development, Philadelphia, 1966, W. B. Saunders Co.

Nellhaus, G.: Head circumference from birth to eighteen years, Pediatrics 41:106, 1968.

Rawlings, G., Reynolds, E. O., Stewart, A., and Strang, L. B.: Changing prognosis for infants of very low birth weight, Lancet 1:516, 1971.

Sinclair, J. C., and Coldiorn, J. S.: Low birth weight and postnatal physical development, Dev. Med. Child Neurol. 11:314, 1969.

Stahlman, M. E., Hedvall, G., Dolanski, E., Faxelius, G., Burko, H., and Kirk, V.: A six-year follow-up of clinical HMD, Pediatr. Clin. North Am. 20:433, 1973.

Stewart, A. L., and Reynolds, E. O.: Improved prognosis for infants of very low birth weight, Pediatrics 54:724, 1974.

Van den Berg, B. J.: Morbidity of low birth weight and/or preterm children compared to that of the "mature." I. Methodological considerations and findings for the first 2 years of life, Pediatrics 42:590, 1968.

Wiener, G.: The relationship of birth weight and length of gestation to intellectual development at ages 8 to 12 years, J. Pediatr. 76:694, 1970.

26

Perinatal mortality

The perinatal period in its broadest definition extends from 20 weeks of completed gestation through 27 days of postnatal life. In 1970 for each 1,000 live births there were 15.1 neonatal deaths and 14.2 fetal deaths, or a 29.3 perinatal mortality per 1,000 live births in the United States (Fig. 25-1). This is a reduction of over 26% since 1950. Estimations are that a more striking reduction is occurring during the seventies. In 1973 the state of Oregon reported a perinatal mortality ratio of 22.5, which included all fetal deaths for which age was not stated.

Obviously this falling mortality rate is the result of widespread improvement in patient care and health practices. As regionalization of perinatal care for the high-risk patient continues to develop, we may also expect concomitant reduction in morbidity, since fewer deaths should indicate fewer perinates who have experienced stress or been damaged short of death.

Infants dying in the first 27 days of life usually reflect perinatal stress, since well over half die in the first day of life. Many fetal deaths, on the other hand, occur after labor has begun.

FETAL MORTALITY

Fetal mortality has shown a similar decline to that of neonatal mortality (Fig. 26-1). Identification of the pregnancy at high risk and better surveillance of the fetus are keeping pace with advances in neonatal care. The 40% of deaths that are primarily preventable now are those which occur in association with maternal disease,

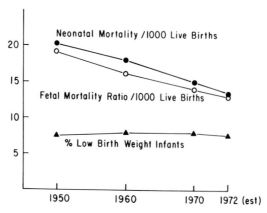

Fig. 26-1. Trends in neonatal and fetal mortality in relation to percentage of low birth weight infants in the United States.

such as diabetes and toxemia, and those resulting from disproportion or malposition. These fetuses are usually over 2,500 gm, are born at term, and as such, contribute thousands of preventable deaths to the perinatal toll. Approximately 40% of fetal deaths, however, are the result of defects of the placenta or cord—factors often silent and undiscovered until delivery unless detected by awareness of interrupted fetal growth. The 15% to 20% of deaths from fetal defects are, in the main, not salvageable.

NEONATAL MORTALITY

States and countries with the lowest mortality are now in the range of ten or below per 1,000 live births. Mortality is inversely proportional to birth weight as shown for the state of Oregon in Table

Table 26-1. Live births (31,213) in hospitals in Oregon* during 1973 matched to neonatal deaths by birth weight groups

Birth weight (gm)	Neonatal death rate per 1,000	Percentage of total births	Death rate per 1,000 live births
Low birth weight			
500 or less	1,000	0.09	0.9
501-1,000	849.1	0.34	2.9
1,001-1,500	341.2	0.54	1.9
1,501-2,000	87.7	1.09	1.0
2,001-2,500	29.9	3.86	1.0
Term birth weight			
2,501-3,000	6.8	15.2	1.0
3,001-3,500	2.8	36.7	1.0
3,501-4,000	1.8	30.7	0.5
4,001-4,500	1.0	9.3	0.1
4,501 and up	1.5	2.1	0.03
Total low birth weight	130.0	5.92	7.7
Total term birth weight	2.9	94.0	2.7
GRAND TOTAL†	10.4	100.0	10.4

*Data from Vital Statistics Section of Oregon State Board of Health.
†Excludes seven in which birth weight was unlisted with no deaths.

26-1. Also shown is the percentage of infants born and the mortality rate per 1,000 live births for each birth weight group. Note that 5.9% of all infants (the low birth weight groups) contribute to three fourths of all neonatal mortality. Mortality figures for 1973 are 38% below those reported 9 years ago in the first edition of this book. Progress is being made—neonatal mortality was 9.6 in 1974. Note that over 50% of neonatal mortality now occurs in infants who weigh under 1,500 gm.

Associations of neonatal deaths (Oregon, 1973)

The associations of neonatal death are listed below. The percentage dying of congenital anomalies incompatible with life has increased as asphyxia and related respiratory distress receive improved care or are prevented. Nevertheless, perinatal asphyxia remains the chief factor in death and morbidity. Only one death from hemolytic disease of the newborn is listed for the year.

Congenital anomalies	20.9
Hyaline membrane disease and/or respiratory distress syndrome	20.3
Asphyxia	18.2
Complications of pregnancy and labor	17.3
Immaturity, unqualified	12.4
All other	10.9

LOW BIRTH WEIGHT INFANTS AND MORTALITY

The incidence of small infants (under 2,501 gm) is a practical measure of pregnancy health and comparisons of neonatal mortality and morbidity of any population. Nevertheless, the traditional separation of newborns into "term" and "premature" on the basis of weight above and below 2,500 gm has little biologic significance. In certain populations and races there may be more mature than premature infants weighing under this figure. In some groups in whom fetal growth is optimal, a greater number of prematurely born infants may weigh over 2,500 gm than under. Finally, neonatal mortality rates do not become minimal until after 3,000 gm in birth weight has been reached (Table 26-1). The World Health Organization has been instrumental in introducing the term "low birth weight" for infants less than 2,501 gm in place of the term "premature." The new appellation recognizes the small, mature infants with their special problems and requirements but lessens the emphasis on the prematurely born, per se. Incorrect conclusions can be drawn from so-called premature baby studies, depending on the number included who are undergrown.

Table 26-2 compares the percentage of low birth weight infants born in the United States, Sweden, and Oregon in relation to neonatal mortality. As Geijerstam has pointed out, these differences in mortality are almost entirely due to the variations in percentage of small babies delivered. This is particularly dependent on the number of infants born who weigh under 1,500 gm, who have the highest mortality rates and account for most of the advantage of the North European countries in infant mortality rates. These smaller infants comprise 1.3% of all births in the United States (triple the percentage in Sweden) and account for over 50% of the neonatal mortality, as compared with 38% for Sweden.

Table 26-2. Comparison of percentage of low birth weight infants born to neonatal mortality in the United States, Sweden, and Oregon

	United States, 1972 est.	Sweden, 1973	Oregon, 1973
Percentage of total births			
2,500 gm or less	7.5	3.7	5.9
1,500 gm or less	1.3	0.4	1.0
Neonatal mortality per 1,000 live births	13.7	5.1*	10.5

*Early neonatal mortality (7 days).

The fact that reduction in the prematurity rate (Fig. 26-1) in the United States has not kept pace with the steady improvement in perinatal mortality suggests that better maternity and nursery care has superseded improvements in social, educational, and economic conditions—factors related to the incidence of low birth weight infants in any area.

SUMMARY

The low birth weight infant contributes a major share to all perinatal mortality and morbidity. The high rates of jeopardy for each low birth weight group are apparent. Often overlooked is the fact that, in terms of numbers, up to 30% of all perinatal deaths occur after 38 weeks of gestation has been achieved and, in terms of weight, after 2,500 gm has been reached. Forty percent of these deaths occur in the immediate period before birth. As pointed out by Gruenwald, death in perinates of this size and maturity is more readily preventable in the present state of our knowledge than that in the smaller and more immature infant.

Much emphasis has been placed in recent years on the more rapid lowering of infant mortality rates in certain other advanced countries of the world over that of the United States. The most recent ranking places the United States in fourteenth place. The poor showing is discomfiting because more money is spent on health per person in the United States than in any of these countries. Medical deficiencies are only one of the factors responsible, however. Although in many areas of medical sophistication the United States is second to none, it is estimated that 25 million Americans receive inadequate or little, if any, health care at all.

Reduction of immaturity by the advancement of fetal age—when this is possible—must be the initial aim in management. Assuming a normally developing fetus, neonatal mortality in infants born at 28

Table 26-3. Neonatal mortality by gestation for 40,000 middle-class Caucasian pregnancies in Portland, Oregon*

Weeks' gestation	Mortality (%)		
28		70.2	
30		38.5	↓73
32	76↓	19.0	
34		9.2	
36		4.3	↓96
38	96↓	0.35	
40		0.17	
42		0.15	
44		0.43	

*Note percentage decrease in mortality on advance in gestation of 4 weeks.

weeks could be lowered 73% by increasing the gestational age from 28 weeks to 32 weeks (Table 26-3). Moreover, an extension of maturity would also sharply reduce the likelihood of physical handicap in the survivors. This goal will be difficult to achieve because the cause of early birth often is unknown or cannot be prevented belatedly. On the other hand, certain complications of pregnancy still require early delivery if fetal death is to be avoided.

The second goal is the reduction of the overall perinatal mortality and the improvement in the quality of survivors by the optimum use of physician and nursing skills, particularly in the recognition and management of acute and chronic fetal stress. Expansion of regional perinatal centers for the intensive care of the fetus and newborn at risk for the best treatment possible is urgent. Certainly, mere survival is no longer good enough.

The final and obviously the most important goal is the reduction of the number of low birth weight infants born—both preterm and undersized. Social and educational advancement, encouragement of welcome and well-born infants, and prevention of unwanted pregnancies are necessary correlates to reaching this goal. Continued research in human reproduction and behavior is urged. Embryologists, pathologists, sociologists, psychologists, cultural anthropologists, and many others must join in the quest.

SELECTED REFERENCES

Battaglia, F. C., Frazier, T. M., and Hellegers, A. E.: Birth weight, gestational age, and pregnancy outcome, with special reference to high-birth-weight–low-gestational-age infants, Pediatrics **37**:717, 1966.

Behrman, R. E., Babson, S. G., and Lessel, R.: Fetal and neonatal mortality in white middle-class infants, Am. J. Dis. Child. **121**:486, 1971.

Erhardt, C. L., Joshi, G. B., Nelson, F. G., Kroll, B. H., and Weiner, L.: Influence of weight and gestation on perinatal and neonatal mortality by ethnic group, Am. J. Public Health **54**:1841, 1964.

Geijerstam, G.: Low birth weight and perinatal mortality, Public Health Rep. **84**:939, 1969.

Gruenwald, P.: Perinatal death of full-sized and full-term infants, Am. J. Obstet. Gynecol. **107**:1022, 1970.

Lilien, A. A.: Term intrapartum fetal death, Am. J. Obstet. Gynecol. **107**:595, 1970.

Lubchenco, L. O., Searles, D. T., and Brazie, J. V.: Neonatal mortality rates: relationship to birth weight and gestational age, J. Pediatr. **81**:814, 1972.

Public health aspects of low birth weight, WHO Techn. Rep. Ser. No. 217, 1961.

Thompson, J.: Perinatal mortality in retrospect and prospect, Scot. Med. J. **14**:89, 1969.

Usher, R.: Clinical implications of perinatal mortality statistics, Clin. Obstet. Gynecol. **14**:885, 1971.

Wallace, H. M.: Factors associated with perinatal mortality and morbidity, Clin. Obstet. Gynecol. **13**:13, 1970.

27

Prevention of prematurity and high-risk pregnancy

In the United States perinatal mortality before and after birth accounts for 90,000 deaths each year, or nearly 3% of all established pregnancies that have reached 20 weeks' gestation. The Committee on Perinatal Welfare of the Massachusetts Medical Society in a 1971 study held that one third of these deaths were preventable. Maternal factors were responsible in 30%, obstetric problems in 46%, and pediatric factors in 40%. With the developments in perinatal care already established in the 1970s, Schneider maintains (as reported at the Sixty-Sixth Ross Conference, held in 1974) that two thirds of neonatal deaths and half of fetal deaths are now preventable, as indicated by his studies in the Wisconsin perinatal program. A similar avoidability probably applies to perinatal morbidity, an important factor in that significant handicaps develop in 7% of the infant survivors of the neonatal period.

The residuals of having been born too soon or too small have been widely publicized and include cerebral palsy, mental retardation, and sensory defects. The enormity of this problem is now apparent, and the need for attacking the factors relating to prematurity, fetal undergrowth, and defective development is urgent. Adverse effects of pregnancy and birth too often have reduced the normal infant to an inferior one, physically and mentally. The damage may be slight or imperceptible clinically, but it may explain the difference between

siblings one of whom may be a dexterous athlete, and the other an "awkward clod."

One goal, at least for the United States, is the extension in regionalization of perinatal care (Chapter 12). Cooperation between practicing physicians and health experts has developed organized levels of care in a number of states, with the result that neonatal mortality has been reduced to less than 10/1,000 deliveries.

Another goal is a reduction in the percentage of live-born neonates who weigh under 1,500 gm. This group accounts for over half the neonatal mortality now in many areas of this country; yet it represents only 1% of all live-born infants. The fact that Sweden, on a percentage basis, has less than half the number born in this weight group may indicate the social advantages of the Scandinavian population.

What should the share of the tax dollar be for full maternity and nursery care programs, with their emphasis on the "quality of life," compared to that now spent for rehabilitation services, such as mental health and retardation centers and crippled children's programs, services so often necessary as the result of deficiencies in some part of pregnancy experience?

As an aid to sharper development of goals, we should examine the working programs of Norway. The objectives of the Family and Child Welfare Services there have been described to be "for the protection and support of families and the rising generation" or, more specifically, "keeping down infant mortality, preventing illness and death in pregnancy and during delivery, ensuring children's healthy development and helping protect mothers from the many strains of bearing and rearing children."*

Our objective in this book has been to lessen such frequent and unfortunate events by detailed care of the fetus and neonate. These last pages summarize the broad approach necessary to prevent prematurity and high-risk pregnancy.

GENERAL MEASURES
Improvement in socioeconomic status

Better education and employment opportunities have improved the lot of underprivileged persons and reduced the number of the poor and incompetent among them. A rise in the living standard will improve the general health of a population and will sharply decrease the percentage of low birth weight infants.

Position in society, with its many implications, has been the most important factor pertaining to the availability and quality of obstetric-pediatric care in the United States. The knowledge of needs and desires and how they can best be met is a primary determinant in the receipt of medical service.

SOCIOMEDICAL MEASURES

1. Ensure the emotional and physical health of adolescents. Adolescent medicine, a potential subspecialty, seeks to improve the fitness of teenagers. Preparation for marriage and family life must be a feature of this new medical function.
2. Promote desirable attitudes toward

---

*From Evang, K.: Health services in Norway, Oslo, 1960, Norwegian social policy; Loughholm, M.: Family and child welfare in Norway, Oslo, 1961, Norwegian Joint Committee on International Social Policy.

family life and parentcraft. The physician should assume responsibility for the well-being of girls and boys during and soon after puberty, when long-standing habits and basic convictions develop, and mothers- and fathers-to-be set their life-style in community living.
3. Guide the young in sexual behavior, pregnancy responsibility, and family planning. Family planning is far more than "birth control." It also includes an understanding of reproductive physiology and pathology, infertility, and social aspects of sex; premarital and genetic counseling; breast and genital cancer detection; pregnancy timing and its spacing; therapeutic abortion and sterilization; demography; and research in human reproduction. Ideally, these and related educational services should be available in every community.
4. Extend immunization programs in anticipation of pregnancy. Immunization of all individuals against rubella before puberty will virtually eliminate this critically teratogenic disease. Early poliomyelitis and measles immunization must continue.

OBSTETRIC MEASURES

The high-risk obstetric patient calls for very special knowledge by physician and nurse, sophisticated laboratory facilities, and trained, available technical assistance, as well as interdisciplinary collaboration. The success of complete maternity care is to be measured not only by the salvage of life and the improvement in standards of health of mothers and babies, but also by diminished fears, difficulties, and discomforts that have to be faced to some extent by every woman who embarks on motherhood. The following measures to prevent prematurity and high-risk pregnancy should be taken:
1. Improve the timing, quality, and

quantity of preconceptional care. Preventive medicine anticipates and corrects problems to avoid complications. Logically, the patient and her husband should be in the best possible health before starting a family. Problems to be controlled or treated range from diabetes mellitus to genital disorders and generative tract abnormalities. Correction of nutritional deficits includes attention to anemia, obesity, and underweight. These conditions are frequent and too often remain uncorrected even when pregnancy is well advanced.

2. Encourage earlier prenatal care. The advantages for the unborn may be identified through secondary education, reinforced at the time of the premarital examination and reinforced when the diagnosis of pregnancy is established.

3. Identify high-risk patients early (before pregnancy, if possible) for "planning for pregnancy," evaluation, treatment, and sympathetic counseling. Many of the handicaps have been discussed and include poor previous pregnancy outcome; undersized or oversized babies; overnutrition and undernutrition of the gravida; very early or advanced age and pregnancy; out-of-wedlock pregnancy; infertility and endocrinopathy; and women who are under stress, anxious, etc.

4. Effect therapeutic abortion in women who do not want the pregnancy and those with serious problems that are likely to be aggravated by gestation. Other indicators for interruption of pregnancy include health and mental disorders and serious familial metabolic diseases and chromosomal aberrations such as Down's syndrome, which may be discovered by tissue culture obtained at amniocentesis.

5. Offer counseling services when family defects are known or have occurred. Many couples will voluntarily limit conception when crippling hereditary disease is likely.

6. Strictly limit cigarette smoking, particularly in the high-risk obstetric patient. Smoking must be suspect and discouraged, although it is still uncertain whether it is the smoke itself or some other factor associated with smoking that increases fetal jeopardy and results in undersized neonates.

7. Deliver better obstetric care through expanded medical resources of referral, diagnosis, consultation, and treatment. The team approach is required for the proper avoidance and control of fetal casualty and serious residuals and sequelae of many serious conditions that occur in pregnancy. Such disorders include urinary tract infection, cardiopathies, eclamptogenic toxemia, and many others that may require hospital admission and readmission for study, therapy, and rest.

8. Expand regional centers for specialized and complete maternity and nursery services, particularly for the perinate in jeopardy. The establishment of such centers should have the highest priority. The following benefits would accrue: (1) training of specialized personnel, who are in short supply in this field, (2) demonstration and participation in specialized perinatal care for the physician and nurse in the regional care area, and (3) cooperation between regional centers and local hospitals for the transfer of pregnant women (and sometimes their infants) who are at high risk (twinning, toxemia, etc.) to lower perinatal mortality and morbidity.

9. Implement care to include migratory, underprivileged persons. There

are many patients who do not "belong" but who need medical attention or special care. Seasonal farm workers and alienated youth are examples.

10. Diagnose twinning by the twenty-sixth week of gestation for institution of enforced rest.

11. Supervise adequacy of diet. Controlling the quantity and quality of nutrients is important to support fetal health. Avoid undernutrition during the third trimester, even in obese women.

12. Obtain homemaker assistance; bed rest is important for cardiac, multiple pregnancy, and chronic abortion patients. Many threatening disorders of pregnancy are associated with uterine hyperirritability. Bed rest may be both prophylactic and therapeutic during pregnancy.

13. Cure abortogenic infections, that is, syphilis, listeriosis, mycoplasma infections, brucellosis, and malaria. Eliminate bacteriuria, vaginitis, and cervicitis.

14. Institute expectant, informed management of midtrimester and third trimester uterine bleeding problems. Far more mischief results from radical as compared with conservative treatment of antepartum bleeding. Maternal hemorrhage or premature birth is a high price to pay for an impulsive direct diagnosis of placenta previa, for example.

15. Avoid ill-timed, early induction of labor or cesarean section. The duration of pregnancy is often uncertain. If dates alone are used to time the termination, an immature neonate may be delivered. With the tests now available to determine fetal maturity and size, elective termination of a preterm infant should not occur.

16. Administer $Rho(D)$ immune globulin to all Rh-negative unsensitized mothers at risk after each delivery or abortion.

PREVENTION OF THE UNWANTED— "TO BE WELCOME AND WELLBORN"

Although improvement in general health and more sophisticated obstetric care carry a high priority, the prevention of unwanted pregnancy is most important. Unwelcome pregnancies contribute significantly to the current increase in population problems and proportionately more to perinatal death and morbidity than do planned and expected pregnancies.

The National Fertility Study in 1965 indicated that 17% of births among the nonpoor were unwanted compared to 42% of births among the poor, or nearly one fourth of all infants born in the United States. We believe that these figures are a very conservative estimate. Approximately 90% of teen-age pregnancies have been found to be the result of an admitted mistake. Reversing these figures could significantly improve the product of conception, the safety of the intrauterine environment, and the quality of life.

1. Sequelae of unwanted pregnancy
   a. An increase in congenital anomalies, prematurity, and undersized newborns results from unwanted gestation. Eighty-five percent of all small babies of white mothers admitted to the neonatal Intensive Care Center of the University of Oregon Health Science Center were unplanned and unwanted. Rejection appeared to persist in 36% of these cases, even with professional counseling. Data covering infants with major congenital malformations are similar.
   b. The battered child, whether the victim of psychologic or physical trauma, is more likely to be the result of an unplanned and unwanted pregnancy. The part parental rejection may play in underachievement, delinquency, and the like may be considerable.

2. Associations of unplanned pregnancy
   Unplanned pregnancy stems from the failure to use a contraceptive method effectively. Factors that relate to these failures are numerous but include
   a. Lack of knowledge
   b. Unconcern for the consequences of sexual intercourse
   c. Religious beliefs
   d. Difficulty in obtaining, or unavailability of, contraceptives
   e. Early dating and emotional immaturity
   f. Poor relationships with parents
   g. Personality conflicts
   h. Efforts to hold the male's affection
   i. Drug abuse, principally alcohol
   j. Personal irresponsibility
3. What can be done
   Some of the positive methods to be considered for the reduction in the number of unplanned pregnancies are as follows:
   a. Education of children and adolescents by specially trained teachers of family life on human responsibility, sexual behavior, drug abuse, venereal disease, etc. to supplement and support information gained in the home.
   b. Education (school, news media, etc.) of parents in family living, for themselves as well as their children; these presentations should include
      1. Each parent's responsibility as an individual and as a member of society
      2. The advantage of planning a family at an optimum time, considering parental age, child number, and spacing
   c. Wider availability and dissemination of knowledge of contraceptives and birth control techniques; training of more public health nurses and paramedical personnel in these details; establishment of Planned Parenthood type of clinics in each community.
   d. The establishment of clinics that offer free testing for early pregnancy, particularly for the teen-ager; the early identification of pregnancy will encourage
      1. Appropriate early prenatal care
      2. Guidance in an unwanted or ill-advised pregnancy
   e. Liberally applied and available abortion; this often questioned procedure has gained popular support and may be necessary even after better techniques in birth control are developed and people are willing to accept and use them.
   f. Financial advantages aimed at reducing the incidence of unwanted pregnancy but benefiting the wanted child.
   g. More easily available sterilization.

Sophistication about sexual behavior, the wider use of contraception and abortion, and the high standard of living in the Scandinavian countries may be the reasons for the reduced number of infants who weigh under 1,500 gm.

The advancement of science, and medicine in particular, has been a major factor in the control of disease and pestilence, which upset the balance of nature in population control of man. Medical personnel must be more forceful in helping to solve the tragedy of overpopulation.

The overcrowding of cities and the increasing public and private costs of rearing and educating children have emphasized the urgency of reproductive restraint and the responsibilities of parenthood. It is the first time in human history that we are totally dependent on the quality of care, nutrition, and education, rather than on sheer quantity.

Families should be created purposefully and intentionally, not accidentally or regretfully. Our world is too small and too complex for any but wanted children who will be loved.

As said in Shakespeare's *Julius Caesar:*

> How many ages hence
> Shall this our lofty scene be acted over
> In states unborn and accents yet unknown.

SELECTED REFERENCES

Abernethy, V., and Abernethy, G. L.: Identification of adolescent girls at high risk for unwanted pregnancy, Am. J. Orthopsychiatry **44:** 442, 1974.

Benson, R. C.: Direction, innovation, exploration: an obstetric tryptych, Am. J. Obstet. Gynecol. **110:**15, 1971.

Gold, E. M., and Ballard, W. M.: The role of family planning in prevention of pregnancy wastage, Clin. Obstet. Gynecol. **13:**145, 1970.

Hunscher, H. A., and Tompkins, W. T.: The influence of maternal nutrition on the immediate and long-term outcome of pregnancy, Clin. Obstet. Gynecol. **13:**130, 1970.

Page, E. W.: Pathogenesis and prophylaxis of low birth weights, Clin. Obstet. Gynecol. **13:** 79, 1970.

Shakespeare, W.: Julius Caesar, Act III, Scene 1.

Vaux, K.: Who shall live? Philadelphia, 1970, Fortress Press.

Wallace, H. M.: Factors associated with perinatal mortality and morbidity, Clin. Obstet. Gynecol. **13:**13, 1970.

APPENDIX A Definitions and terms

abortion the termination of pregnancy before the fetus becomes viable (prior to the twenty-fourth week). An early abortion is one that occurs before the sixteenth week; a late abortion is one that occurs from the sixteenth to the twenty-fourth week.

dysmature refers to infants of any gestational age who show malnutrition at birth, with evidence of dry and scaly skin.

early neonatal period the time interval from birth through 7 days of age.

excessive-sized neonate a newborn who weighs more than 4,500 gm (over 9 lb 15 oz).

fetal death the death of a product of conception prior to its complete expulsion (stillbirth), irrespective of the duration of the pregnancy.

early fetal death death with a pregnancy duration of less than 20 weeks' gestation or an abortus.

intermediate fetal death death in which the pregnancy had a duration of between 20 and 28 weeks.

late fetal death death that occurs from the twenty-eighth week of gestation on.

fetal death ratio I the number of fetal deaths at 28 weeks' gestation or more per 1,000 live births.

fetal death ratio II the number of fetal deaths at 20 weeks' gestation or more per 1,000 live births.

gestational period the number of completed weeks of pregnancy, calculated from the first day of the last menstrual period to the date of delivery. Since conception occurs approximately 2 weeks after the first day of the last menstrual period, a time seldom known, the definition of gestational period includes these 2 prior weeks.

gravida the number of times a patient has been pregnant.

immature infant a live-born preterm infant with a weight at birth of 1,000 gm (2 lb 3 oz) or less.

live birth the complete expulsion or extraction of a product of conception from its mother, irrespective of the duration of pregnancy, which after such separation breathes or shows any other evidence of life such as beating of the heart, pulsation of the umbilical cord, or definite movement of the voluntary muscles, whether or not the umbilical cord has been cut or the placenta is attached; each product of such a birth is considered live-born.*

low birth weight infant any live-born infant with a weight at birth of 2,500 gm (5½ lb) or less.

neonatal death the death of an infant within the first 27 days of life.

neonatal mortality rate the number of neonatal deaths per 1,000 live births.

neonatal period the time interval from birth through the first 27 days of life.

parity the number of infants live or dead that a woman has delivered, excluding abortions.

perinatal mortality rate the combined fetal and neonatal death rate per 1,000 live births.

perinatal period I the time interval from 28 weeks of completed gestation through the first 7 days of life.

perinatal period II the time interval from 20 weeks of completed gestation through 27 days of age.

postmenstrual age the gestational period (fetal), as measured from the first day of the last menstrual period, plus the postnatal age (neonatal). This term allows comparisons of infants on the basis of their total life (fetal and neonatal) independent of the time of birth.

postterm infant (postmature) a live-born infant with a gestational period of over 42 weeks of completed gestation.

preterm infant (premature) a live-born infant with a gestational period of less than 38 completed weeks, regardless of birth weight. Some definitions place this period below 37 weeks.

term infant a live-born infant with 38 to 42 weeks of completed gestation.

undergrown, small-for-dates, and intrauterine growth-retarded infants infants who are significantly undersized for their period of gestation.

---

*Statistical paper, Series M, No. 19, New York, 1953, Statistical Office of the United Nations.

282

APPENDIX B Perinatal record forms

APPENDIX B Perinatal record forms

UNIVERSITY OF OREGON MEDICAL SCHOOL
HOSPITALS AND CLINICS

ANTEPARTUM RECORD

M S W D Sep.___ G____ P____ Ab____
Age_____   Occupation _____
Telephone _____
Address _____

Date _____ Bldg. ____ Fl. ____ Rm. ____

Unit No.
Name
Birthdate

PAST OBSTETRIC HISTORY

Year of Termination	Length of Labor	Gestation	Type of Delivery	Anesthesia	Infant-sex wt., present condition	Complications

PAST MEDICAL HISTORY

Cardiovascular — Respiratory
Gastrointestinal — Renal
Gynecologic — Endocrine
Operations — Allergies
Medications — Injuries
Childhood illnesses (Rubella) — Other

FAMILY HISTORY

Diabetes — Multiple Pregnancy
Cancer — Bleeding Disorder
Congenital — Epilepsy
Other

PHYSICAL EXAMINATION

	Normal	See Remarks		Normal	See Remarks
HEENT			Abdomen		
Funduscopic			Skin		
Thyroid, neck			Neurologic		
Breasts			External Genitalia		
Heart			Cervix		
Chest			Uterus		
Back, extremities			Ovaries		

Remarks

PELVIC MEASUREMENTS

Diagonal conjugate — Sacrum — Spines
Sacral notch — Sidewalls — Posterior sagittal
Bi-ischial — Arch
Summation of pelvis: (Adequate borderline or contracted?)
Inlet — Midpelvis — Outlet

Continued.

2.5-Rev. 7-7/71

2

283

ANTEPARTUM RECORD
PART II

LMP_____ PMP_____ EDC_____ Quickening _____

G_____ P _____ Ab _____ Rubella titer _____

Blood type _____ Serology_____ Comments: _____

Urine culture_____

Pap_____ Chest x-ray_____

Wt before preg. _____ Blood sugar _____

Hct										
Hst										
Visit #	1	2	3	4	5	6	7	8	9	10
Date										
Gestation (dates)										
Gestation (clinical)										
Weight										
BP										
Urine A/G										
Position										
Station										
FHT										
Fundal Ht.										
Edema										
Fetal Size										

COMPLICATIONS and CONDITIONS TO BE NOTED AT TIME OF ADMISSION FOR DELIVERY

_____
_____
_____
_____
_____
_____
_____
_____
_____
_____
_____
_____
_____
_____
_____
_____

DIAGNOSTIC SUMMARY_____

_____
_____
_____
_____
_____
_____
_____
_____
_____
_____
_____

Resident or Faculty Signature

UNIVERSITY OF OREGON MEDICAL SCHOOL
HOSPITALS AND CLINICS

ANTEPARTUM RECORD
PART III

REMARKS

Date   Bldg.   Fl.   Rm.

Unit No.

Name

Birthdate

Visit #	Date	

2

2.5A-7/71

Continued.

University of Oregon Medical School
Hospitals & Clinics

MATERNAL—CHILD NURSING ASSESSMENT CARE PLAN

Date   Bldg.   Fl.   Rm.

Unit No.

Name

Birthdate

Age	Marital Status M S W D Sep	Religion	Ht	EDC		LMP

G	P	AB	CIRC if boy Y N	Blood Type Rh	No. of Children at home

Labor & Delivery Progress, Problems, Behaviour

Spouse (baby's father)	Name	Address	Age	Ht	Wt	Race

Allergies	Previous Hospitalization	Medications on now

Baby   Weight   Status

Describe Usual Bowel Routine	Describe Usual Sleep Patterns

Self-Care Instructions & Observations (check when instructed)

- [ ] Breast self-exam
- [ ] clean catch
- [ ] Breast care for breast feeding
- [ ] peri care
- [ ] heat lamp

Has patient been observed doing these correctly?

Y   N Explain.

Future Plans (outcome of Preg, home situ, job, life style)

Will pt. need follow-up help with any of above?

PRENATAL CLASSES attended:

- [ ] Anatomy, physiology, hygiene
- [ ] family planning, baby care
- [ ] Nutrition, breast & bottle feed.
- [ ] labor, delivery PP, Anesth.
- [ ] Exercises, Group
- [ ] other

Individual Prenatal Instruction—check when pt. instructed

- [ ] warning signs of pregnancy
- [ ] prenatal Lit given

20-28 weeks
- [ ] Breast feeding
- [ ] bottle feeding
- [ ] Breast care
- [ ] bottle sterilization
- [ ] Methods of Prepared Childbirth Referral___
- [ ] Doing breathing & relaxation exercises
- [ ] Room for infant
- [ ] Sibling preparation
- [ ] Clothing for infant

36-40 weeks   **Referrals Made**
- [ ] signs of labor and what to do
- [ ] someone at home to help
- [ ] family planning
- [ ] post-partum & well baby care

Mothering Tasks:

- [ ] Mother has looked over baby completely. If no, why?

Mother observed doing tasks:

	+ correct	— needs help
[ ]	diapering	[ ] holding
[ ]	feeding	[ ] burping
[ ]	other	

Does this mother or family need help in any above area?

NURSING CARE PLAN

(General Observations, Concerns of Patient or Family/and/or problems observed by staff, knowledge and attitudes concerning childbirth and care, restrictions to visitors, etc.)

Date	Area of Concern/Problem list	Intervention (Plan of action)	Progress	Signature

2.5A-1

2.5A-1–3M—10/72

Nursing Care Plan

Date	Area of Concern/Problem List	Intervention (Plan of Action)	Progress	Signature

Discharge Planning

1. Has the baby's father come to visit the baby and/or mother _____
2. Who is at home to help this mother _____
3. These have been discussed: ☐ Bathing baby ☐ Sibling rivalry ☐ Baby's crying ☐ Circumcision care
   ☐ Naval care ☐ new routine at home ☐ other _____
4. Where will she take baby for well baby care and PKU test _____
5. Any problems anticipated when she goes home _____
6. Consults or referrals while in hospital or upon discharge _____

Date of Discharge _____   Signature _____

PERINATAL HISTORY

NAME: _____ HOSPITAL #: _____ HOSPITAL PHONE: _____

HOSPITAL: _____ CITY: _____ STATE: _____

ATTENDANT AT BIRTH: _____ INFANT'S PHYSICIAN: _____ PHONE: _____

MOTHER'S NAME: _____ HOSPITAL #: _____ AGE: _____ PHONE: _____

MARITAL STATUS: _____ RACE: _____ RELIGION: _____ PRIVATE ☐ CLINIC ☐

FATHER'S AGE: OCCUPATION	LABOR Spontaneous ☐ Induced ☐
RELEVANT FAMILY HISTORY (RE BABY)	Induction indication _____
	Method _____
	DRUGS GIVEN DOSE ROUTE TIME

TYPE Rh ANTIBODIES	

PAST OBSTETRIC HISTORY

GRAV _____ LOW BIRTH WT. (<2500g) _____	ANESTHESIA AGENTS USED/DETAILS
PARA _____ PREMATURES (<37 wks) _____	None ☐
	Pudendal ☐
AB. _____ FETAL DEATHS (>20 wks) _____	Paracervical ☐
	Spinal ☐
NEONATAL DEATHS _____ CONGEN. ANOM _____	Epid./Caudal ☐
	Inhalation ☐
LIVING CHILDREN _____	FIRST STAGE _____ HOURS
	SECOND STAGE _____ MINUTES
DETAIL ABNORMALITIES:	MEMBRANES RUPTURED _____ HOURS/DAYS

FETAL DISTRESS   MONITOR:

Not Noted ☐	Meconium ☐	Yes ☐	No ☐
Heart < 100 ☐	Acidosis ☐	Decelerations:	
Heart > 160 ☐	Nuchal cord ☐	Type:	
Heart Irreg ☐	Prolapsed cord ☐		

DELIVERY   Time _____ Date _____

Presentation _____

CURRENT PREGNANCY L.M.P. _____	Spontaneous ☐ Operative ☐
SEROLOGY E.D.C. _____	Breech Ext. ☐ Forceps: Mid ☐ C Section ☐
Rubella _____ S.T.S. _____	Breech Assist. ☐ Low ☐ Vacuum Ext. ☐
Cigarettes/D _____	
COMPLICATIONS:	Indication:
Include details of all drugs/meds: dose, duration and gestational period; recent infections (state bacterial, viral); other prenatal complications.	
DETAILS:	
	AMNIOTIC FLUID Appearance: _____
	Volume _____ ml. Normal ☐ Reduced ☐
	Excessive ☐ Not noted ☐
	PLACENTA Weight _____ Vessels _____
	Abnormalities:

288

NEONATAL   Singleton ☐

Multiple (Birth Order) _____

APGAR SCORE

Min.	H	R	T	S	C	Score
1						
5						
10						

First gasp_____min.

Regular resps. established _____min.

RESUSCITATION

Nil required ☐   Antagonist ☐
O_2 Mask/Catheter ☐   Alkali ☐
O_2 with Pos Press ☐   Cardiac Massage ☐
     by Mask ☐   DETAILS AND RESPONSE:
     Endotracheal ☐

INITIAL EXAMINATION *   At Age

Weight _____   Gestation _____

Length _____   Clin. Gest _____

Head C. _____   Sex _____

DETAIL ABNORMALITIES

Nutrition ☐
Color ☐
Tone ☐
Reflexes ☐
Resps ☐
Head/Face ☐
Eyes ☐
Palate ☐
Chest ☐
Heart ☐
Abdomen ☐
Umbilicus ☐
Hips ☐
Femorals ☐
Genitalia ☐
Limbs ☐
Skin ☐

Vitamin K given: Yes ☐   No ☐
* (✓) indicates item normal to exam.

PROGRESS
Please include all medications and fluids

First Feeding: Age (Hours)_____
Route:_____
Fluid/Formula _____
Last voided _____
Last stooled _____

Signed:_____
ATTENDING PHYSICIAN

REMINDER: We will require
  1. Mother's blood (5 - 10 ml clotted)
  2. Cord blood (when available)
  3. Placenta (when available)
  4. Relevant X-rays, Lab. data, Xerox copies of case notes, mother and baby
  5. This Transfer Record completed in DETAIL.
  6. Consent for Transport.

Adapted from a form in use at National Women's Hospital, Auckland, New Zealand.

APPENDIX D Incubator air temperatures

Temperatures given at right are recommended for use as an initial guide when relative humidity is approximately 50%. A lower humidity would require higher temperatures. Various other factors in the thermal environment and the individual infant's requirements will justify a temperature that is higher or lower than the following.

First 24 hours*

Birth weight			Temperatures (median ± range)	
Gm	Lb	Oz	°C	°F
	1'	0"	35.5 ± 0.5	96.0 ± 0.9
500			35.5 ± 0.5	96.0 ± 0.9
	2'	0"	35.0 ± 0.5	95.0 ± 0.9
1,000			34.9 ± 0.5	94.9 ± 0.9
	3'	0"	34.2 ± 0.5	93.6 ± 0.9
1,500			34.0 ± 0.5	93.2 ± 0.9
	4'	0"	33.7 ± 0.5	92.7 ± 0.9
2,000			33.5 ± 0.5	92.3 ± 0.9
	5'	0"	33.3 ± 0.7	92.0 ± 1.3
2,500			33.2 ± 0.8	91.8 ± 1.4
	6'	0"	33.1 ± 0.9	91.6 ± 1.6
3,000			33.0 ± 1.0	91.4 ± 1.8
	7'	0"	32.9 ± 1.1	91.2 ± 1.9
3,500			32.8 ± 1.2	91.0 ± 2.1
	8'	0"	32.8 ± 1.3	91.0 ± 2.3
4,000			32.6 ± 1.4	90.7 ± 2.5
	9'	0"	32.5 ± 1.4	90.5 ± 2.5

*From Segal, S., editor: Manual for the transport of high-risk newborn infants: principles, policies, equipment, techniques, Vancouver, 1972, Canadian Paediatric Society; adapted from data published by Scopes and Ahmed (1966) and Oliver (1965).

APPENDIX E Drug dosages

Drug or blood replacement	Dosage	Route
Antibiotics (Chapter 9)		
Adrenergics		
Epinephrine (1:10,000 solution)	0.5 ml in single dose; repeat as indicated	IV, IM, or cardiac
Isoproterenol	0.4-0.8 mg/100 ml as infusion at approximately 0.2 µg/kg/min	IV
Anticonvulsants		
Phenobarbital	10 mg/kg for single dose—repeat once if necessary; then follow with 5 mg/kg daily	IM
Diazepam (Valium) (seizures)	0.5 mg-1 mg—repeated once	IV (slowly)
Blood derivatives		
Blood products		
Whole blood	10-15 ml/kg	IV (slowly)
Packed cells	5-10 ml/kg	IV (slowly)
Plasma	10-15 ml/kg	IV (slowly)
Albumin	1 gm/kg	IV (slowly)
Plasmanate	10-15 ml/kg	IV (slowly)
Cardiovascular drugs		
Digoxin	Total digitalizing dose (IM) Preterm infant first week of life, 0.02 mg/kg Preterm infant 2 weeks to 3 months, 0.025 mg/kg Full-term infant first week of life, 0.033 mg/kg Full-term infant 1 week to 3 months, 0.045 mg/kg Oral dose approximately 50% greater Give half of total dose stat, the rest in quarter doses q 8 hr Maintenance one fourth to one third of total digitalizing dose	
Diuretics		
Meralluride (Mercuhydrin)	0.1 ml/5 kg body weight	IM
Furosemide (Lasix)	1 mg/kg	IV
Miscellaneous		
Calcium gluconate (10% solution)	1-2 ml/kg given slowly	IV (slowly) occasionally intra-cardiac

Continued.

Drug dosages—cont'd

Drug or blood replacement	Dosage	Route
Dexamethasone (Decadron)	0.5-2 mg/kg daily, divided into four doses; gradually reduce	IV or IM
Gentian violet (1% aqueous)	Twice daily to skin or mouth	Locally only
Heparin	100 units/kg/4 hr	IV (infusion pump)
Hydrocortisone	5-15 mg q 6 hr; reduce gradually	IM or IV
Iron		
Elemental iron	Prophylaxis: 1-2 mg/kg/24 hr Treatment: 10-30 mg/kg/24 hr	PO
Dextran iron complex (Imferon)	0.5 ml, injected every other day, four times	IM (deep) Use "Z" technique
Levallorphan (Lorfan)	0.05 mg	IM or IV
Magnesium sulfate (50%)	0.1 to 0.2 ml/kg	IM
Nalorphine (Nalline)	0.1-0.2 mg	IV
Sodium bicarbonate	2-4 mEq/kg (diluted)	IV (slowly)
Chlorpromazine hydrochloride (Thorazine)	0.5 mg/kg q 6 hr	IM or PO
Paregoric	4-6 drops q 4-6 hr	PO
Phenylephrine hydrochloride (Neo-Synephrine), 1%- 2.5%	1 drop into each eye	
Vitamin K₁	0.5-1 ml	Subcutaneous

APPENDIX F Perinatal emergency transportation equipment checklist

Maternal equipment

Blood pressure cuff and stethoscope
Clipboard
Doppler fetal pulse rate detector and coupling jelly
Tank of O_2 with tubing and nasal prongs
Examining gloves, povidone-iodine (Betadine)
Ambulance gurney
Vital signs sheets, yellow progress sheet
Ambu bag, trichloroethylene (Trilene mask), endotracheal tube (Nos. 34 and 36), laryngoscope with blade
Plastic bags
Bedpan
IV pole on stretcher
Emergency delivery pack
  In a stainless steel placenta basin place the following:
    4 striped towels
    1 suction bulb wrapped in 4 × 4 sponge
    1 cord scissors
    2 curved Kelly hemostats (cord clamps)
    1 baby receiving set with baby blanket on top (fan-fold both edges to center, then fold ends up to make square)
    1 Hollister clamp
    Wrap box style in 36 × 40 wrapper
Pudendal block kit
  1 Luer Lok 10 ml syringe with 3-ring control handle, separate barrel from syringe, wrap in 8 × 4 sponge
  Needles: 1 No. 20 6-inch, 1 No. 22 2-inch, 1 No. 23 1-inch; check, sharpen, and protect needle tips; stick needles through brown paper
  1 metal medicine glass
  1 Iowa Trumpet guide or straight guide (the No. 20 6-inch needle should stick out the end of the trumpet 0.75 cm)
  Separate syringe, wrap in sponge; place needles side by side through brown paper, as directed above; wrap in striped towel, envelope style; wrap in 22 × 22 wrapper

Umbilical catheter set
  Emesis basin
  2 blue striped towels
  1 20 ml syringe
  1 medicine glass with 4 sponges
  3 hemostats
  2 mosquito clamps
  1 Kelly clamp
  1 No. 15 knife blade in Lee White tube
  1 plain cord tie
  1 circular drape, altered
Umbilical catheter tray
IV equipment
  Solutions: 1 L D_5W, 1 L 10% alcohol, and 1 L lactated Ringer's solution
  IV tubing, extension tubing
  No. 16 Jelco or Angiocath venous cannula
  Nos. 19 and 21 butterfly needles
  Adhesive tape (paper and cloth)
  Alcohol swabs
  4 × 4 gauze squares
Syringes: 30, 10, 5, and 3 ml
Needles: Nos. 18 and 21
Medications (order through pharmacy)
  Oxytocin (Pitocin), 5 ampules
  Methylergonovine maleate (Methergine), 5 ampules
  Magnesium sulfate (both IV and IM), 10 gm
  Calcium gluconate, 4 ampules
  Prochlorperazine maleate (Compazine), 2 ampules
  Diazepam (Valium), 2 ampules
  Atropine, multidose vial
  Levarterenol bitartrate (Levophed), 1 ampule
  Ephedrine, 2 ampules
  Epinephrine (Adrenalin), 2 ampules
  Morphine, 15 mg
  Meperidine hydrochloride (Demerol), 100 mg
  Hydroxyzine hydrochloride (Vistaril), 50 mg
  Lidocaine (Xylocaine), 1%, 50 ml
  Mepivacaine hydrochloride (Carbocaine), 1%, 50 ml

Procaine, 1%, 50 ml
Phenobarbital, 2 gm (120 mg)
Hydralazine hydrochloride, 2 20 mg ampules
Dexamethasone (Decadron), 10 mg
Promethazine (Phenergan), 100 mg
Heparin, 10,000 units
Bicarbonate, 2 ampules
Thiethylperazine maleate (Torecan) tablets, 10
  mg, 4 tablets
6 extra packs 30 chromic catgut
Flashlight with extra batteries

Newborn equipment

Incubator
Chemical hot packs
Plasmanate, 250 ml D_sW
IV solution (also Normosol)
Sodium bicarbonate
Neonatal resuscitation equipment
  Bulb syringe
  DeLee suction
  Laryngoscope
  Endotracheal tubes
  O_2 tank and tubing
  Penlon bag

APPENDIX G Neonatal emergency transportation equipment checklist*

Medications

Calcium gluconate, 100 mg/ml (2)
D$_{50}$W, 50 ml, D$_{10}$W, 250 ml
Digoxin (Lanoxin), 100 μg/ml (2)
Epinephrine (Adrenalin), 1 mg/ml (3) (1:1,000)
Furosemide (Lasix), 10 mg/ml (2)
Isoproterenol (Isuprel), 0.2 mg/ml (4) (1:5,000)
Kanamycin (Kantrex), 333 mg/ml
Gentamicin sulfate, 40 mg/ml
Normal saline solution, 30 ml
Phytonadione (AquaMephyton), 10 mg/ml
Phenobarbital (Luminal), 160 mg/ml
Plasma protein fraction (Plasmanate), 50 ml (5%)
Sodium ampicillin
Sodium heparin, 1,000 units/ml
NaHCO$_3$, 1 mEq/ml, 2 bottles
Sterile (bacteriostatic) water, 30 ml

Miscellaneous

Clear tape, ½ and 1 inch
Adhesive tape, ½ and 1 inch
Elastoplast
No. 4-0 silk on cutting needle (1677)
No. 4-0 silk on taper needle (K-831)
Needle holder
Spongette (10)
Cotton tip applicators (6)
Tongue blade
Dextrostix
Thermometer
Benzoin, 5 ml
Cotton balls (1 package)
Ampule file
Needles: Nos. 25, ⅝ (4), 23, 1 (4), 18, 1 (4), 18 × 1 blunt, and 20 × 1 blunt
Syringes, plain with needle: TB (4), 3 ml (4)

*Basic support items are listed in Chapter 11.

Syringes, Luer Lok without needle: 3 ml (3), 6 ml (3), 12 ml (3), 20 ml (2), 35 ml (2), and 60 ml
Laryngoscope with Miller 7 and 10 cm blades
Band-Aids, small (6)
Band-Aids, large (6)
K-Y jelly (2)
No. 11 blade (2)
Nasogastric tube connector-adapter
O$_2$ tube connector-adapter
Safety pins
Rubber bands
Blood tubes, red top and pink top
Oral airway No. 00
Laryngoscope batteries (2), C
Laryngoscope light (2)
Scissors
Telethermometer battery, O
Small Bennett mask No. 2
ECG leads (2)
Nasogastric tube, Fr 8 (2), Fr 5 (2)
DeLee suction catheters (2)
Sterile gloves: 6½, 7, 7½, 8
Suction catheters, Fr 5 (2), Fr 8 (2), Fr 10 (2)
Argyle catheter, Fr 3½, Fr 5
Holter pump extension tubing A (9105), B (9106), C (9107), D (9108)
Extension IV tubing
Metriset
Scalp vein needles, Nos. 23 and 25
3-way stopcock (2)
Endotracheal tubes, 2.5, 3, 3.5, and 4 mm
Adapters (Ambu), 2, 3, 3.5, and 4 mm
ECG monitor cord
4 × 4 gauze squares
Sterile drape
Blood culture flask
Betadine, 1:1

APPENDIX H Acid-base nomogram

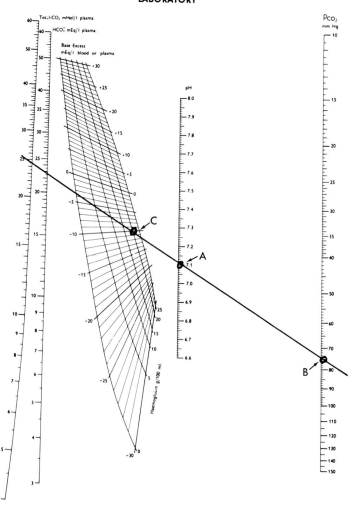

Acid-base nomogram (adapted from Siggaard-Andersen; copyright Radiometer), with an example of plotted data from a sick infant. Base excess can be computed when hemoglobin and any two of the following parameters are known: blood pH, P_{CO_2}, plasma bicarbonate, or total carbon dioxide content of plasma. The values (pH at point **A** and P_{CO_2} at point **B** in this example) are plotted on their scales, and a straight line is drawn through these points across all columns. The base excess is read on the grid line representing the amount of the patient's hemoglobin (**C**). (From Korones, S. B.: High-risk newborn infants: the basis for intensive nursing care, St. Louis, 1972, The C. V. Mosby Co.)

Index